Practical Techniques in Molecular Biotechnology

A well-designed research-based experimental laboratory course is critical for students interested in research in biotechnology and related disciplines, and this book will help immensely in developing these kinds of courses. At the graduate level, this book is a good reference for instructors interested in developing innovative theoretical and practical courses related to biochemistry/biophysical chemistry/biotechnology fields and also for designing research-based courses for the molecular biology lab, or for instruction in cellular biology, nanotechnology, and neurobiology.

Practical Techniques in Molecular Biotechnology engages students in the learning of laboratory and practical research skills by focusing on the solution of some real-world scientific problems. This approach helps students learn biochemical techniques in a context, and allows better integration with research projects. The text intends to familiarize students with the basics of experimental biotechnology science for their use and application in research. While providing the fundamentals of biochemistry, it focuses primarily on concepts and practices related to biotechnology. Theoretical principles underlying experimental techniques, procedures, assignments, and data analysis are presented with adequate examples. The book is designed in such a way that it exposes students to the practice of general biochemical and biophysical techniques, which lay the groundwork for future courses and research projects in biotechnology and its related fields. In addition, the book contains information on data analysis, statistics, units, safety, and best practices.

Bal Ram Singh is Director, Institute of Advanced Science, Dartmouth, USA. He has served on the Blue-Ribbon Panels for National Institutes of Health (NIH) on Biodefense Research, and has also worked in several NIH study section reviewer panels. He is a member of American Chemical Society, American Society for Microbiology, American Association for the Advancement of Science, and American Society for Biochemistry and Molecular Biology. He has published more than 180 papers in peer-reviewed journals.

Raj Kumar is an Associate Professor at the Institute of Advanced Science, Dartmouth, USA. Kumar has served in a study section of the NIH reviewer panel. Other than scientific articles in peer-reviewed journals he has contributed several chapters to books on biochemistry and biophysics. He is the author of the book *Protein Toxins in Modeling Biochemistry*. His areas of research include nanoparticles, biotechnology, drug delivery, cellular biology, MD simulation, protein biochemistry, and drug screening.

Practical Techniques in
Molecular Biotechnology

Bal Ram Singh

Raj Kumar

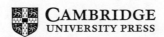

CAMBRIDGE
UNIVERSITY PRESS

CAMBRIDGE
UNIVERSITY PRESS

University Printing House, Cambridge CB2 8BS, United Kingdom

One Liberty Plaza, 20th Floor, New York, NY 10006, USA

477 Williamstown Road, Port Melbourne, VIC 3207, Australia

314–321, 3rd Floor, Plot 3, Splendor Forum, Jasola District Centre, New Delhi–110025, India

103 Penang Road, #05–06/07, Visioncrest Commercial, Singapore 238467

Cambridge University Press is part of the University of Cambridge.

It furthers the University's mission by disseminating knowledge in the pursuit of education, learning and research at the highest international levels of excellence.

www.cambridge.org
Information on this title: www.cambridge.org/9781108486408

First published 2021

Printed in India by Avantika Printers Pvt. Ltd.

A catalogue record for this publication is available from the British Library

Library of Congress Cataloging-in-Publication Data

Names: Singh, Bal Ram, author. | Kumar, Raj (Biochemist), author.
Title: Practical techniques in molecular biotechnology / Bal Ram Singh, Raj Kumar.
Description: Cambridge, United Kingdom ; New York, NY : Cambridge University Press, 2021. | Includes bibliographical references and index.
Identifiers: LCCN 2021013816 (print) | LCCN 2021013817 (ebook) | ISBN 9781108486408 (hardback) | ISBN 9781108659161 (ebook)
Subjects: MESH: Molecular Biology--methods | Biotechnology--methods | Chemistry Techniques, Analytical--methods | Tissue Engineering--methods | BISAC: MEDICAL / Biotechnology | MEDICAL / Biotechnology
Classification: LCC QP801.B69 (print) | LCC QP801.B69 (ebook) | NLM QU 34 | DDC 572/.33--dc23
LC record available at https://lccn.loc.gov/2021013816
LC ebook record available at https://lccn.loc.gov/2021013817

ISBN 978-1-108-48640-8 Hardback

Contents

Figures

Tables

Preface

Over the last 50 years, the development of far superior understanding of genomics and proteomics, has spurred the growth of biotechnology to a level where the revenues the sector generates are now of the order of about $430 billion a year and growing at approximately 8.3%. Directed manipulation of cell genes and development of recombinant technologies are allowing research institutions and industry to create fresh platforms for development of new technologies, products, markets, and indeed expectations. All this is contributing to ever increasing the pervasive influence of the biological organism in our everyday life.

Use of biotechnological processes is not new. For centuries some of these techniques have been used in the manufacturing of wines, beers, milk-based products, bread, and so many others. Although how biological mechanisms worked exactly was not well understood, the optimized biotechnological processes involved for such manufacturing were well established.

A fascinating aspect of biotechnology is its multidisciplinary nature, which draws upon concepts, theory and practices from a gamut of different fields including biology, chemistry, biochemistry, molecular biology, genetics, microbiology, and process engineering.

Although there are several books available on bioanalytical techniques, cellular biology, molecular biology, biotechnology, and so on, there is no readily available source of information that comprehensively yet concisely presents the techniques employed in biotechnology. Accordingly, a book covering the range of principles and applications of biotechnology should be handy for research students.

One of the goals of a science education is to inculcate scientific literacy in such a way that students should be free of any bias while making decisions on day-to-day scientific problems. In this case, the purpose of such education is that students imbibe adequately, the principles, the theory and applications thereof, to develop laboratory and practical research skills focused on the solution of a real scientific problem. This book, on biotechnology, intends doing just that.

Our intention is to familiarize students with the basics of some of the well-known experimental biotechnology processes and practices, for their use and application in research. By referring to this book, students will find the contents useful in strengthening their basic skills in their field of interest and applying their learning to real-world problems. In the experience of the authors, a focus on practical problems helps students learn biochemical techniques in a context, and allows better integration with research projects. This book, at the graduate level (for biotechnology, chemical biotechnology, molecular biotechnology and cell biology courses), should be invaluable for learning the basics of biochemical and biophysical techniques, and would help build a strong foundation for further biomedical courses.

It consists of detailed treatment and study of the fundamental principles and techniques of biotechnology, essential for the understanding of biochemical/biophysical phenomena. Theoretical principles behind experimental techniques and procedures, have been explained extensively and this has been reinforced with assignments and data analysis. This book is replete with examples and questions posed for a better grasp of the topics. In addition, the book contains information on data analysis, statistics, units, safety, and best practices. Unique features of this book include new pedagogical approaches (such as questions to ponder over and protocols), real-world relevance, clear illustrations, and integrated biochemical and biotechnological concepts. All the while, the focus has been on basic concepts combined with some key applications.

Using this book, an instructor can design an experimental course for biochemistry, molecular biology, cellular biology, or biophysics. Instructors may use this book as a quick guide to prepare their lectures and laboratory assignments. Further, this book provides instructors with references. These may be made use of to develop innovative theoretical and practical courses for the fields of biochemistry, biophysical chemistry, and biotechnology.

A well-designed research-based experimental laboratory course is critical for research students interested in following biotechnology and related disciplines, and this book will help immensely in developing such courses.

Conceptualizing this book involved years of work and interaction with several experts in the area of biochemistry and biotechnology. The book has been developed through extraction of topics, experiments, and experience from several courses that were taught by the authors over a long a period of time. These courses included, Biochemistry Laboratory, Physical Biochemistry, Introduction to Biomedical Engineering and Biotechnology, Chemical Biology and Technology, Biological Spectroscopy, Fluorescence Spectroscopy for Biochemists, and Instrumental Methods of Analysis.

We would like to extend our gratitude to Dr. Toby Dills, Dr. Maolin Guo, Dr. Emmanuel Ojadi, Dr. Tim Su, Dr. Valeri Barsegov, Dr. Robert Weis, Dr. Fen-Ni Fu, Dr. Shuowei Cai, Dr. Li Li, Dr. Brian Blanchette, Dr. Yu Zhou, Dr. Roshan Kukreja, Dr. Tzuu-Wang Chang, Dr. Tom Feltrup, Dr. Anne-Marie Bryant, Dr. Ghuncha Ambrin, and many students, including Mario Oliveira, Robin Nunes, Yuhong Hu, for interacting, collaborating, contributing, and supporting the development of the many ideas discussed in this book.

We would especially like to mention Dr. Brian Blanchette, who as teaching assistant in one of the courses, organized several experiments some of which are included in the book. Several staff members at the University of Massachusetts Dartmouth and the Institute of Advanced Sciences, including Mr. Paul Lindo, Mr. Steve Riding, and Ms. Jenny Davis played significant roles in advancing experimental parts of techniques included in this book.

Finally, we are grateful to the Department of Chemistry and Biochemistry, University of Massachusetts Dartmouth, and the Institute of Advanced Sciences for providing opportunities and support for our academic research and teaching to the level required for completing this work, for furthering the knowledge of future students and researchers.

Bal Ram Singh
Raj Kumar

June, 2021

1

Introduction

1.1 Biotechnology – Its Background and History

The office of Technology Assessment of the U.S. Congress defines biotechnology as "any technique that uses living organisms or their products to make or modify a(another) product, to improve plants or animals, or to develop microorganisms for specific uses." In its broadest terms, such a definition includes human beings, making biotechnology to be as old as the development of human skills such as to grow crops, harvest them, and use them as ingredients to cook their meals. In fact, a term Biotechnik, originally referring to social biology by Goldscheid in 1911, was used in the *Nature* journal of 1933 to print an editorial on Biotechnology (Bud, 1989; Goldcheid, 1911). Ironically, time has come a full circle as scientists are now examining gene expression patterns under different social conditions (Cole, 2014).

Biotechnology as a system of knowledge and application probably goes back to Vedic times, when the system of Ayurveda (literally meaning knowledge of life) was developed. Reference to the use of herbs for treating medical conditions are to be found in the earliest literature of India, over 14,000 years ago. According to BioREACH (which stands for Biotechnology Resource for Educational Advancement of Curriculum in High Schools at Arizona State University) some forms of biotechnology were being practiced by the ancients in Babylon, Egypt, and Rome in their selective breeding practices with livestock, over 10,000 years ago. There are instances where people around 6000 BC used fermentation to make wine and beer; and when the Chinese used lactic acid producing bacteria to produce yogurt around 4000 BC.

The modern term 'biotechnology' was first coined by a Hungarian engineer, Karl Ereky (1878–1952), in 1919. He defined biotechnology as general processes of converting raw materials into useful products, such as on industrial farms, using living organisms. A previous term 'zymotechnology' was used in the nineteenth century for using microorganisms to produce products like bread, wine, tofu, and so on. In the early twentieth century zymotechnology also included biological chemistry and covered usage of biological molecules such as enzymes, amino acids, and proteins for industrial production.

Modern biotechnology took root after the discovery of genetic material and the central theme of the gene progression route, namely DNA → RNA → Proteins, during the 1930s to the 1950s. With better fundamental understanding of the macromolecular structure–function, recombinant technology, advancements in microbiology, and chemical engineering, with the use of instrumental tools for synthesis and analysis of molecular characteristics, the field of biotechnology has made giant strides, especially since the 1980s. Armed with advances in cell and tissue engineering, biotechnologists have developed several bold concepts about designer proteins, targeted drug delivery, novel bio-macromolecules, and a variety of bio-based pharmaceuticals, especially after the discovery of designer organisms (Table 1.1); and the detection and diagnostics of diseases, genetically modified plants and food, synthesis of a variety of pharmaceuticals, agriculture and crop protection drugs, and even organic rejuvenation of the Earth and its environment. Biotechnology has become a source of basic and applied research, employing and integrating with other major fields of study such as chemistry, biochemistry, physics, engineering, social sciences, humanities, business, medical care, and environmental protection.

Table 1.1   Events that shaped modern biotechnology.

In Ancient Times

8000–4000 BCE	Humans domesticate crops and livestock.
2000 BCE	Development of fermentation technology for beer, bread, production of cheese, and wine.
500 BCE	First antibiotic – Moldy soyabean curds used to treat boils (in China).
100 CE	First insecticide – powdered chrysanthemums (in China).

During Medieval Times (Prior to the 20th Century)

1663	Robert Hooke gave the first description of living cells.
1677	Detailed description of bacteria and protozoa by Antonie van Leeuwenhoek
1798	First viral vaccine (for smallpox) by Edward Jenner.
1802	The word "biology" first appears.
1830–1833	Proteins are discovered; first enzyme is discovered and isolated.
1857–1862	Bacterial origin of fermentation explained by Louis Pasteur. He later proposed the germ theory of disease. • Theory of evolution proposed by Charles Darwin.
1863–1870	The laws of inheritance was proposed by Gregor Mendal. Identification of DNA.
1871–1880	Discovery of an artificial sweetner. • Development of a staining technique for identification of bacteria. • Discovery of chromatin.
1881–1890	Vaccines developed against cholera, anthrax and rabies.
1893	Immunotherapy was used for the first time to treat a cancer patient.

During the First Half of the 20th Century

1915	Discovery of phages – viruses that only infect bacteria.
1917	Discovery of a beneficial strain of *E.coli*.
1919	First use of the term "biotechnology."
1927	Herman Muller discovers that radiation causes defects in chromosomes.
1928	Discovery of the first antibiotic, penicillin, by Alexander Fleming.
1944	DNA is proven to carry genetic information.

Contd.

Table 1.1 *contd.*

Post 1950

1952	First continuous cell line (HeLa); developed by George Otto Gey
1953	Watson and Crick discover and explain the double-helix structure of DNA.
1954	First kidney transplant between identical twins conducted by Joseph Murray.
1955	Amino acid sequence of insulin discovered.
1957	Scientists reveal that sickle-cell anemia occurs due to an alteration in a single amino acid in hemoglobin cells.
1958	DNA created in a test tube by Arthur Kornberg for the first time.
	• Moore–Stein amino acid analyzer developed.
	• First X-ray diffraction depiction of protein crystal and myoglobin structure.

The 1960s

1960	Discovery of messenger RNA (mRNA).
1961	Concept of Operon developed by François Jacob and Jacques Monad.
1962	Discovery of green fluorescent protein (GFP) by Osamu Shimomura in the jellyfish *Aequorea victoria*. He went on to develop a cellular visualization technique from this.
1963	Measles vaccine developed by Samuel Katz and John F Enders.
	• Independent groups in the USA, Germany and China produce insulin, a pancreatic hormone.
1964	Discovery of reverse transcriptase.
1966	Genetic code for DNA cracked.
1967–71	First American vaccine for mumps developed by Maurice.
	• First vaccine for rubella developed
	• Measles/mumps/rubella (MMR) vaccine developed.
1968	Har Gobind Khorana synthesizes DNA in a test tube. Discovery of protein synthesis process in cells

The 1970s

1970	Discovery of restriction enzymes.
1972	Dicovery of DNA ligases and its uses.
	• The DNA composition of humans was found to be 99% similar to that of chimpanzees and gorillas.
	• First use of reverse transcriptase to prepare complementary DNA from mRNA in a test tube.
1973	rDNA techniques developed by Stanley Cohen and Herbert Boyer.
	• Blotting technique for DNA (Southern blot) developed by Sir Edwin Mellor Southern.
1974	The NIH formed a Recombinant DNA Advisory Committee to supervise recombinant genetic research.
	Chicken pox vaccine developed in Japan.
1975	Development of monoclonal antibodies technology.
1976	NIH publishes the first guidelines for rDNA research.
	• Employment of molecular hybridization for prenatal diagnosis of alpha thalassemia.
	• Yeast genes expressed in *E. coli* bacteria.

Contd.

Table 1.1 *contd.*

1977	Procedures developed to swiftly sequence long sections of DNA.

- Protein, somastatin, cloned using recombinant gene technology. *A landmark year: 1977 is held by many to have heralded the arrival of the "age of biotechnology."*
- First vaccine for pneumonia developed by R. Austrian *et al.* at the University of Pennsylvania.

1978   Boyer synthesizes a version of recombinant human insulin gene.
- The first test-tube baby, Louise Brown, is born in the UK.
- The first vaccine for meningococcal meningitis is developed.

The 1980s

1980   US Supreme Court rules that genetically altered life forms can be patented, creating vast possibilities for commercially exploiting genetic engineering.
- First patent of this nature awarded to the Exxon oil company to patent an oil-eating micro-organism. *This would later be employed in the 1989 cleanup of the Exxon oil spill at Prince William Sound, Alaska.*
- S. Cohen and D.H. Boyer receive US patent for gene cloning.
- First automatic gene machine developed in California.
- Establishment of Amgen, which would grow to become the world's largest biotechnology based medicine company.

1981   Frst vaccine for hepatitis B developed by Baruch Blumberg and Irving Millman.
- First transgenic animals created.

1982   FDA supports the first recombinant protein.

1983   Isolation of AIDS virus by Luc Montagnier of the Pasteur Institute in Paris.
- Demonstration of polymerase chain reaction (PCR) by Kary Mullis.
- FDA sanctions monoclonal antibody-based diagnostic analysis to identify *Chlamydia trachomatis.*
- Production of the first artificial chromosome.
- Discovery of genetic basis for disease inheritance.

1984   Release of DNA fingerprinting technique.
- Release of the first genetically engineered vaccine for hepatitis B.
- Entire genome of the human immunodeficiency virus (HIV) virus cloned and sequenced.

1985   Genetic fingerprinting becomes court admissible.
- Development of genetically engineered plants resistant to viruses, insects and bacteria.
- Successful cloning of the gene encoding human lung surfactant protein. *This was a major step toward reducing premature birth problems.*
- NIH releases guidelines for executing trials of gene therapy on humans.

1986   Use of antibodies and enzymes for therapeutics by Peter G Schultz from University of California, Berkeley.
- FDA approval for first monoclonal antibody treatment to fight kidney transplant rejection.
- FDA sanctions the first biotech-derived interferon drugs to treat cancer.
- FDA sanctions the first genetically engineered human vaccine to prevent hepatitis B.

Contd.

Table 1.1 *contd.*

1987	FDA approves genetically engineered tissue plasminogen activator to treat heart attack.

- Synthesis of yeast artificial chromosomes (YAC) by Maynard Olson and colleagues at Washington University. These are expression vectors for large proteins.
- Discovery of linkage between reverse transcription and PCR to augment messenger RNA sequences.
- DNA microarray technology developed.
- Indentification of genes whose expression is altered by interferon from pools of DNA.
- FDA approval for serum tumor marker test for ovarian cancer.

1988   Congress decides to fund the Human Genome Project.

1989   Amgen releases its first biologically derived human therapeutic.

- FDA approves oil-eating bacteria; which was employed later to clear up the Exxon Valdez oil spill.
- Discovery of the cystic fibrosis gene.

The 1990s

1990   The first gene therapy treatment is conducted.

- The Human Genome Project is launched.
- FDA approves first hepatitis C antibody test.
- FDA approves bioengineered form of the protein interferon gamma to treat chronic granulomatous disease.
- FDA sanctions a modified enzyme for enzyme replacement therapy to treat severe combined immunodeficiency disease. It is the first successful application of enzyme replacement therapy for an inherited disease.

1992   The US Army collects and collates blood and tissue tests from all new recruits as part of a genetic dog-tag plan to better identify bodies of soldiers killed in combat.

- FDA approves the first genetically engineered blood-clotting factor. It is a recombinant protein used to treat hemophilia A.
- FDA sanctions a recombinant protein to treat renal cell cancer.
- American and British researchers reveal technique for analyzing embryos in vitro for genetic abnormalities, e.g., cystic fibrosis and hemophilia.

1993   FDA approves a recombinant protein to treat multiple sclerosis.

- A rough map is created of all 23 pairs of human chromosomes by a research team led by Daniel Cohen from the Center for the Study of Human Polymorphisms, Paris.

1994   FDA approves a recombinant protein to treat growth hormone (GH) deficiency. .

- Discovery of the first breast cancer gene, BRCA1 by Mary-Claire King at University of California, Berkeley.
- FDA sanctions a modified enzyme to deal with Gaucher's disease.
- Identification of a number of genes, human and otherwise, with explanation of their functions. These comprise of: Ob, a gene connected to obesity; BCR, a breast cancer receptiveness gene; BCL-2, a gene linked to apoptosis (programmed cell death); Hedgehog genes (named because of their shape), which synthesize proteins that direct cell differentiation in complex organisms; and Vpr, a gene regulating the reproduction of the HIV virus.
- Genetic linkage studies recognize the role of genes in a variety of disorders, including bipolar disorder, cerulean cataracts, melanoma, dyslexia, prostate cancer, thyroid cancer, hearing loss, sudden infant death syndrome and dwarfism.
- FDA approvesa genetically engineered human DNase.

Contd.

Table 1.1 *contd.*

1995	First baboon-to-human bone marrow transplant conducted on an AIDS patient.
	• First vaccine for hepatitis A is developed.
	• Researchers at the Institute for Genomic Research complete the first full gene sequence of a living organism for the bacterium *Haemophilus influenzae.*
	• A European study group determines that a genetic defect is the most frequent cause of deafness.
1996	Researchers at the Department of Biochemistry at Stanford University and Affymetrix develop the gene chip, a small glass or silica microchip that contains thousands of individual genes that can be examined simultaneously. This is a major scientific breakthrough in gene expression and DNA sequencing technology.
	• Research groups sequenced the complete genome of a complex organism, *Saccharomyces cerevisiae*, otherwise known as baker's yeast. The accomplishment symbolizes the entire sequencing of the largest genome to date.
	• A novel, economic diagnostic biosensor test is developed to hasten the detection of a toxic strain of *E. coli*, the bacteria responsible for food-poisoning outbreaks.
1997	Discovery of the first human artificial chromosome.
	• Synthesis from a mixture of natural and synthetic DNA, of a genetic cassette that could possibly be adapted and employed in gene therapy.
	• FDA sanctions a recombinant follicle stimulating hormone to deal with infertility.
	• FDA permits the first bloodless HIV-antibody analysis, based on cells from patients' gums.
	• Researchers at the Institute for Genomic Research sequenced the entire genome of the Lyme disease pathogen, *Borrelia burgdorferi*, along with the genome for the organism associated with stomach ulcers, *Helicobacter pylori*.
	• Researchers at the University of Wisconsin–Madison sequence the *E. coli* genome.
	• FDA permits the first therapeutic antibody to treat cancer in the USA. It is employed for patients with non-Hodgkin's lymphoma.
	• Dolly, the first cloned animal is born.
1998	For the first time, Human skin is created in the laboratory.
	• Two research groups culture embryonic stem cells. Embryonic stem cells can be employed to regenerate tissue and produce disorders mimicking diseases.
	• Researchers at the Sanger Institute in the UK and at the Washington University School of Medicine in St Louis, USA, sequence the first whole animal genome for the *caenorhabditis elegans* worm.
	• Creation of a rough draft of the human genome map displaying the sites of more than 30 000 genes.
	• The first vaccine for Lyme disease is developed
	• FDA approves treatment of Crohn's disease by using a novel monoclonal antibody.
	• Employment of a monoclonal antibody therapy against breast cancer.

The 2000s

2000	Kary Mullis adds value to Har Gobind Khorana's findings by amplifying DNA in a test tube, to create a thousand times more DNA than the original amount.
	• First cloned sheep, Dolly, is displayed by Sir Ian Wilmut.

Contd.

Table 1.1 *contd.*

	• Craig Venter sequences the human genome; the first publicly accessible genomes would later be those of James Watson and Venter.
	• Successful completion of a rough draft of the human genome by researchers at Celera Genomics and the Human Genome Project.
2001	The human genome sequence is reported in journals *Science* and *Nature.*
2002	Conclusion of an era of very rapid shotgun sequencing of major genomes during which those of the mouse, chimpanzee, dog and hundreds of other species were all sequenced.
2003	Celera and the NIH successfully conclude the sequencing of the human genome.
2004	FDA approves the first monoclonal antibody with antiangiogenic properties (i.e., inhibiting blood vessel formation or angiogenesis) for cancer therapy.
	• FDA approves a DNA microarray analysis system.
2006	FDA approves a recombinant vaccine against the human papillomavirus.
	• Discovery of the three-dimensional (3D) structure of HIV.
2007	Researchers discover how to use human skin cells to produce embryonic stem cells.
2008	Venter replicates a bacterium's genetic structure completely from laboratory chemicals, taking a step nearer to generating the world's first living artificial organism.
2008	Development of first synthetic DNA for gene therapy by Japanese researchers.
2009	Discovery of three new genes connected with Alzheimer's disease.
	• FDA approves the first clinical trial by means of embryonic stem cells.
2010	FDA sanctions modified prostate cancer medicine for enhancing the capability of a patient's immune cells to distinguish and attack cancer cells.
	• FDA approves osteoporosis treatment based on genetic investigation.
	• Replication of a synthetic genome demonstrated by Craig Venter. He showed duplication can be done alone.
2011	First stem cells developed organ (trachea) is transplanted into a human recipient.
	• 3D printing technology is used for "skin-printing" for the first time.
	• FDA approves the first cord blood therapy.
2012	FDA issues Draft of Regulations for bio-similar drugs.
2013	CRISPR-Cas is used in human genome editing.
2014	Integrative Microbiome Project launched.
	• Embryonic stem cells for human skin are cloned for the first time.
2015	Oncology oriented gene therapy is approved in both US and Europe for the first time.
2017	Completion of the Human Microbiome Project.
2018	Human eggs are grown in a laboratory for the first time.
	• USFDA approves first-ever drug based on RNAi.
	• Chinese scientist announces existence of gene-edited babies for the first time.
2019	CRISPR technology used to edit human genes to treat cancer.
	• Prime editing technology for gene edition is introduced.
2020	RNA and DNA based vaccines against Corona virus approved by the United States, United Kingdom and other countries

(Table 1.1 is a modified version of that from Bhatia, 2018)

The scope of biotechnology ranges from tools and techniques for examination of the biological system itself for health, basic mechanism, refitting, and so on, to the creation of new molecules, drugs, cosmetics, and much more. Biomimicry is becoming an important source of technology for bio-engineering. DNA sequencing and other biomarker technologies have become part of the criminal justice system. One's individual genome is being used for devising medical treatment.

Plant extracts are being used to prepare nanomaterials from metals for medical, agriculture, and information technology applications. Biotechnology is limited not just to utility applications, but is also an integral part of basic research on biological systems. Its application ranges from dealing with subtle mental issues to whole bodies and on to environment concerns. Thorough understanding of the basic principles is thus vital to practical applications of such technologies and their future development.

Technology of every kind is basically the application of techniques and biotechnology (also being a field of technology) is all about techniques and their applications. However, given its source and use in biological science, it encompasses physics, chemistry, biology, engineering, computer, socio-economics, business, and the environment. Therefore, it is not sufficient to learn only techniques in a unidimensional way. Proficiency in biotechnology demands holistic learning. This book, therefore, presents not only practical technological protocols, but also fundamental principles. While it has not covered the entire spectrum of biotechnology, it still explores in depth, adequate aspects of the subject to enhance student learning and practicing.

1.2   Technology and Laboratory Practice

Biotechnology and associated courses like biochemistry, molecular biology, or cell biology include laboratory courses at the undergraduate and graduate levels. These are essential in developing proper understanding of chemical analysis and biological processes. Typical laboratory courses utilize "cookbook" experiments to introduce handling, analysis and interpretation of biological experiments using techniques borrowed from chemistry. Several variations have been introduced whereby more than one set of experiments have been integrated to teach protocol preparation, assay design, and interconnectedness of techniques (Hannan et al., 1999; Wolfsen et al., 1996). However, real research-based biotechnology laboratory courses have yet to fully develop. In the experience of the authors, this focus allows students to learn biotechnology skills in a context, and so it trains them for a better integration of chemical and biological techniques with research projects.

The biochemistry aspect of biotechnology encompasses a vast number of chemical processes involved in any biological phenomenon. Students generally need a high level of concentration and critical thinking to correlate several interconnected topics. While biological processes easily attract students' attention and enthusiasm out of, both, curiosity to learn about ourselves (as living beings) and a likely opportunity to improve the quality of life for society, the delicate nature of biological samples generally requires greater hands-on attention for students to learn and perform chemical analysis of biological samples. Generally, all chemical techniques are applicable to biological samples but they usually require substantial modifications and adaptations to be applied to, sufficiently, understand significant biological processes. Therefore, an advanced biochemistry laboratory course is necessary to introduce chemical techniques that are commonly used to analyze biological samples.

Biochemistry and/or biotechnology laboratory courses, especially at the undergraduate level, tend to be limited in their depth and are scattered in terms of their content, primarily because of the vast number of biochemical processes involving a wide range of substances (e.g., lipids, nucleic acids, carbohydrates, proteins) which are further complicated due to variations in organisms (e.g., bacteria, plants, animals). Biotechnology/biochemistry laboratory textbooks, currently available, describe experiments such that a given "cookbook" experimental system is deemed enough for demonstrating a particular technique. For example, in a standard experimental biochemistry textbook, an enzyme kinetics experiment may involve egg lysozyme, hut for enzyme inhibition analysis it may be lactate dehydrogenase. In the same book, the gel filtration technique may consist of using immunoglobulin G as a biological sample. In such cases, while students may succeed in the "cookbook" exercise because a given biological system is the most suitable sample to demonstrate a technique, they lose the connection between different experimental exercises. Their ability to understand the design and execution of experiments remains limited, and their potential to utilize these techniques to solve any real-world problem remains minimal. An additional problem with biochemistry/biotechnology laboratory and biotechnology courses is that the lecture class material is not always easy to directly practice in the laboratory because the sophisticated instruments required are simply not there and neither is the substantial amount of time needed to complete experiments. One way to alleviate this is to teach a laboratory course based on a research topic that involves several commonly used cellular, molecular biological, immunochemical, and biochemical techniques. This book provides access to not only those techniques but also to the fundamental principles behind those techniques to enable a student to independently design research and learning projects. A brief summary of techniques employed in the various chapters, follows.

Chapter 2 on recombinant DNA and protein technology outlines the basic methods of genetic cloning, gene expression in various organisms, protein purification, and estimation. In addition to presenting the detailed scientific principles behind each of the technologies, advantages and pitfalls have also been pointed out to allow a student to assess their suitability for specific situations and/ or examine the experimental data in view of those. Further strategies are pointed out to address any difficulties.

Chapter 3 on enzyme kinetics, proteomics, and mass spectrophotometry is primarily devoted to the characterization of proteins. The enzyme kinetics segment forms the bulk of this chapter, as this is one common functional technique that a biotechnologist must master, not simply to perform enzymatic activity assays but to understand various features of enzymes for practical applications, such as to devise inhibitor/activator use in bio-processing, conducting comparative evaluation of their function under different environmental conditions, and to understand the basic mechanics of operation for structure–function analysis. Adequate mathematical treatment and experimental precautions have been described in detail to provide students with the information they need for independent design and operation of a biochemical or biotechnological project. Proteomics is a field that examines proteins in space and time for their behavior and changes that may occur due to the biological processes. Mass spectrophotometry is a set of very highly sensitive methods for protein detection and identification, and thus has been detailed separately.

Chapter 4 covers analytical techniques that are readily available to examine biological molecules, both, small (pigments, hormones, metabolites, and such) as well as large (proteins, genetic material, and such). Such techniques can be used to either examine the characteristics of the molecules or their interactions in biologically relevant conditions. Numerous sedimentation, calorimetric, spectroscopic (UV/Vis, fluorescence, circular dichroism, and Fourier Transform Infrared or FT-IR) and electrophoresis techniques have been described in detail to understand the principles and applications for structure, stability, size, mobility, interactions, and biological activity. Examples of practical demonstrations are also provided for the instructors to engage students in the learning process.

Chapter 5 deals with molecular biology, which is perhaps a misnomer for molecular genetic biology, as biochemically speaking all the biological systems are based on molecules. However, recognizing that the genetic material is in fact the ultimate basis of all other molecules, biology of the genetic molecules is referred to as molecular biology. These molecules were also the first examples of molecular manipulation in the laboratory, and thus became a popular part of molecular biology. Techniques for molecular structures of DNA and RNA in isolated or complexed state with other biological molecules such as proteins: replication, transcription, mutations, recombinant gene expression, polymerase chain reaction (PCR), and reverse-transcription (RT) PCR for duplication and detection, genetic hybridization, electrophoretic mobility, blotting, nucleic acid sequencing, and such, have all been covered. Background information on genetic material, genes, and their discovery and role has been emphasized to enhance student ability to link the basic knowledge with the current experimental practices for developing projects.

Chapter 6 focuses on cell culture, which has emerged as a very useful technique for biotechnological exploration into microbial, plant, and animal systems. Cells provide an in situ environment to examine biological activities, for natural synthesis of biological molecules, cell–cell interactions, assays, organelle studies, metabolic experiments, developmental studies, and toxicity studies of therapeutics or poisons. Cell cultures of both prokaryotic and eukaryotic cells are possible now, including those of nerve cells. In eukaryotic cells, cancer cell lines are available as perpetual cultures convenient for most studies, but primary cell cultures are also possible to imitate natural cell growth and differentiation. Stem cell based development of cell culture allows preparation of cells and tissues of various kinds conveniently. Modern tools of light microscopy, electron microscopy, confocal microscopy, fluorescence microscopy, and atomic force microscopy allow detailed examination of cell structures, delivery of external molecules, and cell–cell tight junctions. Cell microchips with co-culturing options are becoming very useful for assays of drugs and for understanding cell–cell interactions, both physically and biochemically.

Chapter 7 on antibody technology primarily covers experimental uses of antibodies in immunochemical analysis and characterization encompassing topics ranging from immunoassays to immunotherapy. Basic information on antibodies, including monoclonal antibodies, is provided to let the reader grasp the variety of features special to these molecules which have been useful in unraveling the many facets of biological systems for detection, diagnostics, and therapy.

1.3   Pedagogical Strategy of Biochemical Technology Practice

There are numerous techniques in these six chapters which may be adopted for either a single experiment or as a series of related scientific questions. Such a series provides more realistic replication of real-life situations. For true imbibing of techniques, one has to attempt to use them to answer specific scientific questions, and each lab experiment needs to be part of that learning goal.

A Model

To illustrate, consider a research-based biochemical technology laboratory course that engages students in learning laboratory skills that are focused on solving a real science problem. A research problem can generally be chosen which is related to a significant biological question that can easily be understood by students with one semester of biochemistry and cell biology knowledge. And so, the project now being taken up relates to the analysis of glutathione-S-transferase (GST) of marine organisms from a local harbor which had been contaminated with polychlorinated biphenyls. In real-life, New Bedford harbor (in Massachusetts, USA) was a super-reservoir site for PCB pollution.

The enzyme exists in several isomeric forms which differ in isoelectric points that can be exploited for ion-exchange chromatography. Finally, it is inhibited by several polyaromaric hydrocarbons (PAHs), thus allowing varying kinetic analysis. We used the different biochemically relevant features of this enzyme to teach several biochemical techniques and to provide students with independent research projects for evaluating glutathione-S-transferases from different marine animals such as clams, oysters, quahogs, scallops, and other organisms. The availability of different organisms here, allows new projects to be formulated every year. By collaborating with a biology faculty to coordinate with one of their laboratories that ran a biochemistry laboratory course, we were able to conduct nucleic acid chemistry experiments on glutathione-S-transferases from local marine animals, and so, to understand the role of marine pollution in the genetic expression of this enzyme as well. Most students taking this course were quite enthusiastic about this approach. The approach can be applied in any part of the world because GST is ubiquitous in all organisms ranging from prokaryotes to mammals, and its gene expression is responsive to environmental conditions including pollution (Mannervik and Danielson, 1998; Prestera et al., 1993; Rushmore and Pickett, 1993; Vandkevaa et al., 1993). The great enthusiasm shown by students for this approach stemmed not just because they learnt laboratory techniques, but also because they felt they were contributing to solving a real local environmental problem.

Design

The course is designed to focus on the GST which is a detoxifying enzyme involved in the metabolism of PAHs, pesticides, herbicides, and other electrophilic xenobiotic compounds. The enzyme is known to catalyze the conjugation of glutathione to xenobiotics, which makes them water soluble so that they can be easily disposed of through further metabolism and excretion (Singh, 1999).

About two-thirds of the laboratory course incorporated ten advanced biochemical techniques. Since this project was connected to the PCB pollution that had drawn great publicity from local media, it caught the absolute attention of the students involved.

Strategy

The enzyme (GST) has several desirable features that make it particularly suitable to be used for an undergraduate/graduate project in a biochemical laboratory set-up. It is a relatively small protein (25 kDa) that exists as a dimer in solution. It is an enzyme whose genetic expression is induced by organic pollutants, including PCBs. It specifically binds to glutathione so that affinity chromatography (focused to analyze various chemical characteristics of the glutathione-S-transferase (GST)) may be used for its purification. The remaining third of the semester time, students could work on a project that involved application of all the newly acquired techniques to solve a biochemical problem that encompassed the same detoxifying enzyme. One particular year, students decided to analyze the enzyme from a local shellfish species, quahog, obtained from a superfund site for

PCB (polychlorinated biphenyls) pollution. Because of the link of the course to the local superfund environmental site-related problems, students found the whole course exciting and relevant.

In deciding such a project one has to keep several points in mind. Glutathione-S-transferases are well known to be important for biomedical reasons because of their relationship to cancer in animals and humans; and for environmental reasons, as GSTs are responsible for a large part of xenobiotic metabolism. The enzyme being a protein allows application of all protein techniques to study its characteristics. In literature, GSTs are classified based on their isoelectric points, thus providing students with further interesting reasons to determine the enzyme's isoelectric point (pI) so that they can classify it. Of course, pI is also used to strategize ion-exchange chromatography. The enzyme exists as an oligomer which allows students to observe differences in the molecular size determined with the use of sodium dodecyl sulfate polyacrylamide gel electrophoresis and size-exclusion chromatography. GSTs are two-substrate enzymes, and are inhibited by a variety of biological metabolites such as bilirubin, hemin, anthocyanin, and suchlike providing ample opportunity to explore various enzyme kinetic issues.

To integrate it further with student learning, a biology professor (Professor Robert Leamnson) who taught cell biology laboratory courses was roped in to introduce GST activity, gene cloning, and its expression. This exposed students to the genetic aspect of the protein, leading to greater familiarity with the subject, and to develop curiosity about the biochemical techniques regarding the enzyme.

Students need exposure to various techniques with different systems, and an integrated approach that includes analysis of systems provides contextual learning of the techniques. In the process, not only do students master the techniques that may be employed, but also learn how to interpret data for a biological system.

Table 1.2   Course outline and tentative schedule of a biochemical technology course

---

Week 1: *Introduction to the laboratory and literature search and buffer preparation*

Objective: Library literature search to obtain biochemically relevant information on glutathione-S-transferases.
Examples: Group 1-Metabolic substrates of glutathione-S-transferases; Group 2-Effect of environmental factors on glutathione-S-transferases; Group 3-Role of glutathione-S-transferases in human or animal ageing; Group 4-Plant senescence and glutathione-S-transferases.

Week 2: *Spectroscopic determination of protein pK*

Objective: Demonstrate the use of absorption spectroscopy for pKa determination. Observe variation in the p.Ka of Tyr side chains in a protein (glutathione S-transferases) compared with those in free aqueous solution. Calculate the number of ionized Tyr residues in glutathione-S-transferases.

Week 3: *Protein estimation*

Objective: Use three different common methods of protein assay (Bradford, Lowry and spectroscopic) to determine absorption extinction coefficient of a protein, glutathione-S-transferases.

Week 4: *Discussion and catch-up*

Contd.

Table 1.2 *contd.*

Week 5: *Polyacrylamide gel electrophoresis*

Objective: Use sodium dodecyl sulfate-polyacrylamide gel electrophoresis (SOS-PAGE) to estimate molecular weight of a protein, glutathione-S-transferases.

Week 6: *Isoelectric focusing of protein(s)*

Objective: Use isoelectric focusing-polyacrylamide gel electrophoresis (IEF-PAGE) to estimate p/ of a protein, and classify the given glutathione S-transferases.

Week 7: *Size exclusion chromatography*

Objective: Determine the native molecular weight of a protein, glutathione-S-transferases, using size exclusion column chromatography, and compare your results with the molecular weight obtained from SOS-PAGE.

Week 8: *Affinity chromatography*

Objective: Purification of glutathione-S-transferases using glutathione agarose affinity column chromatography. Obtain pure homogeneous glutathione S-transferases (GST) from oat plants or Tetrahymena (examples).

Week 9: *Immunochemical technique ELISA*

Objective: Examine the relationship between glutathione-S-transferases from two sources with a polyclonal antibody using enzyme linked immunosorbent assay (ELISA).

Week 10: *Enzyme kinetics*

Objectives: Estimate Km and V""'" of glutathione S-transferases using glutathione (GSH) and 1-chloro-2,4-dinitrobenzene (CDNB) as substrates.

Weeks 11–15: *Isolation and biochemical characterization of glutathione-S-transferases from scallops, oats, quahogs or cranberries (examples)*

Objectives: Utilizing all the techniques learnt in the course, isolate, purify and characterize glutathione S-transferases for its absorption extinction coefficient, subunit structure, pl, enzyme kinetic parameters, and relationship to glutathione-S-transferases from other sources. Write your results in the form of a manuscript.

Problems and Solutions

While students have enjoyed the "integrated research approach" to the teaching of the biochemistry laboratory course in the past two years, they have repeatedly suggested that more time was required to complete the research project portion of the course. I have observed myself that while the "cookbook" set of course experiments works very well, application of the same techniques in the research project (where students have to design all the details themselves with only minimum input from the instructor) does not produce successful results, at least from students' first attempts. With limited time available in the semester, students in the past have been able to succeed in applying their techniques only when they continued their experiments over part of the summer months. Therefore, a second semester of the course not only allows students to conclude their incomplete projects but also allows for additional techniques to be taught to expand their learning. Several critical aspects of modern biochemistry, nucleic acid analysis and manipulation through molecular biology techniques that are not covered in a single semester biochemistry laboratory course due to the lack of time can be included with an additional semester of the course. To elaborate, techniques such as DNA isolation, cloning, polymerase chain reaction, and recombinant gene expression have become common in workplaces as well as in graduate research. The monomeric subunit of the GST has a size of 25–30 kDa, which is small enough to present advantages for genetic manipulation. Additionally, since the GST gene expression is responsive to environmental conditions, experiments related to gene expression can be designed using this system.

1.4 Laboratory Safety

General Laboratory Practices and Procedures

Due to the wide variety of experiments listed in this text it would be cumbersome to roster each specific chemical danger here. Therefore, dangers inherent to each exercise will be listed in the experiments in each chapter. The following safety precautions are a generalized list that will be encountered in each of the exercises. Individuals involved in biochemical experimentation should be intimately familiar with the below mentioned precautions.

General Precautions

1. Wear safety goggles at all times in the laboratory. For biochemical experimentation regular eyeglasses do not provide sufficient protection from either chemical hazards or broken glassware. Recently, the American Chemical Society has approved the use of contact lenses but only when worn in combination with safety goggles. The contact/goggle combination is important because most modern eyewash stations are not able to remove chemicals trapped behind contacts.
2. Proper clothing should be worn in the laboratory at all times. Long sleeve shirts, long pants and full shoes are the best choice. Skin protection will be at a maximum if such garments are covered with a full lab coat/apron.
3. Make use of the fume hoods for handling volatile and/or hazardous chemicals. When handling the chemicals, gloves should be worn to protect the hands.
4. Dispose of solid and liquid waste in containers, which are properly labeled. Notify the instructor if any of the waste containers are full or damaged. If you are not sure where to dispose of the waste ask your instructor for help.
5. Get acquainted with the layout of the lab, paying special attention to the fire extinguishers, emergency eye wash stations, first aid kits and the nearest emergency phone. Knowledge of the location of this apparatus may help save your life and prevent injury to others.

6. Never eat or drink in the laboratory area. Contamination of food or drink can take place without your knowledge. Dropping a reagent bottle on the lab floor may cause a toxic substance to spatter into your food or drink. Because the biochemistry lab usually involves long hours of analysis it is sometimes unavoidable for lab time to overlap with meal-time. If you must eat or drink something during the laboratory period leave the food or drink outside the laboratory. A short break to eat or drink will not be detrimental to the outcome of your experiments.

General Laboratory Courtesy

Like most teaching laboratories, the biochemistry laboratory can be a confusing crowded place for the new student. A lack of experience with the chemicals involved in the biochemistry laboratory can cause time consuming mishaps. Therefore, all biochemistry laboratory students, experienced or inexperienced, should observe the following laboratory courtesies:

1. Prior to the laboratory period the student should read the experimental protocol thoroughly, noting any questions for the instructor. As confusing as the biochemistry laboratory is to the new student it becomes many fold more confusing when the student has no idea what comes next.
2. When preparing reagents for your use from a common stock solution, be sure to return the stock solution to its proper storage place. Many chemicals used in biochemistry experiments degrade rapidly below 4°C. If you are preparing a mixture from a purchased chemical stock, check the label on the reagent bottle for the proper storage procedures.
3. After using common laboratory equipment, micropipettes, distilled water bottles, timers, etc., return them to their proper place immediately after cleaning. Many biochemistry laboratory courses do not have enough funding to provide equipment such as micropipettes to each student. Therefore, it is imperative for events to flow smoothly during the experiments; that common equipment be cleaned and returned as soon as possible.
4. Use only as much of the chemicals supplied to you as you need. In order to cut costs and produce less environmental waste many instructors prepare only required quantity of the common reagents for the experiment at hand. Use of excessive amounts of common reagents may cause a delay in the experiment for the others in the course, while they wait for more reagents to be prepared by the instructor.
5. Never insert the tip of your pipet/micropipetter into a common reagent bottle. This practice can easily spread contamination throughout laboratory, thus ruining many hours of work by yourself and other students.
6. After each lab period, clean your work area and any glassware that you used. After cleaning used glassware and rinsing with tap water rinse the glassware with distilled water and place it in a strainer to dry overnight.

1.5   Biosafety and Biosafety Levels

Biotechnology practices necessarily involve biological samples, which could be hazardous to health. Therefore, biosafety protocols have been developed by various organizations, including the US Centers for Disease Control and Prevention (CDC). The biosafety information provided here is largely based on CDC protocols.

Biosafety

The definition of biosafety is as follows: It includes the set of safety precautions which reduce a laboratorian's risk of exposure to potentially hazardous chemicals and infectious microbes. Additionally, it limits the contamination of the work environment and, ultimately, the community.

Biosafety Levels (BSLs)

There are four biosafety levels consisting of measures for containment of microbes and biological agents. Levels of biosafety are determined by infectivity, severity of disease, and transmissibility of microbes and biological samples. This also include: the nature of the work conducted, origin of the microbe, the agent and route of exposure. Based on these criteria BSL-1 to BSL-4 are defined (Figure 1.1). Each biosafety level builds on the controls of the level below it.

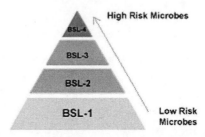

Fig. 1.1   Biosafety levels.

Every microbiology laboratory, regardless of biosafety level, follows standard microbiological practices, such as no mouth pipetting, labeling all the reagents, washing hands, sterilizing equipment, disinfecting the work areas, and so on.

Each biosafety level has its own specific containment controls that are required for the following:

BSL-1 Laboratory

A lab is designated a BSL-1 when the microbes there are not known to consistently cause disease in healthy adults and present minimal potential hazard to laboratorians and the environment. An example of a microbe that is typically worked with at a BSL-1 is a nonpathogenic strain of *E. coli*.

Specific considerations for a BSL-1 laboratory include the following (Figure 1.2):

Laboratory Practices

- Standard microbiological practices are followed.
- Work can be performed on an open lab bench or table Ⓐ.

Safety Equipment

- Personal protective equipment Ⓑ, (lab coats, gloves, eye protection) are worn as needed.

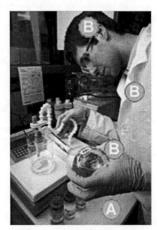

Fig. 1.2   BSL-1 type open workplace and personal protective equipment (PPE).

Facility Construction

- A sink must be available for hand washing.
- The lab should have doors to separate the working space from the rest of the facility.

BSL-2

BSL-2 builds upon BSL-1 for a lab that works with microbes that pose moderate hazards to laboratorians and the environment. The microbes are typically *indigenous* and associated with diseases of varying severity. An example of a microbe that is typically worked with at a BSL-2 laboratory is *Staphylococcus aureus*.

In addition to BSL-1 practices, BSL-2 laboratories have the following containment requirements (Figure 1.3):

Laboratory Practices

- Access to the laboratory is restricted when work is being conducted.

Safety Equipment

- Appropriate personal protective equipment (PPE) Ⓐ is worn, including lab coats and gloves. Eye protection and face shields can also be worn, as needed.

- All procedures that can cause infection from aerosols or splashes are performed within a biological safety cabinet (BSC) Ⓑ.

- An autoclave or an alternative method of decontamination is available for proper disposals.

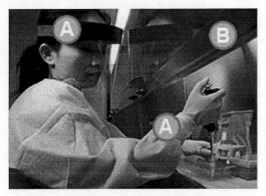

Fig. 1.3   BSL-2; working with personal protective equipment (PPE) in a safety cabinet.

Facility Construction

- The laboratory has self-closing doors.
- A sink and eyewash are readily available.

BSL-3

BSL-3 builds upon the containment requirements of BSL-2 for working with the microbes that can be either indigenous or exotic, and that can cause serious or potentially lethal disease through respiratory transmission. Respiratory transmission is the inhalation route of exposure. One example of a microbe that is typically worked with in a BSL-3 laboratory is *Mycobacterium tuberculosis*, the bacteria that causes tuberculosis.

In addition to BSL-2 requirements, BSL-3 laboratories have the following containment requirements (Figure 1.4):

Laboratory Practices

- Laboratorians are under medical surveillance and might receive immunizations for microbes they work with.
- Access to the laboratory is restricted and controlled at all times.

Safety Equipment

- Appropriate PPE must be worn, and respirators might be required Ⓐ.
- All work with microbes must be performed within an appropriate biological safety cabinet or BSC Ⓑ.

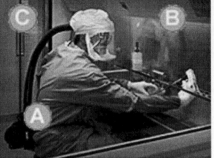

Fig. 1.4 BSL-3 type workplace - note extra PPE and contained safety cabinet.

Facility Construction

- A hands-free sink and eyewash are available near the exit.
- Exhaust air cannot be recirculated, and the laboratory must have sustained directional airflow by drawing air into the laboratory from clean areas towards potentially contaminated areas.
- Entrance to the lab is through two sets of self-closing and locking doors Ⓒ.

BSL-4

BSL-4 builds upon the containment requirements of BSL-3 and is the highest level of biological safety. There are a small number of BSL-4 labs in the United States and around the world. The microbes in a BSL-4 lab are dangerous and exotic, posing a high risk of aerosol-transmitted infections. Infections caused by these microbes are frequently fatal and without treatment or vaccines. Two examples of microbes worked within a BSL-4 laboratory include Ebola and Marburg viruses.

In addition to BSL-3 considerations, BSL-4 laboratories have the following containment requirements (Figure 1.5):

Laboratory Practices

- Change clothing before entering.
- Shower upon exiting.
- Decontaminate all materials before exiting.

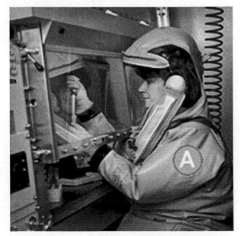

Safety Equipment

- All work with the microbe must be performed within an appropriate Class III BSC, or by wearing a full body, air-supplied, positive pressure Ⓐ suit.

Fig. 1.5 BSL-4 workplace - note positive pressure body suit (PPE) in a Class III BSC.

Facility Construction

- The laboratory is in a separate building or in an isolated and restricted zone of the building. The laboratory has dedicated supply and exhaust air, as well as vacuum lines and decontamination systems.

References

Bhatia, S. (2018). History, scope and development of biotechnology. *Introduction to Pharmaceutical Biotechnology*, 1.

Bud, R. (1989). The history of biotechnology. *Nature*, 337: 10.

Cole S. W (2014). Human Social Genomics. *PLOS Genetics*, 10(8): e1004601. https://journals.plos.org/plosgenetics/article?id=10.1371/journal.pgen.1004601.

Harman, J. G., Anderson, J. A. Nakashima and Shaw, R. W. (1995) An integrated approach to the undergraduate biochemistry laboratory. *Journal of Chemical Education*, 72 (7): 641–645.

Mannervik, B., Helena Danielson, U. and Ketterer, B. (1988). Glutathione transferases—structure and catalytic activit. *Critical Reviews in Biochemistry*, 23(3): 283–337.

Prestera, T., Holtzclaw, W. D., Zhang, Y. and Talalay, P. (1993). Chemical and molecular regulation of enzymes that detoxify carcinogens. *Proceedings of the National Academy of Sciences*, 90(7): 2965–2969.

Rushmore, T. H. and Pickett, C. B. (1993). Glutathione S-transferases, structure, regulation, and therapeutic implications. *Journal of Biological Chemistry*, 268(16): 11475–11478.

Singh, B. R. (1999). A single protein research integrated advanced biochemistry laboratory course: design and general outline. *Biochemical Education*, 27(1): 41–44.

Vandewaa, E. A., Campbell, C. K., Oleary, K. A. and Tracy, J. W. (1993). Induction of Schistosoma mansoni glutathione S-transferase by xenobiotics. *Archives of Biochemistry and Biophysics*, 303(1): 15–21.

Wolfson, A. J., Hall, M. L. and Branham, T. R. (1996). An integrated biochemistry laboratory, including molecular modeling. *Journal of Chemical Education*, 73(11): 1026.

2

Recombinant DNA and Protein Technology

2.1 Introduction

To understand cellular structures and their functions, comprehensive knowledge of proteins and the mechanisms of their action is needed. For better understanding of cellular processes, the protein component needs to be extracted from a complex mixture. Earlier, proteins were extracted in a purified form either by using large amounts of animal or (a variety of) plant tissues or biological fluids. With the advent of recombinant protein technology, most biochemical projects start with conceptualizing purification of the target protein in a recombinant form. The capabilities of this technology allows biochemists to design, clone, extract, and purify a protein for its biochemical characterization, better understanding, and research/commercial applications.

Protein purification is a series of steps required to isolate a target protein from a complex mixture of biomolecules. Protein purification may be preparative or analytical. Preparative purification aims to produce relatively large amount of protein for their use, such as soy protein extract and insulin. Analytical purification aims at obtaining just sufficient amounts of protein required for the specific research. In general, recombinant protein purification steps are straightforward. The process starts from identifying the gene of interest, which is a clone and transform into a proper host, and after induction of gene expression the designed protein is ready for further experimentation, such as development of purification protocols and its biochemical characterizations. However, these experiments involve several steps that can go wrong, such as inappropriate transformation, poor growth conditions, inclusion body formation, degradation of the target protein, inactive protein, and even no expression.

Inside tissue, some proteins are present in enough amounts that can be isolated from their host directly. But for getting larger amounts of proteins, scientists need to enhance their expression by using an appropriate host and develop protocols for their purification. There are four main steps involved: a gene of interest, an optimized vector that contains that gene, an appropriate expression host, and a complete purification procedure. Cloning, expression, and purification are the three major steps in getting the desired amount of pure protein.

2.2   Cloning

Gene cloning employs a series of molecular biology methods that culminate with the insertion of the gene of interest into a host cell and replicating this in many other cells under appropriate conditions of the expression of that gene. This technique allows biochemists to design, allow expression and produce sufficient

> **Questions to ponder over**
>
> 1. What cloning strategy will be suitable?
> 2. Which organism to use for gene expression?
> 3. What kind of promoters, tags and selection markers would enhance efficient expression?
> 4. How much protein would be required?
> 5. What would be the best purification strategy?

quantities of the gene of interest. After identifying such a gene of interest, the most critical step is to select the appropriate cloning method for inserting the selected gene into an expression vector. For this step, optimization of codon for the expression host is very important. However, proteins are so varied that expression in hosts other than natural host becomes the critical parameter, and it is nearly impossible to select a precise method for expression of protein, and the appropriate conditions in which an expressed protein is soluble and active.

For cloning, a cDNA is first synthesized and used as a PCR template. After using appropriate primers, the selected gene is amplified and cloned in an appropriate vector. Three major points need to be considered at this point: (a) reduction of leaky expression of the gene of interest because this may lead to toxicity and render it difficult for the host to produce target protein, (b) selected vectors may have low copy numbers due to larger sizes of expression vectors, and (c) designing errors in PCR primer (this tends to be common). To circumvent these problems, a primary cloning method is used in which the selected gene is first cloned into a non-expressing vector of small size and higher copy number. This also improves expression and purification.

To start cloning, one needs a proper cloning vector. Cloning vectors are vehicles which are used to transport the optimized clones into appropriate biological hosts. Bacteriophages and bacterial plasmids are two natural vectors that can be used to insert foreign DNA into bacterial cells. There are other forms of vectors as well, but they all share four common properties:

(a) They are able to promote autonomous replication.
(b) For proper selection, they contain a genetic marker.
(c) Contain a unique restriction site(s) for cloning and inserting the selected gene.
(d) For optimized cloning, they have the least amount of nonessential DNA.

2.3   Types of Cloning Vectors

Various types of cloning vectors are used as per the requirements of cloning experiments. Selection of cloning vectors is mainly based on the size of DNA to be cloned.

2.3.1   Plasmid Vectors

Extra chromosomal DNA present in the bacterial cells can replicate independently. These DNA are referred as plasmids and organized as a small double-stranded circular DNA (Figure 2.1A). The size of plasmid vectors are ~ 1.2–3 kb. They contain a gene sequence, known as replication origin

(ORI) sequence which allows replication of DNA in the cell. Additionally, in plasmids, there is a gene, which is used for selection, that encodes the enzyme β-lactamase (e.g., AmpR or Amp^r), which inactivates antibiotics. Endogenous genes can be inserted into the MCS (multiple cloning site) (Figure 2.1B).

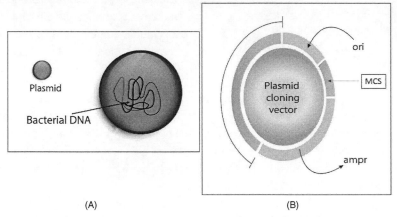

(A)   (B)

Fig. 2.1   Plasmid in bacterial cells (A) and general organization of a plasmid vector (B). Plasmid vectors contain a replication origin (ORI) sequence, and a targeted gene (exogeneous DNA) which is inserted at the multiple cloning site (MCS) and an antibiotic selection gene (AmpR). Antibiotic selection genes provide antibiotic resistance which inactivates antibiotics. For example, the Amp^r gene inactivates ampicillin.

The selective markers and antibiotic resistance genes allow selection and maintenance of plasmids inside cells. Genes that confer resistance to various antibiotics can be used, such as ampicillin, carbenicillin, neomycin, kanamycin, or chloramphenicol. Cloning vectors contain a DNA segment with several unique sites for restriction endo-nucleases located next to each other (at MCS; Figure 2.2). Restriction enzymes are used to cut the plasmid at the respective restriction sites. Cutting plasmid is done just to insert the DNA. Inserting the DNA does not disrupt the organization of other parts of the vector, and essential features of the plasmid remain intact.

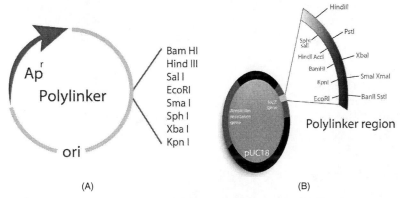

(A)   (B)

Fig. 2.2   Plasmid vectors with multiple cloning sites (A). Several unique sites for restriction enzymes which are next to each other will be used for inserting the recombinant gene of interest. One of the common plasmid vectors used for cloning (B).

DNA ranging in size from a hundred to thousands of base pairs (100 bp – 10 kbp) can be cloned using plasmid vectors. Some common plasmid vectors are ColE1 based pUC vehicles.

2.3.2 Bacteriophages or Phage Lambda

Bacteriophages are viruses that infect only bacteria. Viruses are composed of protein and nucleic acid molecules. In viruses, nucleic acid molecules are surrounded by a protective coating. The nucleic acid, inside the coating, called the phage genome which encode most of the gene product in a bacteriophage, is made of single-or double-stranded DNA or RNA. The phage genome can replicate and make more phages. The genome can be either circular or linear. The structure of a typical phage consists of three units: head (capsid), tail, tail fibers (Figure 2.3). The DNA has cohesive sticky end, known as cos site, located at both ends and can be hybridized to each other. Lambda tail fibers bind to the cell surface receptors allowing DNA to be injected inside the cell. At the cos site, circularization of the DNA allows its replication to begin the life cycle of the phage inside the host. The genetic map of phage lambda is shown in Figure 2.3.

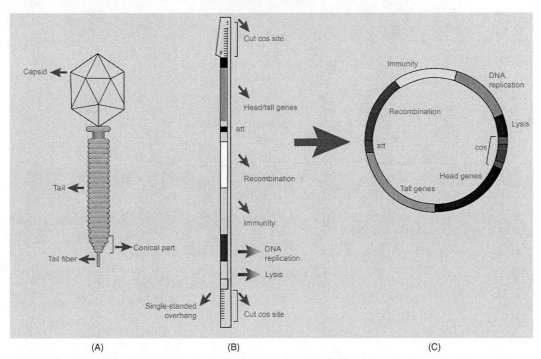

(A)   (B)   (C)

Fig. 2.3   (A) Structure of Lambda bacteriophage. They have an isomeric head (Capsid: ~ 55 nm), tail tube (~ 135 nm), conical region (~ 15 nm) and tail fiber (~ 23 nm). (B) DNA organization in bacteriophage head. (C) At the cos site at both ends, DNA is circularized and the phase starts replicating. [See color plates]

Bacteriophage lambda can affect its host in a number of ways. In **virulent** form it can enter the lytic cycle in which it replicates aggressively to produce more phages, and destroys its bacterial host. Another mode (**benign**) of their growth is lysogenic growth in which it integrates its DNA into the bacterial chromosome. **Temperate** phages are those that can go to either lytic mode or lysogenic mode. Prophage is a type of phage in which the phage genome is integrated into the bacterial genome. When prophage is present, then the host is called a lysogen.

Some reasons why bacteriophage lambda could be a good cloning vehicle are given below:

(a) Very large pieces of foreign DNA (~ 20 kbp) can be integrated into the phage.
(b) Through genetic engineering, it is possible to construct a lambda phage that contains only one or two restriction sites.
(c) Reconstitution of bacteriophage is very easy. They can be reconstituted by mixing phage DNA with phage proteins.

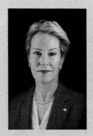   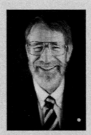   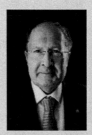

Frances H. Arnold
California Institute of
Technology USA

George P. Smith
University of Missouri
USA

Sir Gregory P. Winter
MRC Laboratory of
Molecular Biology, UK

The 2018 Nobel Laureates in Chemistry discovered the concept of directed evolution. They were inspired by the concept of evolution based on genetic changes and selection and uses of this concept to develop better enzymes and proteins.

Dr. Frances Arnold, in 1993, conducted experiments to demonstrate the first directed evolution of enzymes. She established a method which is now routinely used to create new and better enzymes.

Dr. George Smith, in 1985, developed the elegant method of phase display. Phase display is a technique where bacteriophage – a virus that infects bacteria – can be used to produce proteins.

Dr. Gregory Winter used the phage display to study the directed evolution of antibodies. Using his techniques several antibodies are produced that can neutralize toxins, counteract autoimmune diseases and be used in immunotherapy treatment in cancer. First approved therapeutic antibody based on this method is adalimumab which is used for rheumatoid arthritis, psoriasis and inflammatory bowel diseases.

2.3.3 Cosmids

Cosmids (cos sites + plasmids) are plasmid vectors that contain cos sites (Collins and Hohn, 1978). COS is an abbreviation of cohesive end sites. They are engineered vectors with characteristics of both plasmids and phages. The presence of a cos site is the only requirement for DNA to be inserted into a phage particle. Organization of a cosmid is shown in Figure 2.4. Cosmids are difficult to maintain in a bacterial cell because they are somewhat unstable. In cosmids, the genome from λ virus is used as a vector by removing the central region of the genome. A large DNA insert can be inserted into this region.

Cosmids are constructed by including the cos site which are originally from the lamda phage. Cloning cosmids is similar to normal cloning protocol. It involves digestion of exogeneous DNA with a restriction enzyme, cutting the vector with a compatible restriction enzyme and ligation. One of the advantages of cloning into cosmids is that larger DNA fragments, such as 32–47 kbp, can be inserted into the vector.

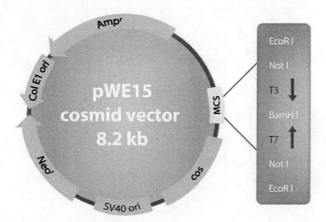

Fig. 2.4   Organization of cosmids. Cos sites and suitable antibiotic resistance genes are inserted into the plasmid. MCS (multiple cloning sites) provide several options for the insertion of foreign DNA.

2.3.4   Yeast Artificial Chromosomes (YACs)

Yeast artificial chromosomes are special linear DNA vectors that resemble normal yeast chromosomes. Basic structural features of YACs include containing telomers to stabilize chromosome, centromeres that ensures chromosome partitioning between two daughter cells and selective marker genes (Figure 2.5).

YACs are double-stranded circular DNA sequence carrying the blagene that has β-lactamase activity and the bacterial pMB1 (origin of replication). ARS1 (Autonomously Replicating Sequence; carry the sequence that enables *E. coli* vectors to replicate in yeast cells and acts as an origin of replication) associated with CEN4 (Centromere; involved in chromosome segregation) and URA3 (a gene involve in uracil biosynthesis) are the marker of YAC plasmid. Other markers are TRP1 (a gene involved in tryptophan biosynthesis), His3 and Tel (Yeast Telomere). A few of the restriction enzyme sites are HindIII, BamH1 and XhoI. Some YACs also contain SUP4 suppressor of a tyrosine transfer RNA (tRNA) gene.

In addition to cloning, YACs have a wide range of other applications. YACs can be used in identifying essential mammalian chromosomal sequences by generating DNA libraries of the organisms. These have been used as hybridization probes, regulation of gene expression, and generation of transgenic mice.

Apart from all the above mentioned vectors some other vectors are also used for various cloning purposes. P1 derived artificial chromosomes, bacterial artificial chromosomes and retroviral vectors are some of the examples of unconventional cloning vectors. Cloning vector that are unable to express a protein which is cloned into the vector, serve the purpose of carrying it to the host. Expression of the desired protein is generally performed by an expression vector. Once these vectors are inside host cells then the desired protein can be produced by using host cell transcription and

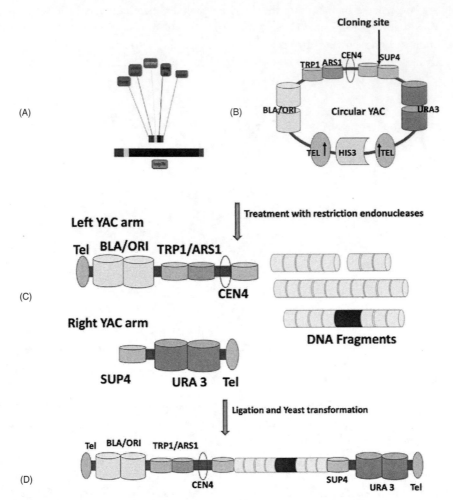

Fig. 2.5 (A) Basic YACs organization. (B) A circular YAC. (C) From source DNA, DNA fragments with compatible ends are designed and prepared. Using restriction endonucleases, YAC vector is digested. The digested vectors are separated into two chromosomal arms: TRP1 on the left and URA3 on the right arm. (D) Ligation of the separated chromosomal arms is done with DNA and transformed into an appropriate yeast strain. [See color plates]

translational machinery. For an efficient transcription, the plasmid can be engineered to include regulatory sequences that include enhancers and suitable promoters (see Section 4.1). Therefore, for a vector to be used as an expression vector, it should contain a strong promoter region along with a host-optimized codon for translation initiation and terminator sequence.

Expression vectors require sequences that encode: (a) polyadenylation tail, which is an added sequence at the end of pre-mRNA that protects the mRNA from exonucleases and stabilizes mRNA production; (b) minimal UTR (Untranslated Region) length, for optimal expression, because UTR contains specific characteristics which may impede transcription or translation; (c) Kozak sequence, which assembles the ribosomes for a translation of mRNA; and (d) a tag, for the easier affinity purification process.

Other than YACs, there are a few other types of yeast plasmid vectors available as well. This includes Yeast integrating plasmids (Yip), Yeast episomal plasmids (YEps), Yeast replicating plasmids (YRps) and Yeast centromere plasmids (Ycps).

2.4 Expression Systems

Expression systems are systems engineered to express multiple copies of a desired protein within a host cell. This is accomplished by inserting (process of insertion into bacteria is termed as transformation, whereas process of insertion into mammalian cells is termed as transfection) an expression vector into a host cell. The inserted vectors are designed in such a way that they contain the necessary genetic information to encode proteins of interest, regulatory elements, origin of replication, the antibiotic resistance gene, ribosome binding sites (RBS), and start and stop codon (Figure 2.6). The most critical issue here is to choose an appropriate method for expression for desired yields with acceptable purity. Therefore, selection of an appropriate expression host is vital to avoid misfolded or poorly expressed target protein, lack of post-translational modifications or any other unwanted changes. There are various types of expression systems (Table 2.1):

(a) Bacterial: plasmids, phages
(b) Yeast: plasmids, yeast artificial chromosomes (YACs)
(c) Insect cells: baculovirus, plasmids
(d) Frog oocytes: injected mRNA
(e) Mammalian expression systems
(f) Plant cell systems

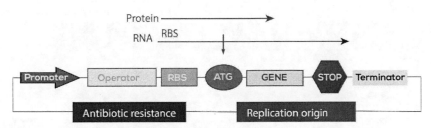

Fig. 2.6 Organization of expression vector. RBS is ribosome binding site and ATG is start codon. Ribosome recognizes and binds to RBS and initiates expression. Target protein expression starts at ATG codon (shown by an arrow) and stops at the stop codon. Antibiotic resistance genes allow only those bacterial cells to grow and multiply which have plasmids with such resistance genes.

Table 2.1 Comparison of various expression systems.

Characteristic	Bacteria	Yeast	Baculovirus	Mammalian
Cell growth	Rapid (30 min)	Rapid (90 min)	Slow (18–24 h)	Slow (24 h)
Media complexity	Minimum	Minimum	Complex	Complex
Cost	Low	Low	High	High
Expresssion	High	Low-High	Low-High	Low-Medium

2.4.1 Bacterial Expression Systems

The most popular bacterial expression system is *Escherichia coli* (*E. coli*) (Figure 2.7). *E.coli* systems have several advantages which include very fast doubling time, rapid and simple methods of transformation, growth, and expression. Additionally, rates of translation and folding are also very fast compared to eukaryotic cells. The disadvantages include accumulation of aggregated particles (inclusion bodies, insoluble proteins), and difficulties in coping with higher molecular weight proteins. Several approaches have been described to avoid aggregation or misfolding.

(a) The most straightforward method involves lowering the temperature during the expression period.

(b) One of the preferred approaches for increasing protein stability is by co-expressing the recombinant protein with molecular chaperones.

(c) Another method to promote stability of the expressed proteins is achieved by designing the recombinant protein with a soluble fusion tag, either the N-terminus or C-terminus. Fusion partners known to increase solubility of recombinant proteins include His-Tag, glutathione-S-transferase (GST), thioredoxin, maltose-binding protein (MBP), small ubiquitin-modifier (SUMO), and N-utilization substrate (NusA). GST, MBP, and His-Tag have an additional advantage because tagging proteins with these fusion partners allows protein to be purified using affinity purification (Section 2.6.3).

(d) One of the disadvantages of using *E. coli* as an expression system is its inefficiency in promoting the correct disulfide bonds formation. Normally disulfide bond formation is catalyzed by the Dsb (Disulfide bond formation system) system and occurs only in the periplasm. However, a major disadvantage is the significant reduction in production yield.

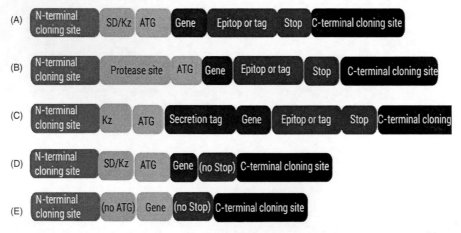

Fig. 2.7 Various combinations of protein genes commonly inserted into an expression vector. (A) Protein expression motifs with aepitope tagged on c-terminal (for antibody detection or purification). (B) For removal of tag, a protease site is introduced at the N-terminal with a epitope at C-terminal (this scheme could be reversed in which protease site and epitope tag would be at the C-terminal and N-terminal, respectively. (C) In another scheme, a secretion signal can be introduced at the N-terminal and C-terminal epitope and tag. (D) Also, a protein can be encoded without stop codon. (E) Expression vector will supply both the translation start and stop codon; so the insert does not need start and stop codons (Kz for Kozak; SD for Shine–Dalgamo sequences).

(e) Finally, efficiency of *E. coli* post-translational modifications is very limited compared to eukaryotic organisms. *E. coli* does not support enzyme-mediated N-linked glycosylation, O-linked glycosylation, amidation, hydroxylation, palmitation, or sulfation. Although, co-expression with kinases can produce phosphorylated protein.

In bacterial expression, a plasmid can produce up to 30% of the total protein.

2.4.2 Yeast Expression Systems

The yeast expression system has two major advantages: (a) it combines advantages from both prokaryotic and eukaryotic expression systems and (b) it does not produce toxins. Yeasts are eukaryotes. Although they contain complex cell structures, they are easy to manipulate as bacterial expression systems. Other advantages of yeast expression systems include: allow post-translational modifications, facilitate faster and easier growth, cost less than eukaryotic expression systems, are well-defined genetically, and are highly versatile DNA transformation systems with higher expression levels. In genetic engineering, this expression system is one of the most preferred.

S. cerevisiae is the commonest expression system used for a variety of purposes. The utility of this species of yeast in brewing and bread industry has been known for thousands of years. However, compared to the modern yeast systems, the *S. cerevisiae* expression system has some major disadvantages, such as inability to handle high density culture, lack of a stringent regulation promoter and low secretion efficiency (< 30 kDa). To overcome some of these disadvantages scientists developed fission yeast and methanol yeast expression systems. Examples of methanol yeast expression system are *H. polymorpha*, *Candida bodini* and *Pichia pastoris*.

2.4.3 Baculovirus Expression Systems

The insect expression system is one of the popular eukaryotic ones. It can cope with protein levels up to 500 mg/L. Baculovirus genome is a single closed circular double-stranded DNA with a size of ~ 80–160 kb. It can thus accommodate large fragments of foreign DNA and have greater flexibility in replication. The major advantages of baculovirus systems include: expression of the protein with complete biological function (such as correct folding and disulfide bond), post-translation modifications, high level of expression, can accommodate large inserts, and can express multiple genes simultaneously. There are a few disadvantages of this expression system which include viral infection and varying levels of glycosylations.

2.4.4 Mammalian Expression Systems

Mammalian cells are generally more difficult to work with than the bacterial expression systems, because they are more fragile and expensive. However, the major advantage is that they produce correct folding, post-translational modifications (such as disulfide bond and N-linked glycosylation), and expression of intact macromolecules that provide the native structure. Depending on the temporal and spatial difference in protein expression, this expression system can be divided into three systems: transient, stable and induced.

A transient expression system has no selection pressure and protein expression is short. Exogenous vector is gradually lost during cell division. The advantage of this system is its simplicity and short expression time.

A stable expression system implies that the carrier DNA, replicate facilitated by selection pressure, expresses for a long duration (i.e. stably) in the host cell. However, it is time consuming and laborious.

In an induction expression system, the target protein is expressed when the relevant gene is induced by foreign molecules. This method has some advantages, including increased protein production by using heterologous promoters, enhancers and amplifiable genetic markers (Figure 2.8).

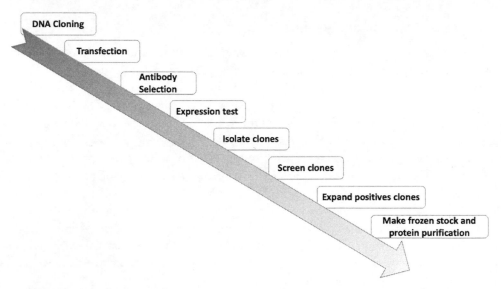

Fig. 2.8   Steps in mammalian expression system for exogeneous protein production.

2.4.5   Cell Free Expression Systems

Cell free expression systems are one of the more viable and valuable methods for expressing recombinant proteins. As the name suggests, this is a tool for protein production without using any kind of cell. Instead, this system uses necessary translation machinery including ribosomes, factors (such as initiation, elongation and termination), t-RNA, and aminoacyl-tRNA synthetases. There are mainly two formats of cell free expression system: (a) the mRNA-based translation system and (b) the DNA-based transcription and translation system. mRNA-based systems are either used in vitro with transcribed mRNA or mRNA isolated from tissue. In DNA-based systems, either plasmid DNA or a PCR template are used for transcribing and translating the recombinant DNA.

Advantages of cell free systems include:

(a) Expression of toxic, membrane, viral and unstable proteins.
(b) Capability for incorporating isotopic labeling addition of non-natural amino acids to the proteins.
(c) Rapid and economical production of protein.

The disadvantages include low yield and short duration of expression. There are two modes to perform cell free protein expression: (a) Batch mode: transcription and translation are performed in a vessel which contains all the necessary components. Due to rapid depletion of energy, degradation of nucleotides and other components, the reaction in this mode reaches saturation in about 1–2 hours. Yield by this mode can be up to 500 μg/ml. (b) Dialysis mode: transcription and translation reactions are carried out in a small chamber separated by a dialysis membrane from a larger reservoir containing low molecular weight reagents (such as ions, energy substrates, nucleotides and amino acids). This allows reaction to go on for longer duration (typically 20–24 hours) and produce more protein (up to 5 mg/ml).

2.5 Promoters

Promoters are upstream DNA sequences which regulate the transcription of genes (Figure 2.9). They are typically located at the end of the transcription initiation sites where RNA polymerase or other necessary transcription factors bind, initiate and direct transcription. Promoters are classified into three classes: (a) constitutive promoters can express independently without getting affected by any transcription factors and their activity is dependent on the RNA polymerase holoenzyme, (b) tunable promoters which can adjust the expression depending on the concentration of biotic or abiotic factors, and (c) bidirectional promoters which are able to regulate transcription in two opposite directions enabling rapid multi-gene co-expression. Constitutive promoters produce at a constant rate and are involved in regulating expression of basal genes, such as housekeeping genes or genes of glycolytic pathways. Whereas, tunable promoters can be fine-tuned (either activating or repressing), depending on either concentration or competitive properties of modulating substances. Bidirectional promoters are regulated at multiple points and can produce diverse types of transcripts.

Proper promoter selection is very important in designing an expression system. Strong promoter properties include high rate of transcription initiation and express 10–30% of target protein, and are located upstream of the ribosome-binding site (RBS). All promoters are designed such that they are under strict regulatory control (to avoid any toxicity due to unwanted expression) and their regulatory units are either located on a plasmid or within the host chromosome. The strict regulations allow the target protein to express in an appropriate time and thus, the host will be under minimal stress when expressing exogeneous proteins. Initially, the promoter is completely repressed. For transient induction, an inducer is added at an appropriate growth stage, when expression is desired for optimal yield. The *lacZYA*, *araBAD*, and *rhaBDA* are the most-studied promoters. These operons are responsible for regulating sugar metabolism. The most commonly used promoters are *Lac*, *Trp*, *Tac*, *pL*, and T7. All of these promoters bind to the σ^{70} factor for transcription. The wild type *lac* promoter is of moderate strength and is considered as a better option for membrane protein expression. Various transcription initiation factors (σ factor) for *E. coli* are tabulated in Table 2.2. Some expression vectors have wild type *lac* promoter, while others have modified *lac* promoters, such as, when two mutations are present – the *lacUV5* promoter itself, plus one at the -10 region of the *lac* promoter, and (b) at the catabolite gene activator protein (CAP) binding site which presents in the -66 region. These mutations are beneficial for increasing the promoter strength relative to wild type *lac* promoter, and the catabolite repression is comparatively less.

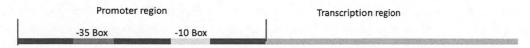

Fig. 2.9 A simple promoter. A typical promoter consists of two short DNA sequences located -35 (consensus region) and -10 (TATA box) from the start site. These two regions are separated by 16–18 base pairs (most commonly 17 base pairs).

Table 2.2   Various sigma factor of *E. coli*.

Sigma Factor	Function
σ^{70}	Housekeeping genes
σ^{32}	Heat shock
σ^{24}	Extreme heat shock, periplasmic stress
σ^{28}	Flagellar-based motility
σ^{38}	Stationary phase adaptations
σ^{54}	Nitrogen-regulated genes
σ^{fecl}	Ferric citrate uptake

2.5.1   The Lac Promoter

The lactose (*lac*) system is an intensively studied operon. It is based on the *E. coli lac* operon. Such operators are also found in some enteric bacteria. The lac system contains gene coding which is translated to the proteins responsible for transporting lactose to the cytosol and digesting it into glucose. Three of the enzymes are grouped into *lac* operon: *lacZ*, *lacY* and *lacA* (Figure 2.10A). *lacZ* encodes for an enzyme, β-galactosidase, which produces glucose and galactose by digesting lactose; *lacY* is a permease and helps transport lactose to the cytosol; while *lacA* is trans-acetylase.

Lac repressor binds tightly to the operator when there is no lactose in the media. Repressor binding to the operator prevents RNA polymerase from binding to promoter and stop transcription (Figure 2.10B). The lac repressor (*lacI*) changes conformation in the presence of lactose or inducer, such as isopropyl-β-d-1-thiogalactopyranoside (IPTG). Conformational changes in *lacI*, prevent its binding to the operator which allows RNA polymerase to initiate transcription (Figure 2.10C).

The second aspect of *lac* system is a CAP site. CAP is an allosteric regulator of the *lac* operon known as catabolite activator protein and is located very close to the promoter. Binding of CAP protein to cAMP allows tighter binding of RNA polymerase to the promoter and leads to high transcription. The concentration of cAMP is inversely proportional to the glucose concentration. When glucose is low, adenylate cyclase is able to produce cAMP from ATP. This is why high level of lactose and low level of glucose promotes high transcription at high cAMP (Figure 2.10D). The modified *lac* operator is used to optimize *E. coli* protein expression. In response to high glucose, the mutation in lacUV5 renders it to be insensitive to repression and allows rich media to be used for the growth of the expression strain.

2.5.2   The tac and trc Promoters

Historically, **tac** and **trc** are the most commonly used promoters. These promoters are hybrid promoters of *lac* and tryptophan (trP). These promoters are designed to be comparatively stronger and more tightly regulated promoters. In addition to the tight regulation these are very active promoter systems and this is the main reason why they still have some basal expression in the uninduced state. Both promoters are very efficient promoters in vitro, but comparatively *trc* is less efficient than the *tac* promoter, in *E. coli*. Examples of commercially available vectors containing *tac* promoters are PinPoint, pMAL, and pGEX. pThioHisABC, pTrcHis TOPO, pTrcHis ABC, and pHB6 are some of the available *trc* vectors.

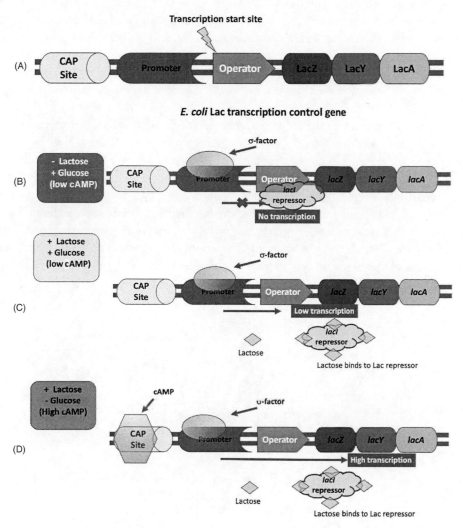

Fig. 2.10 (A) Lac promoter system. (B) When there is no lactose, the lac repressor binds to the operator, so no mRNA transcription. (C) With both glucose and lactose present, σ-factor binds to the promoter region resulting in low mRNA transcription. (D) In presence of lactose (no glucose) both catabolite gene activator protein and σ-factor bind to the promoter and CAP binding site resulting in high mRNA transcription. σ-factor is a transcription initiation factor. [See color plates]

2.5.3   The ara Promoter

The arabinose promoter is more complex than the *lac* system. It is part of a regulated expression system. The arabinose operon (pBAD) contains three genes: araA (arabinose isomerase), araB (ribulokinase), and araD (ribulose-5-phosphate epimerase). Together, these genes encode enzymes which convert arabinose to xyulose-5-phosphate, an intermediate that can be utilized to generate energy. If arabinose is present, pBAD acts as an inducer, while in the absence of arabinose pBAD acts as a repressor gene. Adjacent to the three pBAD genes, there is a regulatory gene, araC (which actively represses protein transcription as well as pBAD gene synthesis). Depending on binding state (bound or unbound) of AraC (a repressor protein) to arabinose, AraC behaves in two radically different manners. In the absence of arabinose, the AraC repressor protein binds to operator site O_2 and l_1 instead of l_1 and l_2 sites. This results in DNA adopting a looped conformation in transcription (Figure 2.11) which prevents binding of the promoter to the RNA polymerase leading to blockage of transcription. However, when arabinose is present, conformational changes in the AraC repressor result in binding of AraC to the adjacent l_1 and l_2 sites. Conformational changes in the AraC repressor lead to the opening of the loop configuration which allows RNA polymerase to bind to the promoter region and start transcription. The ara promoters have a second layer of complexity depending upon the presence or absence of glucose. Levels of cAMP are high in low glucose cases, activating the cAMP receptor protein (CRP). Activated CRP then binds to the CAP (catabolite activator protein) site leading to the complete induction of the arabinose genes. This results in the expression of araBAD genes to approximately 300 folds more than their uninduced level. The major disadvantage of this system is the autoregulation of AraC which increase the level of AraC. Increased concentration of AraC causes its binding to the O_1 operator and prevents mRNA transcription. The major advantages of this promoter system include partial induction and tight repression depending on the concentration of arabinose.

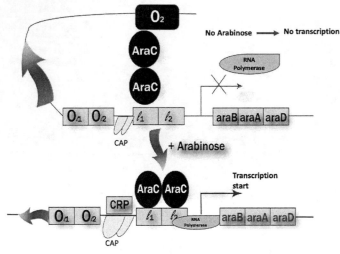

Fig. 2.11 Model representing the arabinose operon regulation mechanism. As described in the text, the opening of loop configuration, due to configurational changes, is induced by adding arabinose which leads to RNA polymerase binding at the promoter site to start transcription.

2.5.4 The T7 Promoter

One of the most common bacterial expression systems is the pET series (plasmid for expression by T7 RNA polymerase). The T7 RNA polymerase (T7 RNAP) is very active and selective, and widely used in expression of proteins in bacteria. This is the reason T7 promoter system is recognized for its capacity to generate high level of expression. Recent developments allow this expression to modulate the level of transcription. The main advantage of this system is that it does not utilize the host polymerase, due to which basal expression of toxic gene products cannot occur in absence of T7 RNAP.

There are two ways to induce expression in T7 RNAP-dependent systems: (a) by infection with the T7 phage, and (b) incorporating T7 RNAP gene in the host strain. The former method provides complete repression in the absence of induction, while the later method results in some basal expression. "Co-overexpression" of phage T7 lysozyme can minimize basal expression by degrading T7 RNA polymerase. pLysS and pLysE plasmids available from Novagen utilize this strategy. By creating a lag time between induction of the RNA polymerase and maximum induction of the protein, these plasmids allow increase in the amount of RNAP to overcome the inhibition by the lysozyme.

The T7 promoter systems are available from Novagen as the pET (plasmids for expression by T7 RNAP) series.

2.5.5   The Lambda Promoters

The lambda promoters have better efficiency than the *lac* promoter (even ten times more). The *XcI* gene is the regulatory element in these promoters which can repress transcription. These promoters are temperature sensitive and can be turned on or off by simply changing the temperature. The temperature sensitivity is achieved by a mutation in the repressor gene, *cI857*. This repressor is active at 28°C, and inhibits transcription. But at 42°C, the repressor is inactivated which induces the promoter to start transcription. Lambda promoters are better in large-scale protein production, compared to lac promoters which require chemical inducers. Moreover, in large-scale protein production, chemical inducers (such as IPTG) can be toxic and expensive. Since these promoters can be activated by increasing temperature, they can also increase the proteolytic activity during the heat-shock response, and may induce folding change or destabilize protein.

2.5.6   Cold-shock Promoters

Cold-shock promoters are alternative promoters which can circumvent issues associated with the heat-shock response. One example is the cold-shock protein (CspA) which is a promoter of *E. coli*. This is repressed at and above 37°C and active at 10°C. A disadvantage is its lower expression of target protein.

2.5.7   Non-promoter Regulatory Elements

For achieving high level expression, there are some other factors which may require tweaking to regulate or affect expression. Sequences in the vicinity of transcriptional and translational sites are important. Such optimized GC content and gene codons result in up-regulation of protein and mRNA content. Upstream (UP) elements interact with the α-subunit of RNA polymerase and increase transcription. They also increase the strength of the promoters (> 300-fold increase in transcription). It should be noted that expression can vary significantly when the same gene is cloned into two different vectors. Although the choice of promoter could be one factor, this difference in expression level could be due to the differential interaction of vector with inserted sequence.

Finally, depending on the requirement scientists use various tag with recombinant protein to facilitate identification and purification. Table 2.3 lists all the available tags.

Table 2.3   Available recombinant protein tags and their size and purification methods.

Tag	Size (no. of amino acids)	Purification
His-tag	5–15	Under native or denaturing condition by affinity chromatography
FLAG	8	mAb purification
SterptagII	8	Proteincan be eluted using biotin
HA-tag	9	Ab-based purification
Softag1, Softag3	13,8	Polyol-responsive m Ab
c-myc	10	mAb-based purification
T7-tag	11–16	mAb-based purification
S-tag	15	S-protein resin affinity purification
Elastin-like peptides	18–320	Organic or centrifugation or aqueous back-extraction
Chitin-like peptides	52	Binds only insoluble chitin
Thioredoxin	109	Affinity purification
Xylanase 10A	163	Glutathione or GST-Ab affinity
Maltose binding protein	396	Amylose affinity purification
NusA	495	Affinity purification
GFP	238	Antibody or affinity purification

Sometimes in plasmid design for recombinant protein, some protease nicking sites are included to remove tags. Some of the available fusion cleavage sites are given below (Table 2.4).

Table 2.4   Common nicking sites.

Enzyme	Recognition Site	Comments
Thrombin	LVPR/GS	Less specific
Factor Xa	IEGR/	Less specific
Enterokinase	DDDDK/	Very specific

2.6   Protein Purification Methods

Getting a pure protein is one of the important steps in any biochemical study. Questions to be considered are: Intended use of the purified protein? Availability of starting material and their regulatory requirements? What is the expected yield and purity of the purified protein? Scale of purification? Requirements and scope for scale-up on the chosen purification techniques? Economic constraints and availability of resources?

In general, more than one purification step is required to achieve the desired quality of protein. Notably, each step will incur some loss in the product. For example, if each step yield is 80% and it requires eight steps to purify protein then the yield of the final product is ~ 20%. So, one of the goals of protein purification is to have a simple protocol with minimal steps.

In general, the three main steps of purification process are: capture, intermediate, and polishing steps. The capture step consists of isolation, concentration, and stabilization of the target protein. The intermediate purification step involves removal of bulk impurities and the polishing step is that of removing remaining impurities and achieving maximum purity.

Flow chart of basic purification steps is shown in Figure 2.12.

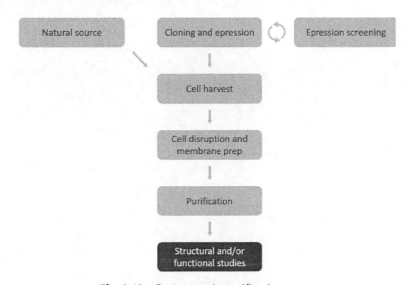

Fig. 2.12 Basic protein purification steps.

Recombinant Protein Purification Protocol

- Obtain cDNA either by amplifying genomic DNA or total gene synthesis. If target protein has codon biases the codon should be optimized before gene synthesis.
- Clone the DNA of interest into an *E. coli* expression vector.
- Use T7 RNA polymerase-drive expression system (BL-21 DE3 competent *E. coli*) cells and N- or C- terminal tag (include cleavage site to remove tag after purification).
- In the competent cells of the *E. coli* strain, the target protein is expressed by inducing a suitable condition with good aeration.
- Immobilized metal affinity chromatography should be preferred as the initial step of purification.
- If additional purification steps are required, then use size-exclusion or ion-exchange columns for final polishing step.
- Activity, fold purification and concentration of proteins should be determined wherever it is necessary.
- Identification of protein should be done by SDS-PAGE (Sodium Dodecyl Sulphate-Poly Acrylamide Gel Electrophoresis) and Western blot.

2.6.1 Cell Disruption

The first step in protein purification is cell harvesting. Pelleted cells need to be suspended in suitable buffer and be disrupted. There are a number of methods available for disrupting cell wall or membrane (Table 2.5). Cell disruption produces a suspension of membrane fragments containing soluble protein and other soluble biomolecules. Cell disruption also produces cell debris, insoluble biomolecules, and other contaminants. These contaminants, other than protein, need to be removed. Table 2.5 also lists various methods for cell disruption with their advantages and disadvantages. While disrupting cells, the cell pellet suspension buffer should contain protease inhibitors (protease inhibitor cocktail or PMSF/Benzamidine), DNase (degrading DNA) and lysozymes (disrupting bacterial cell wall).

Table 2.5   Cell disruption techniques.

Technique	Principle	Advantages/Disadvantages
Presses	Use of high pressure (French press) to disrupt microbial cells.	• Fast and efficient • Good for large volume • Cause heating of sample (cooling is required)
Grinding with abrasive	Cells are lysed when caught between the colliding beads	• Useful for cells that are more difficult to disrupt • Slow process
Sonication	Cell Disrupted by high frequency sound	• Simple • Causes heating of the sample • Not suitable for large volume • Can destroy protein
Osmotic Shock	Disrupt cells by changing from high to low osmotic medium	• Simple, inexpensive • Useful for cells with less robust walls
Freezing and Thawing	Usually combine with enzymatic lysis; use formation of ice crystals to disrupt cells	• Simple, inexpensive • Yield large membrane fragments • Slow • Low yield • May damage sensitive proteins
Enzymatic lysis	Usually combined with other techniques, such as soniciation/freeze-thawing/osmotic shock; Lysozyme is commonly used to disrupt the cell walls; non-ionic detergent or EDTAs are also used.	• Gentle • Yield large membrane fragments • Slow • Low yield when used alone

After disruption, most of the protein is soluble in aqueous buffer. However, to solubilize a membrane protein buffers need to be supplemented with detergent, and in some cases with lipids as well.

2.6.2 Purification Methods

To purify protein, a scientist needs to exploit some of the common properties of protein molecules. Based on their properties there are various ways to purify target proteins. Depending on requirement and the protein itself one can use various combinations of these methods. The principle and its connected specific method are listed as under:

(a) Charge ----------- Ion exchange chromatography
(b) Hydrophobicity -------- Reverse phase chromatography
(c) Affinity ------ Ni-affinity, Glutathione affinity, antibody affinity column
(d) Solubility and stability ----- Salting in/salting out methods
(e) Molecular weight ---- Gel filtration or size exclusion chromatography
(f) Centrifugation methods ---- Analytical centrifugation, CsCl ultra-centrifugation.

One of the widely used purification methods is ion-exchange chromatography. It is based on the interaction of a protein's ionic charges with the stationary phase. The separation is due to interaction between charges on the protein with the charge groups of the ion-exchange adsorbents (stationary phase). Proteins are complex ampholytes molecules (with both positive and negative charge amino acid residues). Their net charge depends on the pH of the solution and isoelectric point (pI). At pHs above the pI level all proteins are negatively charged and below pI all are positively charged. For example, if the protein pI is 5.0 and the buffer in which protein is dissolved, has a pH of 7.0, then the protein's net charge will be negative whereas if the buffer pH is 4.0 the protein's net charge will be positive. Depending on the pH of the solution, arginine, lysine, and histidine provide positive charges to the protein., whereas, aspartate and glutamate amino acids will provide negative charges. Utilizing this property of the protein and changing its solution environment, we can separate proteins by using appropriate charges on the stationary phase, anion exchanger or cation exchanger. A protein must displace the counter ions to attach to the stationary phase. Using stronger counter ion in the mobile phase, attached protein molecules can be exchanged and eluted in that phase. Because of this exchange it is called ion-exchange chromatography. In general, to carry out anion exchange chromatography (AIC) the pH of the solution should be above the pI, whereas for cation exchange the solution pH should be below pI. To achieve good adsorption, the pH of the buffer should be chosen to be at least one pH unit above or below the isoelectric point of the analyte of interest. Different steps of ion-exchange chromatography are shown in Figure 2.13. Table 2.6 provides a list of various stationary resins for ion-exchange chromatography.

Questions to ponder over

1. Name two essential features on an expression vector that are absent in cloning vectors?
2. Three advantages of using GST or other such, in protein/peptide tags in generating the recombinant protein?
3. What is the importance of SDS in SDS-PAGE?
4. For identification of protein, when you perform a Western blot the entire area of the blot is black. What could be the possible reason for this? If it is a mistake, is it possible to correct it? How?
5. You forgot to add SDS in your sample for SDS-PAGE. What happens when you run the gel?

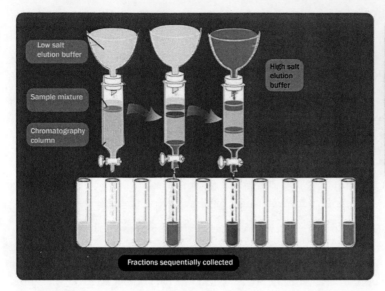
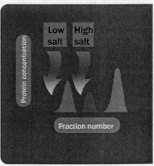

Fig. 2.13   Ion-exchange chromatography.

Table 2.6   Ion-exchange resins

Name	Type	Group	Purification Utility
DEAE-cellulose	Weakly basic	Diethylaminoethyl	Separate acidic and neutral protein
CM-cellulose	Weakly acidic	Carboxymethyl	Separate basic and neutral protein
P-cellulose	Strongly/weakly acidic	Phosphate	Basic protein purification
DEAE-sephadex	Weakly basic cross-linked to dextran	Diethylaminoethyl	Acidic and neutral proteins
SP-sepharose	Strongly acidic cross-linked to agarose	Methyl sulfonate	Basic proteins

$$DEAE: R = -CH_2-CH_2-\overset{+}{N}H(CH_2CH_3)_2$$
$$CM: R = -CH_2-COO^-$$

2.6.3   Affinity Purification

Macromolecules such as proteins, polysaccrides, and nucleic acids generally bind reversibly with other molecule or their substrate. In general, biological interactions are specific and reversible. The complex forms of interaction and resulting protein complex can be utilized for their separation and purification.

Principle of affinity purification is based on an interaction between the immobilized ligand molecules (stationary phase, affinity ligand onto a solid matrix) and the biomolecules in the mobile phase. Their highly specific interactions allow binding of target protein to the column, which can be eluted using stronger affinity counter ions. Several ligands are available to purify respective binding partners. Frequently used molecules and their interactions in affinity chromatography, are as follows:

Enzyme: Substrate, inhibitor, co-factor.
Antibody: Antigen, virus, cell.
Lectin: Polysaccride, glycoprotein, cell surface receptor, cell.
Nucleic acid: Complementary base sequence, histones, nucleic acid polymerase, nucleic acid, binding protein.
Hormone and Vitamin: Receptor, carrier protein.
Glutathione: Glutathione-S-transferase (GST) and GST-fusion proteins.
Metal ions: Poly (His) fusion proteins, native proteins with histidine, cysteine and/or tryptophan residue on their surface.

Ligands based on these interactions are immobilized on a solid support by covalent coupling, and used to prepare a column. As the solution containing the biological molecule, which can react with the ligand, is passed through the column, the components with higher affinity bind to the column whereas the components with no affinity to the ligands in the solid support will pass through the column. The bound components can be eluted from the column by modifying the conditions of mobile phase, such as ionic strength, pH, solvent, or by using dissociating agents. Notably, the conditions of application of sample should be chosen such that the binding between ligand and target analyte is strong.

Successful purification requires understanding the nature of interactions between the target and ligand. In addition, precise knowledge of possible effect on these interactions with change in buffer conditions, such as temperature and pH would be helpful. The following are to be considered:

a) Support material

As mentioned earlier, the important parameter is that the target should bound tightly and specificity should be high. So a support material (stationary phase) should have greater affinity for the ligand and form a suitably strong complex with it. Another important property for the support material to have is that the material should be biologically and chemically inert. This is needed to avoid any non-specific bindings. The support material should be compatible with the medium in which it is operating. In addition, uniformity of particle size, porosity, and easy activation are also desired qualities in the preferred support materials. Many commercial support materials are available: natural (agarose, dextrose, cellulose), synthetic (acrylamide, polystyrene, polymethylacrylate), and inorganic (silica, glass) materials.

b) Ligands

Ligands are molecules that bind to the target specifically and reversibly and this property is the basis of affinity purification. In general, ligands are modified in order to attach to the support material. Therefore it is important to consider that such modification should not affect the specific binding affinity of the ligands. The common ligands are dyes, amino acids, Protein A and G, lectin, coenzymes, metal chelates, antibodies, and so on. Two types of affinity ligands are available: synthetic and biological. Synthetic ligands are produced by de novo synthesis of existing molecular structures (non-natural peptides, dyes, oligosaccharides, etc.). Biological ligands are available from identified natural sources (such as RNA and DNA fragments, nucleotides, coenzymes, lectins, antibodies, etc.).

c) Elution

Elution is the most important step for successful separation of target analyte. For sample application to the affinity column, the column should be equilibrated in the mobile phase with an appropriate pH, ionic strength, and buffer composition. The mobile phase should be compatible with proteins in solution too. In appropriate condition the molecules complimentary to the ligand will bind to the column while other molecules are washed off the column. After properly washing the column, elution is achieved by reducing the ligand-target molecule interaction. The target molecule is generally eluted by using either bio-specific or non-specific elution. To displace target solute from the column, using a bio-specific molecule, which competes with the attached solute, will facilitate the elution of attached molecules. The main advantage of the bio-specific elution is that it is a gentle method for elution. Non-specific elution can be achieved by changing solvent conditions like pH, ionic strength, denaturating agents, detergents, and polarity. Although this elution is faster than bio-specific elution, it is a harsher method and carries the risk of denaturation of target molecule. Therefore, proper conditions must be considered for using non-specific elution to avoid long durations for column regeneration, denaturation of solute, and irreversible loss of ligand activity.

2.6.4   Gel Filtration or Size Exclusion

When proteins are of different sizes or molecular weights, this difference can be exploited for their separation by gel filtration or size exclusion. It is the simplest and mildest technique of purification. To begin with, a gel filtration medium (martix of different pore size) is packed into a glass column and equilibrated with buffer of appropriate pH. The gel filtration medium is a porous matrix made of spherical and inert particles. Porosity of matrix is chosen based on the size of target molecule (Figure 2.14). The porous matrix is stable and inert. When samples are loaded and allowed to flow through the column, molecules greater than the size of the pores are excluded and flow through the mobile phase, while molecules smaller than the pore size enter the pores partially or wholly and are discarded in the elution process. The large molecules are not retained in the column and elute through the column unhindered with the flow of the mobile phase.

Gel filtration is used in the purifications of enzymes, polysaccharides, nucleic acids, proteins, and other biological molecules. It is also used for desalting, separation of sugar and peptides. One of the major advantages of such chromatography is that it is possible to determine the quaternary structure of purified protein or protein complex. The major advantages include resolution within a short period of time, minimal sample loss, narrow band, and good sensitivity.

2.6.5   Salting In/Salting Out

Salt concentration is an important parameter in protein solubility. At low concentrations, because of stabilization of various charged groups on a protein molecule, protein interacts more favorably with

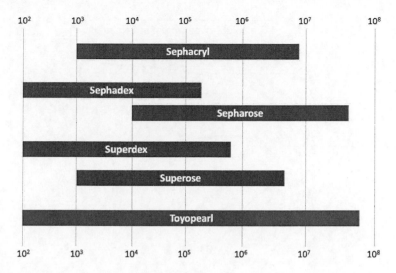

Fig. 2.14 Molecular weight range for different gel filtration media. Numbers, above and bottom, are molecular weights.

the solvent molecules in the solution, enhancing its solubility. This process is known as salting-in. Conversely, increase in the salt concentration allows the solution to reach a point where the stability of protein, in the solution, peaks. Further increment in the salt concentration of solution, implies lesser availability of water molecules to keep protein dissolved. Finally, when the charge on the protein molecule is masked by salt molecules, reducing their interaction with water molecules, protein molecules start to precipitate. This phenomenon is known as salting-out (Figures 2.15 and 2.16). Since different proteins exhibit salting-in and salting-out differently at different salt concentrations, the phenomena can be used to selectively dissolve or precipitate the protein of interest.

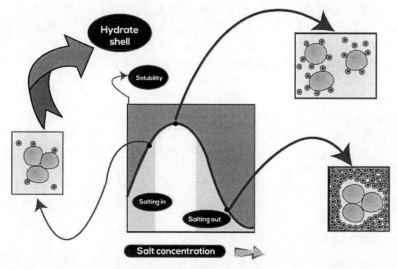

Fig. 2.15 Depicting "salting in" and "salting out" processes. Blue balls represent solvated ions of salt. [See color plates]

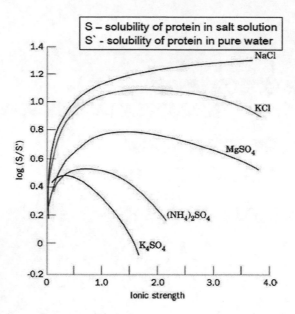

Fig. 2.16 Solubility of a protein in different salts solution. http://www2.vuw.ac.nz/staff/alan_clark/ teaching/index.htm.

2.6.6 Analytical Centrifugation

Biological centrifugation is a technique in which centrifugal force is used to separate the mixture of biological molecules. The smaller the particle the higher the g-forces (see Chapter 4) required for the separation of particles and there can be two types of centrifugation: analytical and preparative. Analytical centrifugation is used to purify macromolecules or isolate supramolecular assemblies. Preparative centrifugation, on the other hand, is used for separation of tissues, cells, subcellular structures, membrane vesicles, and other particles of biological interest.

Biological molecules are in constant random thermal motion. However, their relative distribution in an aqueous solution is not significantly affected by the Earth's gravitational field. By using centrifugal force they can exhibit distinguishable sedimentation patterns which can be utilized for their separation. It should be noted that centrifugal force of the order of 200,000g can be generated by an ultracentrifuge.

Centifugation demands a few fundamental requirements from the sample: (a) it should have a distinct optical property to distinguish it from the mixture, (b) it must have different sedimentation property, and (c) it should be chemically compatible with the matrix which is used for producing the required density gradient.

Analytical ultracentrifugation can be useful in determining the size and shape of macromolecules in solution. The range of analytical centrifugation could be from a few hundred daltons to several hundred, million daltons.

Analytical centrifugation can be used for:

(a) determination of the purity and oligomeric state of macromolecules,
(b) determination of the average molecular mass,

(c) ligand binding studies, and

(d) detection of conformation or conformational changes of the macromolecule.

2.7 Monitoring Protein Purification

In general, protein purification involves more than one step. It is important to determine the efficiency of purification at each step. Normally, proteins are collected in different fractions in each chromatographic step, and individual tubes are tested for identification and purity. If one is purifying an enzyme, then each tube can be individually assayed for the presence of enzyme activity. For a protein whose biological assay cannot be measured easily, other approaches can be employed. If the antibody of that protein is available, then the protein sample can be tested for target protein by using immunoblot techniques. If the antibody is not known, available, then protein samples can be run off SDS-PAGE gel, looking for the appearance of a target band on the gel.

In case of an enzyme, a successful fractionation process is recognized by an increase in the specific activity.

$$\text{Specific Activity} = \frac{\text{total units of enzyme in fraction}}{\text{total amount of protein in fraction}}$$

The amount of enzyme that will convert 1 μ mole of substrate to product in 1 minute, under defined conditions, is termed as a unit of an enzyme.

Therefore, with increasing purity, after every step of purification, the specific activity of protein increases.

$$\text{Fold Purification} = \frac{\text{Specific activity of fraction}}{\text{Original specific activity}}$$

Another important parameter to monitor is the yield of the target protein after each step of the purification. Yield is defined as follows:

$$\text{Yield} = \frac{\text{Units of enzyme in fraction}}{\text{Units of enzyme in original preparation}}$$

2.7.1 Determination of Protein Concentration

Every biological reaction involving protein requires the accurate determination of protein concentration. The determination of protein concentration is a regular activity in any biochemistry laboratory. Most of the methods of measuring protein concentration are colorimetric methods, where a reaction in the protein solution will produce a colored product. This colored product is measured at a specific wavelength in a spectrophotometer. The amount of color can be quantified and is related to the amount of protein present in the solution. However, none of the methods for protein concentration determination are absolute because the amount of color development is dependent on the amino acid composition. In general, BSA (Bovine Serum Albumin) is used to prepare a standard curve because of its low cost, high purity, and ready availability. However, it should be noted that if amino acid composition of the given protein is different from BSA, the measurement of concentration can only be approximate.

2.7.2 Ultraviolet Absorption

This is a non-destructive method and can be employed for continuous measurement of chromatographic column effluents. The aromatic amino acids such as tryptophan and tyrosine, absorb wavelengths at 280 nm and provide an extinction coefficient. Since the number of these amino acids vary, so does the extinction coefficient of a protein. Approximately, protein concentrations of 1 mg/ml will give an absorbance of 1.0 at 280 nm, using a cuvette of pathlength 1.0 cm. This method is sensitive and can detect concentrations as low as 10 µg/ml.

$$\text{Concentration of protein (mg/ml)} = [(A_{235} - A_{320}) - (A_{280} - A_{320})] / 2.51$$

where, A_{235}, A_{280}, and A_{320} are absorbance at wavelengths of 235, 280, and 320 nm respectively.

However, the method may suffer distortion from the presence of nucleic acids. In presence of nucleic acid, a correction factor is applied.

$$\text{Concentration of protein (mg/ml)} = 1.55\, A_{280} - 0.76\, A_{260}$$

The most sensitive wavelength for absorption measurement is 190 nm, because peptide bonds absorb at this wavelength. However due to absorption of oxygen at this wavelength and low output of spectrophotometers at this wavelength, measurements are usually made at 205 or 210 nm. These wavelengths are more sensitive than 280 nm. However, the buffer components may also absorb at these wavelengths making measurement not always practically possible.

2.7.3 Bradford Method

The Bradford assay is very fast and fairly accurate. The assay uses Coomassie Brilliant Blue dye which binds to the protein. At acidic pH, the dye has an absorbance at 470 nm which shifts to 595 nm after binding with protein. Anionic forms of dyes are stabilized by both hydrophobic and ionic interactions, causing a change in color in the visible range. Sensitivity of this assay is up to 20 ug/ml. Disadvantages are that proteins may not dissolve properly in the acidic medium and that dye binding depends of the exposure of the basic amino acids.

2.7.4 Lowry (Folin–Ciocaltaeu) Method

This method is based on the reaction of Cu^{2+} ions with peptide bonds under alkaline conditions. With peptide bonds of protein, Cu^{2+} ions form a complex and reduce to Cu^+, a monovalent ion. Cu^+ then reacts with the Folin–Ciocalteu reagent (a mixture of phosphotungstic acid and phosphomolybdic acid). Although, the exact mechanism is not very clear (although the oxidation-reduction mechanism is widely accepted which involves Cu^+ initiated oxidation-reduction reaction) the reagent is reduced and aromatic residues are oxidized (mainly tryptophan and tyrosine, but to some extent cysteine, too). This reaction produces a blue-purple color which can be quantified by its absorbance at 660 nm. Care must be taken to reduce interference from the other components: Tris, zwitterionic buffers such as Pipes, Hepes, and EDTA (Ethylene Diamine Tetra Acetic Acid) can interfere with this method.

2.7.5 The Bicinchoninic Acid (BCA) Method

This method can be termed as modified Lowry's method. Similar to Lowry's method, this method involves the conversion of Cu^{2+} to Cu^+ under alkaline conditions. The monovalent Cu^+ is then reacted with BCA to give an intense purple color with an absorption maxima at 562 nm. Advantages of this method include the stability of colored product and better tolerance of the interfering compounds than the original Lowry's method.

2.7.6   Kjeldahl Method

This method is based on the determination of nitrogen content of any compound. In the presence of sodium sulphate, the sample is digested by boiling with concentrated sulfuric acid and copper and/or selenium is used as a catalyst for this reaction. The digestion reaction converts all the organic nitrogen present in the protein to ammonia, which is finally trapped as ammonium sulphate. The amount of ammonia is either determined by titration or using a selective ammonium ion electrode. However, this method is best suited for pure protein. Presence of impurities such as DNA or buffer components can lead to inaccurate determination of nitrogen content. In general, nitrogen content in protein is 16% by weight.

Purification Issues and Their Pitfalls

1. Poor lysis

First, step in protein purification is to isolate proteins from the cell. For this proper cell lysis is required. Proper care should be taken to ensure complete lysis. Inclusion bodies should be extracted by using appropriate non-ionic detergents. Sonication cycles and chemical lysis parameters should be optimized.

2. Affinity chromatography related issues

Sometime the optimum binding of target recombinant protein could be an issue in affinity chromatography. The pH of lysis buffers should be 7.5–8.0 for efficient binding. The buffer should not include any chelators, high imidazole concentrations or DTT (Dithiothreitol). The column should be properly charged with metal ions. pH of the elution and washing buffer with imidazole should be adjusted to 7.5. Sometimes adding urea (0.5–1.0 M) will help in the binding.

3. The wrong protein was expressed or purified

It may result due to clone mix-up or when expression is low. Although PCR errors are very rare, but to avoid expression issues, it is essential to optimize the sequence of the expression clones for the host. Sometimes due to size or cellular degradation, target protein expression is low. In these cases, the growth and induction condition should be optimized. Sometimes optimization of lysis conditions are also required.

4. Samples contains impurities after affinity purification

It is very common to find that after affinity purification there will be multiple bands other than your target bands. Carefully using ion-exchange or gel-filtration chromatography will achieve the desired purity.

5. Precipitation of pure protein

Pure proteins often precipitate or fail to concentrate. This may be due to the alternate folded states or the presence of exposed hydrophobic patches on the surface of the target protein. There is no general solution. However, using better stabilizing buffer, maintaining an adequate reduced state, optimal salt concentration, addition of glycerol or arginine, and addition of non-ionic detergents will keep the protein in soluble form.

Rescue Strategies

In spite of all the precautions, biochemists often face some unusual situations in protein purifications. That is why alternative approaches are required.

1. Changing expression conditions

Adjusting the expression conditions sometimes produce desired result. One of the strategies is to reduce the induction temperature. Media such as terrific broth, 2 x YT or auto-induction medium are good for expression. Using different genetically modified *E.coli* strains could also help.

2. Changing tags

Most common tag is the N-terminal histidine tag but is somewhat prone to solubility issues. The solubility of the target protein can be improved by changing the tag. GST (Glutathione S-Transferase) or MBP (Maltose Binding Protein) fusion proteins generally elute as soluble proteins. Other tags to consider are NusA (N-utilization substance protein A), ubiquitin, and SUMO (small ubiquitin-like modifier).

3. Co-expression

Many proteins are multiprotein assemblies and their appropriate folding and stability requires interaction with other proteins in the assemblies. Co-expressing the cognate protein will improve the purification characteristics of these proteins.

4. Other expression hosts

If bacterial expression is associated with generating purified protein, then using baculovirus, yeasts, mammalian, or cell free systems can generate the desired protein.

5. Co-expression of chaperons

For proper folding, vectors such as pG-Tf2 vector (combination of GroEL-GroES and trigger factor) can be co-transformed with the target protein.

6. Refolding

For the insoluble proteins, refolding strategies may be the last resort in which the protein is first denatured and then refolded.

Regeneration of Ni-NTA Affinity Column

1. Remove the fluid in the column containing the His Affinity matrix and wash with 5–10 column volumes (CV) of 1 M NaOH.
2. Wash with 10 CV double distilled (dd) water.
3. For removal of contamination (hydrophobic proteins or lipids or precipitated proteins), wash the matrix with 10 CV each of, 100% ethanol, 8 M urea, or 6 M guanidinium hydrochloride. Thoroughly wash with distilled water.
4. Add 100 mM EDTA (10 CV) to the column and pass through the matrix.
5. Rinse the column again with 10 CVs of dd water.
6. Add 10 CV Wash Buffer to the column and allow the entire volume to flow through the matrix.
7. Rinse the column with 10 CVs dd water
8. Add 10 mM $NiSO_4$ (10 CV) to recharge the matrix.
9. Rinse the column with 10–20 CVs dd water.
10. Add 5 CV of regeneration Buffer nd then wash with dd water.

11. Equilibrate the column with equilibration buffer.
12. Add 10 CV of 20% (v/v) ethanol in equilibration buffer. The matrix is now ready to be re-used.

Regeneration of Protein A Affinity column
1. Wash the column with 10 CV of elution buffer (0.1 M Sodium citrate buffer pH 5.5).
2. Wash with 10 CV of binding buffer (1.5 M Glycine/NaOH buffer, 3 M NaCl, pH 9.0).

Regeneration of Protein G Affinity column
1. Wash the affinity matrix with 5 CV of elution buffer (0.2 M Glycine, pH 3.5–5.0).
2. Re-equilibrate the column with 10 CV of binding buffer (0.1 M phosphate buffer, 0.15 M NaCl, pH 7.4.

Regeneration of ion-exchange column
Regeneration of ion-exchange column stands for displacement of the contaminating ions with H^+ or OH^- ions.

After the completion of elution, wash the column with counter ions and equilibrate the column in low salt equilibration buffer.

Questions

1. Why should induction be done at log phase of bacterial growth?
2. How are Ni-NTA affinity columns recharged?
3. What should be done when a protein is being precipitated during dialysis?
4. What is the easiest and most rapid method of His Tag removal?
5. How to purify protein from inclusion bodies?
6. What are the different methods to concentrate the purified proteins?
7. How is DNA removed from protein solution?
8. In your lab, your project is to purify a protein. You have cDNA of that protein. Place the following steps in the correct order (1 through 6)
   __ Transformation
   __ Ligation
   __ Restriction digestion of expression plasmid
   __Bacterial cell lysis
   __PCR amplification of cDNA
   __Affinity and other chromatographic purifications
9. In a Bradford assay, a scientist generated the alongside curve. Straight line equation is y = 0.9429 x + 0.1196.
   The OD_{595} of the undiluted protein is 1.850
   The OD_{595} of a 1:10 dilution of the protein is 1.525.
   (a) What is the concentration of your protein?
   (b) If you diluted your protein 1:5, what would be the expected OD_{595}?
10. During your PCR reaction, the PCR stops at the second step of the 14th cycle due to power outage? What would you expect in terms of product formation?

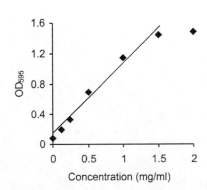

References

Bruschi, C. V., Gjuracic, K. and Tosato, V. (2001). *Yeast Artificial Chromosomes*. https://doi.org/10.1038/npg. els.0000379.

Chen, R. (2012). Bacterial expression systems for recombinant protein production: E. coli and beyond. *Biotechnology Advances*, 30(5), 1102–1107.

Cheng, X. and Patterson, T. A. (1992). Construction and use of λ PL promoter vectors for direct cloning and high level expression of PCR amplified DNA coding sequences. *Nucleic Acids Research*, 20(17), 4591–4598.

Collins, J. and Hohn, B. (1978). Cosmids: a type of plasmid gene-cloning vector that is packageable in vitro in bacteriophage lambda heads. *Proceedings of the National Academy of Sciences*, 75(9), 4242–4246.

De Boer, H. A., Comstock, L. J. and Vasser, M. (1983). The tac promoter: a functional hybrid derived from the trp and lac promoters. *Proceedings of the National Academy of Sciences*, 80(1), 21–25.

Feng, D. X., Liu, D. P., Huang, Y., et al (2001). The expression of human α-like globin genes in transgenic mice mediated by bacterial artificial chromosome. *Proceedings of the National Academy of Sciences*, 98(26), 15073–15077.

G. Qing, L. C. Ma, A. Khorchid, et. al. (2004). Cold-shock induced high-yield protein production in Escherichia coli. *Nature Biotechnology*, 22(7), 877–882.

Hsiao, C. L. and Carbon, J. (1979). High-frequency transformation of yeast by plasmids containing the cloned yeast ARG4 gene. *Proceedings of the National Academy of Sciences*, 76(8), 3829–3833.

Lee, S. B. and Bailey, J. E. (1984). Genetically structured models for lac promoter–operator function in the chromosome and in multicopy plasmids: lac promoter function. *Biotechnology and Bioengineering*, 26(11), 1383–1389.

Orlova, E. V. (2009). How viruses infect bacteria?. *The EMBO Journal*, 28(7), 797–798.

Qing, G., Ma, L. C., Khorchid, A., et al (2004). Cold-shock induced high-yield protein production in Escherichia coli. *Nature Biotechnology*, 22(7), 877–882.

Rosano, G. L. and Ceccarelli, E. A. (2014). Recombinant protein expression in Escherichia coli: advances and challenges. *Frontiers in Microbiology*, 5, 172.

Siegele, D. A. and Hu, J. C. (1997). Gene expression from plasmids containing the araBAD promoter at subsaturating inducer concentrations represents mixed populations. *Proceedings of the National Academy of Sciences*, 94(15), 8168–8172.

Struhl, K., Stinchcomb, D. T., Scherer, S. and Davis, R. W. (1979). High-frequency transformation of yeast: autonomous replication of hybrid DNA molecules. *Proceedings of the National Academy of Sciences*, 76(3), 1035–1039.

Tabor, S. (1990). Expression using the T7 RNA polymerase/promoter system. *Current Protocols in Molecular Biology*, 11(1), 16–2.

3

Enzyme Kinetics, Proteomics, and Mass Spectrometry*

Biochemical analysis techniques are a set of procedures and protocols used by scientists to analyze substances and the chemical reactions underlying life processes. For a complete biochemical analysis, the biomolecules such as proteins, lipids or carbohydrates must be isolated in their pure form from biological samples, characterized for structure–functions. Assays may involve spectrophotometric measurement, gel staining, densitometric analysis, determining the concentration and purity of the protein, and so on. The assays can be simple or tedious, based on the size, shape and net charge, in order to determine different properties and characteristics of the myriad biomolecules involved in different stages of life processes and to understand their role in the biochemical steps involved in maintaining the life.

Since biomolecules generally exist in very minute quantities in the cell, so, many a times it is not possible to employ chromatographic or other such methods to purify them in adequate quantities to carry out chemical and biological analyses. Hence, other approaches, such as proteomics have been devised so as to at least develop a general sense of the types of molecules, changes in their quantities (e.g. during growth), and identify their sequences using such sensitive techniques, such as mass spectroscopy, for comparison with known molecules, aiming at characterization of the biochemical processes in the cells by observing a few biomolecules at a time. This, in combination with the recent developments in understanding gene structures with their expressions, their genetic manipulations, bioinformatic tools, and large-scale automated analysis techniques, enable scientists to analyze cell process in greater depths.

One of the well-known biochemical processes that exists in every cell, and likely is responsible for the development, evolution, and maintenance of life is the enzymatic characteristics of most proteins, with some exception of RNA. Enzymes are used to assay biological activity of cells, tissues, organs, and even the whole organism or animal. Enzyme characteristics are useful tools for understanding structure–function relationship and biological activity at the molecular level. Therefore, a scientist interested in biochemistry generally has a solid knowledge of the principles and practice of enzyme function, including enzyme kinetics.

---

* Ghuncha Ambrin, co-authored this chapter, contributing significantly to the writing of this book.

BASICS OF CHEMICAL KINETICS

3.1   Order and Molecularity

Chemical kinetics is a wonderful tool in understanding the behavior of a chemical reaction. To classify any chemical reaction, two parameters are very important: order and molecularity. Molecularity of any reaction is defined as a number of molecules that can alter the course of any reaction. It is the sum of stochiometric coefficients of reactants in the reactions. For example $A \rightarrow B$ is a unimolecular reaction, and a reaction $A + B \rightarrow P$ is bimolecular reaction.

To define the kinetics of any reaction, the term "order of reaction" is used. It is defined as the number of concentration terms that are required to get a mathematical expression of the rate of reaction. Thus, in a first-order reaction, the rate is proportional to one concentration term, whereas, in a second-order reaction, the rate is proportional to two concentration terms, and so on. For a reaction

$$aA + bB \rightarrow P$$

a rate equation can be written as in Figure 3.1.

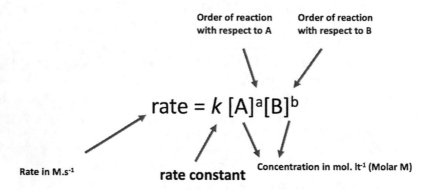

Fig. 3.1   A simple rate equation.

In general molecularity is same as the order of reaction. However, some reactions are a combination of sequences of different molecularity steps. Complex orders are very common in enzyme kinetics. Nonetheless, the concept of reaction order is important in understanding enzyme kinetics because individual steps generally follow simple reaction orders.

3.2   Important Theories Related to Enzyme Kinetics

3.2.1   Collision Theory

In order for a reaction to take place, the molecules of reactants need to collide. It depends on the available energy. The more the energy available to the reactants, the faster they will move around and so, the higher the probability of collision with each other to form new products. Sluggish molecules are less likely to collide whereas energetic molecules easily collide with each other.

Higher temperatures provide more energy and thus favor greater frequency of collision. The rate at which molecules collide, i.e. the frequency of collision, is termed as collision frequency, Z (collisions per unit time).

For a reaction such as $A + B \rightarrow$ product, the collision frequency is defined as

$$Z = N_A N_B \sigma_{AB} \sqrt{\frac{8kBT}{\pi\mu_{AB}}} \qquad \text{(Eq. 3.1)}$$

where, N_A and N_B are the numbers of molecules A and B and are directly related to the concentration of A and B.

The mean speed of the molecules is given by the Maxwell-Boltzmann distribution of thermalized gases.

$$\sqrt{\frac{8kBT}{\pi\mu_{AB}}}$$

μ_{AB} is the averaged sum of the collision cross-section of molecules A and B.

μ is the reduced mass and is given by $\mu = \dfrac{m_A m_B}{m_A + m_B}$

According to the Equation 3.1, for a successful reaction to occur there are two important factors, (a) temperature and (b) the concentration of reactants.

In any reaction, not all the reactant molecules collide and lead to product. Only those molecules take part in the reaction, which have enough energy to overcome the activation energy.

The fraction of collisions able to overcome the activation energy is given by Equation 3.2.

$$f = e^{\frac{-E_a}{RT}} \qquad \text{(Eq. 3.2)}$$

where, f is the fraction of collisions with enough energy to react, E_a is activation energy, R is the gas constant, and T is the temperature in degrees Kelvin.

The fraction of collisions leading to product is directly proportional to the temperature and inversely proportional to the activation energy.

Additionally, for any reaction to happen the reactant molecules should have the right orientation and positioning to interact and may lead to product with desirable geometry and stereo-specificity. This phenomenon is represented by a term called steric factor, ρ.

Therefore, for a reaction to occur there are three important factors: (a) collision frequency, (b) activation energy, and (c) steric factor. Considering the contribution of all these factors, the gas-phase reaction is proportional to the collision frequency (Z), steric factor (ρ), and inversely proportional to the activation energy (E_a).

$$k = Z\rho e^{\frac{-E_a}{RT}} \qquad \text{(Eq. 3.3)}$$

where,

k is the rate constant for the reaction

ρ is the steric factor

$Z\rho$ is the pre-exponential factor, A, of the Arrhenius equation $\mathbf{k = A}e^{-Ea/RT}$. The pre-exponential factor is the frequency of total collisions that take place with the right orientation. In practice, this pre-exponential factor is determined experimentally and then used to calculate steric factor, $\tilde{\rho}$

E_a is activation energy

T is absolute temperature

and, R is gas constant.

Although the collision theory deals with gas-phase reactions, its concept can be applied to the reactions in solution phase as well.

3.2.2 Transition State Theory

A disadvantage of collision theory is its inability to accurately predict the probability factor of the reaction. Collision theory assumes that the molecules are hard spheres rather than structures with varied specific shapes. To provide a more accurate alternative to the collision theory, in 1935, Henry Eyring helped develop the transition state theory (TST).

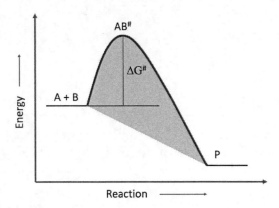

Fig. 3.2   Reaction coordinate diagram for the bimolecular reaction.

According to TST, there is a state known as transition state which is between reactants state and products state. The species in the transition state are referred to as activated complex. Three major factors determine the course of any reaction.

(a) The concentration of the activated complex.

(b) Activated complex disintegration rate.

(c) The pathway taken by the activated complex to break apart: whether it breaks apart to form the reactant or form a new complex or products.

Consider a bimolecular reaction:

$$A + B \rightarrow C$$

$$K = \frac{[C]}{[A][B]} \qquad \text{(Eq. 3.4)}$$

where, K is the equilibrium constant.

In the transition state model, an activated complex $AB^{\#}$ is formed.

$$A + B \rightarrow AB^{\#} \rightarrow C$$

$$K^{\#} = [AB^{\#}]/[A][B] \qquad \text{(Eq. 3.5)}$$

Activation energy is required by the reactant molecules and they need to cross this barrier for the reaction to occur. The transition state complex, $AB^{\#}$, is formed at the maximum energy and is very unstable (Figure 3.2). Once the reactants overcome the energy barrier, the reaction proceeds to yield the product. The equilibrium constant $K^{\#}$ can be calculated by considering fundamental properties (such as bond length, atomic mass, and vibration frequency). Because of this the transition rate theory is also called the absolute rate theory.

The rate of reaction will be given by:

$$\text{rate} = v[AB^{\#}]$$

$$= v[A][B]\ K^{\#} \qquad \text{(Eq. 3.6)}$$

The rate can be also written as:

$$\text{rate} = k[A][B] \qquad \text{(Eq. 3.7)}$$

From Equations 3.6 and 3.7:

$$k[A][B] = v[A][B]K^{\#} \qquad \text{(Eq. 3.8)}$$

$$k = vK^{\#} \qquad \text{(Eq. 3.9)}$$

where,
v is the frequency of vibration,
k is the rate constant, and
$K^{\#}$ is the thermodynamic equilibrium constant
As per statistical mechanics

$$v = \frac{k_B T}{h} \qquad \text{(Eq. 3.10)}$$

where, $k_B T$ is thermal energy and h is Planck's constant.

Applying Equation 3.9 to Equation 3.10:

$$k = \frac{k_B T}{h} K^{\ddagger} \qquad \text{(Eq. 3.11)}$$

Equation 3.11 is often multiplied with M^{1-m}, where M is the molarity of reactant and m is the molecularity of the reaction.

$$k = \frac{k_B T}{h} K^{\ddagger}(M^{1-m}) \qquad \text{(Eq. 3.12)}$$

Thermodynamics of Transition State Theory

For establishing the relationship between the theory and thermodynamics, $K^{\#}$ must be expressed into the term of Gibbs Free Energy, $G^{\#}$.

$$\Delta G0^{\#} = G^0(\text{transition state}) - G^0(\text{reactants}) \qquad (\text{Eq. 3.13})$$

$$\Delta G^{\#} = -RT \ln K^{\#}$$

Therefore,

$$[K]^{\ddagger} = e^{-\frac{\Delta G^{\ddagger}}{RT}} \qquad (\text{Eq. 3.14})$$

Using $\Delta G^{\ddagger} = \Delta H^{\ddagger} - T\Delta S^{\ddagger}$ and Equation 3.12.

$$k = \frac{k_B T}{h} e^{\Delta S^{\ddagger}/R_e - \Delta H^{\ddagger}/RT} M^{1-m} \qquad (\text{Eq. 3.15})$$

Equation 3.15 is known as the Eyring equation. The linear form of this equation is:

$$\ln \frac{k}{T} = \frac{-\Delta H^{\dagger}}{R}\frac{1}{T} + \ln \frac{k_B}{h} + \frac{\Delta S^{\ddagger}}{R} \qquad (\text{Eq. 3.16})$$

The quantitative measurement of $\Delta H^{\dagger}$ and $\Delta S^{\ddagger}$ can be obtained from kinetic data by plotting $\ln k/T$ versus 1/T. Equation 3.16 is a straight line equation which gives slope $\frac{-\Delta H^{\ddagger}}{R}$, and a y-intercept, $\frac{\Delta S^{\ddagger}}{R} + \ln \frac{k_B}{h}$.

3.2.3   Arrhenius Equation

An increase in temperature also increases the rate of any chemical reaction. For example, milk turns sour at room temperature and reptiles/insects are more lethargic on cold days. As temperature rises, molecule collides faster and the probability of bond breaking or molecular rearrangement increases.

Whether it is collision theory or transition state theory, both conclude that rate of reaction is directly proportional to the temperature.

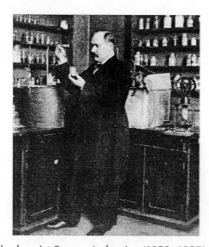

Swedish chemist Svante Arrhenius (1859–1927) in his lab.

In 1899, Arrhenius combined the concept of activation energy and the Boltzmann distribution into a relationship which is famously known as Arrhenius equation.

$$k = Ae^{-Ea/RT} \qquad\qquad\text{(Eq. 3.17)}$$

where,

k is rate constant

A is pre-exponential factor

Ea is activation energy

R is gas constant

T is absolute temperature

RT is average kinetic energy

Equation 3.17 is an exponential decay law in which the magnitude of the rate constant is a function of $-Ea/RT$. The exponent in this law is a ratio of the activation energy Ea to the average kinetic energy RT. This means that higher temperatures and low activation energy favor large rate constants and the rate of reaction is high.

3.3 Enzymes

The chemical reactions that occur in the cell would normally require higher temperature than those existing inside the cell. It is for this reason that each reaction requires a boost in chemical reactivity. This is a crucial requirement as it allows the cell to control the reaction. This control is influenced by the specialized proteins called enzymes, which speed (catalyze) up the chemical reaction without taking a part in it.

Enzymes are a group of biological molecules (proteins and RNA) which catalyze chemical reactions. Enzymes play a key role in living organisms by catalyzing numerous chemical reactions of metabolism, gene replication and expression, signal transduction, and many more. Enzymes are characterized by their biological specificity to catalyze a particular type of chemical reaction. Enzyme-catalyzed reactions are usually interconnected reactions of several steps in which the product of the previous reaction becomes the starting material for next reaction. These reactions enable cells to do their functions. Each enzyme is classified into six groups by the type of chemical reaction that it catalyzes. Each group is further divided into subgroups based on the nature of the involved chemical group and co-enzymes in the reaction.

The six classes are:

(a) **Oxidoreductases:** Transfer hydrogen, oxygen or electrons from one substrate to the other. This group consists of dehydrogenase, reductase, oxidases.

(b) **Transferases:** Transfer whole chemical groups, e.g., kinases, acetyltransferase.

(c) **Hydrolases:** Catalyze hydrolytic cleavage of bonds e.g., esterase, phosphatases.

(d) **Lyases:** Catalyze elimination reactions resulting in the formation of double bonds. This group consists of adolases, adenylyl cyclase, etc.

(e) **Isomerases:** Convert molecules in other isomeric forms by intramolecular rearrangements. Some examples are phosphoglucomutase, glucose 6 phosphate isomerase, etc.

(f) **Ligases:** Catalyze covalent bond formation with the breakdown of adenosine triphosphate (ATP), e.g. DNA ligase.

Enzymes have the following important properties:

1. They are not altered irreversibly during the course of the reaction.
2. They have no effects on the thermodynamics of the reaction.
3. They are required in small amounts.

Since enzymes are not the suppliers of energy of any reaction, therefore, they do not determine the course of reaction whether they are thermodynamically favorable or unfavorable. The catalytic property of the enzyme often depends on co-enzymes or co-factors. They are nonproteins which may be tightly or loosely attached to the enzyme. Examples of co-enzymes include NAD^+ (Nicotinamide Adenine Dinucleotide), $NADP^+$ (Nicotinamide Adenine Dinucleotide Phosphate), FMN (Flavin Mononucleotide), FAD (Flavin Adenine Dinucleotide), heme, Mg^{2+}, Zn^{2+}, etc.

And so we can say that, enzymes accelerate the rate of chemical reactions by lowering the energy of activation without themselves taking part in the reaction. There are two main reasons for enzyme analysis.

(a) Genetic expression, diagnosis of diseases, detection of reagents, and so on. Enzyme levels are estimated by assaying enzyme activity by measuring and monitoring the disappearance of substrate or formation of product. There are different methods available for measuring change in the concentration of substrate or product. These include UV/VIS absorbance, fluorescence, pH, conductivity, and radioactivity. The choice of such methods depends on the substrate, the product of the reaction and the type of chemical reaction.

(b) Enzyme kinetics: Kinetics of enzyme catalyzed reactions allow assessment of the enzyme characteristics for structure and function studies about it, and its mechanism of action. Kinetic parameters such as K_m and V_{max} are computed to compare enzyme activities under various conditions to understand an enzyme's intrinsic catalytic ability.

3.3.1 Catalytic Mechanism

An enzyme reacts with its substrate and reaction takes place at its active site, where it catalyzes the chemical reaction by which products form and dissociate. The product formed by reaction of an enzyme and its substrate is called the enzyme–substrate complex. The roles of the enzymes include binding to its substrate through a hydrogen bond or other types of interactions, lowering the reaction activation energy barrier, providing a nucleophile to attack its substrate, providing components for acid-base catalysis, and stabilization of the transition state.

The activity of the enzyme can be regulated by altering the kinetic conditions and the environment under which the enzyme is operating. These alterations change the amount of active form of the enzyme either by promoting enzyme synthesis/degradation or by chemical modification of the enzyme.

Before describing the steps to conduct enzyme assays and enzyme kinetics, it is important to familiarize oneself with the following commonly used terms to characterize enzymes.

3.3.2 Enzyme Unit

The standard unit, or international unit, of an enzyme recommended by the International Union of Biochemistry Commission on Enzymes is defined as the amount of an enzyme required to convert 1 μmole of substrate to product in one minute at 25°C under optimum conditions (pH, ionic strength and substrate concentration) of the enzyme activity. Enzyme unit is a functional quantification of an enzyme. It can be used to assess the quantitative levels of enzymes even in the crude tissue preparations, which often is the case in biological samples.

3.3.3 Transition States and Reaction Rates

There are several questions about enzyme catalyzed reaction which require answer, such as: (a) What determines the rate of the chemical reaction? (b) How do enzymes achieve effective catalysis? For a chemical transformation to occur, either certain covalent bonds must be broken or be rearranged within the reactants. Sufficient kinetic energy is required to be there to overcome the activation energy (E_A) barrier. In a solution at room temperature, molecules exist in a state of random motion possessing different amounts of kinetic energy. Molecules with higher energy remain in their activated state for a small period of time. Once some have attained sufficient activation energy to cross the threshold barrier, they react to form product molecules. The rate of the reaction depends on the number of reactant molecules and their kinetic energy at any given time.

Transition states are most important in determining the reaction rate, as they determine what happens between the reactants during the reaction which leads to the formation of product(s). In first-order reactions, only some molecules reach an energy state for the reaction to occur, for otherwise, all molecules would have easily reacted. Similarly, in the second-order reaction, the entire reactant does not convert to products as all molecules might not have adequate energy or might not be properly oriented. This leads to the concept of free energy barrier to reaction and activated state or transition state. The transition state may be thought of as a stage through which the reacting molecules must pass. Higher the barrier, lesser number of molecules will have sufficient energy to surmount it. Once the molecule is activated, it can hop to either side of the barrier, reactant side or product side. What does a catalyst do? It reduces the energy barrier of the reaction, thereby increasing the fraction of molecules with enough energy to attain transition state and overcome the barrier, making the reaction go faster (Figure 3.3).

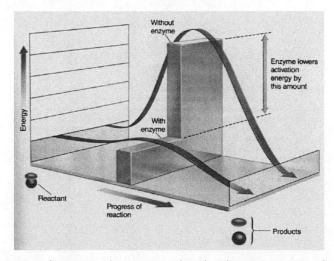

Fig. 3.3 Depiction of energies of enzyme catalyzed and non-enzyme catalyzed reactions.

The reactants must possess sufficient energy to achieve an activated state in which the atomic rearrangement is necessary for the reaction to occur. The amount of energy required is the activation energy (E_A) and is represented by the height of the curve. E_A is not a constant value, and varies with different reactions. It is greatly reduced when it combines with an enzyme catalyst.

> **Questions to ponder over**
>
> 1. How does an enzyme act as a catalyst?
> 2. What are the properties of enzymes?
> 3. What is an enzyme unit?

3.3.4 Initial Velocity

Initial velocity or initial rate of reaction refers to the instantaneous rate of substrate disappearance or product formation with time.

$$\text{Initial Velocity } (v_i) = d[P]/dt = -d[S]/dt \qquad \text{(Eq. 3.18)}$$

where, [P] is the product concentration, [S] is the substrate concentration and "t" is the time. Initial velocity is determined by first recording changes in substrate or product concentration with time, and then calculating the slope of the curve corresponding to the initial linear portion of the curve. This method of initial velocity calculation contrasts with the fixed time measurements in which concentration of substrate or product is estimated at fixed time intervals such as 1, 2, or 5 min. The rate of reaction, v, can be written as follows:

$$v = \Delta[P]/\Delta t = -\Delta[S]/\Delta t \qquad \text{(Eq. 3.19)}$$

However, fixed time measurement is not an appropriate method because at a fixed time the reaction may have reached saturation and may have deviated from the linear relationship between time and (changes in) concentration of the substrate or product.

The hypothetical graph (Figure 3.4) shows an example of time dependence of substrate loss or product formation in a reaction catalyzed by an enzyme. The time scale for the initial velocity measurement depends on the enzyme. The linear portion of the time versus [S] or [P] plot is usually for minutes but may then deviate considerably within seconds. For an accurate measurement of the initial velocity, dilute enzyme concentration should be used so that loss of substrate or formation of product can be conveniently followed.

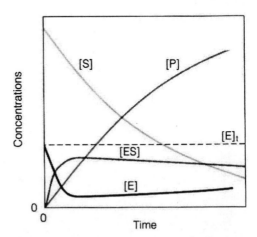

Fig. 3.4 Changes in enzyme, substrate, enzyme–substrate complex or product concentration with respect to time during enzyme catalysis.

3.4 Enzyme Kinetics

As mentioned before, analysis of enzyme kinetics allows characterization of an enzyme for its catalytic ability. In its simplest form, enzyme activity, in terms of initial velocity, is monitored as a function of the substrate or product concentration. This is relatively easy to carry out for enzymes with only one substrate. However, there are several enzymes, which have two substrates. In such cases, the order of the reaction becomes important.

3.4.1 Order of Reaction

As mentioned earlier, the reaction rate is dependent on the substrate concentration. Therefore, a general kinetic expression can be given by Equation 3.21. The reaction may involve one or more substrate(s). Here, n denotes the order of reaction. For a simple reaction of a single substrate with conversion to product see Figure. 3.5.

$$nS \rightleftharpoons P \qquad \text{(Eq. 3.20)}$$

the velocity (v), may be expressed as $v = k[S]^n$
$$\text{(Eq. 3.21)}$$

where, k = rate constant of the reaction
n = order of the reaction

For $n = 0$, $v = k$ = constant. Such a reaction would be a zero-order reaction.

For, $n = 1$, $v = k[S]$, the reaction would be a first-order reaction, unit $(\text{seconds})^{-1}$. A large k means the reaction is rapid and a small k means it is a slow reaction.

For $n = 2$, $v = k[S]^2$, and the reaction would be a second-order reaction. It has a dimension of $(\text{mol/L})^{-1}\text{s}^{-1}$.

Enzymatic reactions are always analyzed in terms in initial reaction rate or velocity for obtaining kinetic parameters such as K_m and Vmax (described later).

Fig. 3.5 Concentration dependent variation of substrate on the reaction order of an enzyme catalyzed reaction.

(Figure labels: Maximal velocity; Zero-order reaction $V_i = K$, constant; First-order reaction; V_i; [S])

Leonor Michaelis (1875–1949) and Maud Menten (1879–1960)

Leonor Michaelis was a German biochemist. Maud Menten, after receiving a degree in medicine from the University of Toronto in 1911, left Canada and joined the Michaelis' laboratory in Germany. Together they published their classical paper, Die Kinetik der Invertinwirkung (the Kinetcs of Invertase activity) in 1913. They presented a kinetic model for an enzyme–substrate reaction to form a complex, which further proceeded to form product(s). Based on their kinetic model they formulated a rate equation for single substrate enzymatic reaction.

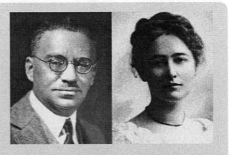

Source: www.carnotcycle.wordpress.com

3.4.2   Michaelis–Menten Analysis

The kinetic steps involved in enzyme catalyzed reactions can be represented as follows:

$$E + S \underset{K_2}{\overset{K_1}{\rightleftharpoons}} ES \underset{K_4}{\overset{K_3}{\rightleftharpoons}} E + P \qquad (Eq.\ 3.22)$$

where,

S = substrate

ES = enzyme–substrate complex

$k_1, k_2, k_3,$ and k_4 are rate constants

The initial reaction velocity (v_i) changes with substrate concentration. The Michaelis–Menten kinetic is based on two assumptions:

- That E, S, and ES are in rapid equilibrium.
- The reaction velocity is proportional to the concentration of ES complex. This assumption ignores the rate constant k_4. For that reason, it is extremely important to ensure that the initial velocity is measured in a concentration in excess of the substrate so that there is no significant P formed during the time of measurement that would make k_4 a significant factor.

From these assumptions, the following equation can be derived.

$$Vo \quad or \quad v = \{V_{max}\ [S]\}/\{K_m + [S]\} \qquad (Eq.\ 3.23)$$

where,

V_o or v = initial velocity or rate of reaction

V_{max} = maximum velocity of the reaction

S = molar substrate concentration

$K_m = \{k_2 + k_3\}/k_1$ = substrate concentration at $\frac{1}{2}V_{max}$

K_m = Michaelis–Menten constant

Both V_{max} and K_m are the defining parameters of an enzyme for its catalytic ability. K_m reflects on the dissociation constant of an enzyme with substrate to form the ES complex

If $k_2 >>> k_3$

then, $K_m = k_2/k_1$ = Equilibrium dissociation constant

$$= [E][S]/[ES] \qquad (Eq.\ 3.24)$$

Thus, K_m can provide information on the affinity of an enzyme for its substrate.

Estimation of V_{max} leads to the calculation of k_3, the turnover number of an enzyme

$$v_i = k_3[ES] \qquad (Eq.\ 3.25)$$

In the presence of excess [S], all the enzyme active sites are saturated, and

$$[ES] = [E_T] \qquad (Eq.\ 3.26)$$

where,

$[E_T]$ is the total enzyme concentration.

Therefore, under conditions of enzyme saturation with substrate

$$V_{max} = k_3[E_T] \tag{Eq. 3.27}$$

and
$$k_3 = V_{max} / [E_T] \tag{Eq. 3.28}$$

k_3 is also known as catalytic constant or k_{cat}, and can be estimated by first estimating Vmax using a known concentration of enzyme and excess concentration of substrate.

For an enzyme with one active site per molecule, k_3 or k_{cat} is the number of substrate molecules transformed into product(s) by one enzyme molecule per unit time (min or s). Catalytic efficiency of an enzyme is defined as k_{cat}/K_m.

3.4.3 The Significance of K_m, k_{cat} and k_{cat}/K_m

K_m is the affinity of the enzyme for the substrate. A large K_m means that the reverse reaction is much greater than the product formation and the enzyme binding to the substrate is very weak. High K_m can be interpreted as either the product is formed very rapidly or the complex dissociates rapidly. To achieve a given reaction velocity, an enzyme with a high K_m requires a higher substrate concentration than an enzyme with a lower K_m.

k_{cat} is the turnover number and gives the direct quantitative measurement of catalytic properties of an enzyme under optimum condition. Unit of k_{cat} is s^{-1}, so the inverse can be thought of as time, i.e., the time required by an enzyme molecule to convert (turn over) one substrate molecule or it is the measure of the number of substrate molecules converted to product per enzyme molecule per second.

k_{cat}/K_m is the measure of enzymatic efficiency. Either a large value of k_{cat} (i.e. rapid turnover) or a small value of K_m (i.e. high affinity of substrates) will make k_{cat}/K_m large. When the substrate concentration is very low.

$[S<<<K_m]$ then, $\qquad V = k_{cat}/K_m [E][S]$

In this situation, the ratio k_{cat}/K_m behaves as a second-order rate constant. This ratio provides a direct measure of specificity and enzyme efficiency. It also allows a direct comparison of the action of any enzyme on different substrates.

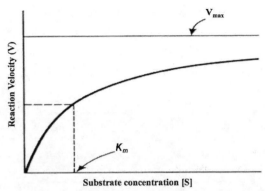

Fig. 3.6 The general enzyme–substrate reaction graph between the reaction velocity with respect to the substrate concentration; according to Michaelis–Menten kinetics. At the point where [S] = K_m, the reaction is exactly half its maximum velocity.

3.5   Graphs of the Michaelis–Menten Equation

3.5.1   Plotting v Against [s]

Figure 3.6 is the simplest plot of enzyme kinetics but this is an unsatisfactory plot for the following reasons: it is difficult, here, to get the accurate details of enzyme kinetics; it is difficult to establish any relationship between a family of enzymes; and it is difficult to detect and analyze any deviation from the expected curve if they occur. To address these issues Michaelis and Menten plotted v against log [S]. The resulting curve is particularly useful in comparing the properties of different isoenzymes that catalyze an enzymatic reaction with different affinities for substrate. However, this plot is not often used in the modern biochemistry. Some useful plots based on Michaelis–Menten kinetics are described below.

3.5.2   The Double-reciprocal Plot

In practice, however, the plot of V_0 versus [S] (Figure 3.7) is not very useful in determining the value of V_{max} because at very high concentrations of substrate, the value of V_{max} can be asymptotic and its determination can be difficult. To address this issue, American chemists H. Lineweaver and Dean Burk developed a plot which employs the double-reciprocal plot of $1/V_0$ and $1/[S]$.

From Equation 3.23,

$$V_0 \quad \text{or} \quad v = V_{max} \, [S]/([S] + K_m)$$

Rearranging this equation will give

$$1/V_0 \quad \text{or} \quad 1/v = K_m/V_{max} \, [S] + 1/V_{max} \qquad \text{(Eq. 3.29)}$$

Slope and intercepts of the straight line given by this plot can give quantitative measurement of K_m and V_{max}, respectively (Figure 3.7).

Questions to ponder over

1.   What is the significance of k_{cat} and K_m?
2.   What is the advantage of Lineweaver–Burk plot vs Michaelis–Menton's equation?

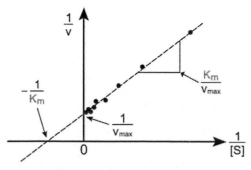

Fig. 3.7   Lineweaver–Burk plot. Slope and intercepts are representing K_m/V_{max} and $1/V_{max}$. Line of this plot can be extended to intersect at x-axis on second quadrant and provides the value of K_m.

3.5.3 The Plot of [S]/v Against [S]

If we multiply both sides of Equation 3.23 by [S], we obtain the following equation

$$\frac{[S]}{V_0} = \frac{K_m}{V_{max}} + \frac{[S]}{V_{max}} \qquad \text{(Eq. 3.30)}$$

Plotting [S]/V_0 against [S] will provide a straight line with slope of 1/$Vmax$ and intercept at K_m/V_{max} on the [S]/V_0 axis. This plot is also referred as Hanes–Woalf plot (Figure 3.8).

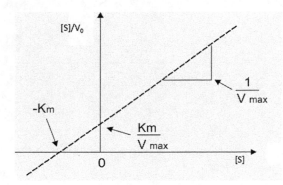

Fig. 3.8 Hanes–Woalf plot. Slope and intercepts represent $1/V_{max}$ and K_m/V_{max}, respectively. Line of this plot can be extended to intersect at x-axis on second quadrant and provides the value of K_m.

This method also gives rapid determination of parameters K_m, V_{max} and V_{max}/K_m. The main drawback of this plot is that neither abscissa or ordinate are independent variables.

3.5.4 The Plot of v Against v/a

From Equation 3.23

$$V_{max} = \frac{K_m V_0}{[S]} + V_0 \qquad \text{(Eq. 3.31)}$$

Rearranging Equation 3.31

$$V_0 = V_{max} - K_m V_0 / [S] \qquad \text{(Eq. 3.32)}$$

Equation 3.32 is again a straight line equation of the plot between V_0 and V_0/[S] with slope $-K_m$, and intercept V_{max} on V_0 axis. Such plots are called Eadie–Hofstee plots (Figure 3.9).

The character of this plot is opposite to the double-reciprocal plot. This plot is very effective in the determination of deviation from Michaelis–Menten behavior. Moreover, the V_0 axis from 0 to V_{max} corresponds to the entire observable range, so poor experimental design and range selection are difficult to hide.

The main drawback of this plot is that both abscissa and ordinate are dependent on reaction velocity, so any error in measurement will be present on both axes.

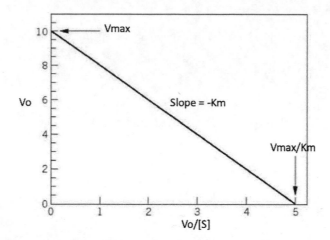

Fig. 3.9 Eadie–Hofstee plot. Slope represents K_m. X and Y-intercepts represent V_{max}/K_m and V_{max}, respectively.

3.5.5   The Direct Linear Plot

The Michaelis–Menten Equation (Equation 3.23) may be rearranged in another way as follows:

$$V\text{max} = V_0 + \frac{V_0}{[S]} K_m \qquad\qquad\qquad (\text{Eq. } 3.33)$$

If V_{max} and K_m are variable and [S] and V_o are constants, this equation will present a straight line with a slope of $V_o/[S]$ and intercept V_o on the V_{max} axis. For any pair of V_o and [S] there is an infinite set of values of V_{max} and K_m. For any value of K_m there will be corresponding value of V_{max}. The straight line will determine all pairs of K_m and V_{max} values of first observation. If a second line is drawn in similar way it will relate different pair of K_m and V_{max} of second observation. However, the value of K_m and V_{max} which satisfy both the observation will be given by the point of intersection. Perpendicular point on ordinate (y-axis) and abscissa (x-axis) represents V_{max} and K_m, respectively.

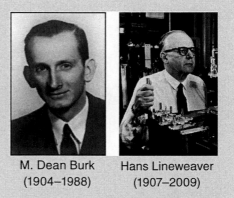

M. Dean Burk   Hans Lineweaver
(1904–1988)   (1907–2009)

Hans Lineweaver with **Dean Burk** developed the Lineweaver–Burk plot to explain enzyme mechanism and quantify kinetic parameters.

In ideal situations, there is perfect intersection of lines (Figure 3.10). However, in reality observations are associated with errors and all lines cannot be expected to intersect at same point. Each intersection point provides an unique sets of K_m and V_{max}. In such cases, median estimate is the best representative of K_m and V_{max}.

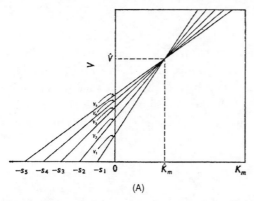
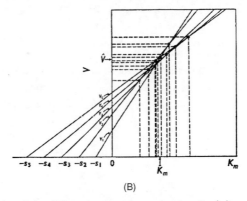

(A)
(B)

Fig. 3.10 Direct linear plot of V against K_m. (A) In ideal situation, all lines intersect at one point. Each line will represent one observation, and is drawn with an intercept of $-[S]$ on the abscissa and an intercept of v on the ordinate. (B) In real experiment, considering experimental error, there is a family of intersection points, each point with separate K_m and V_{max} (Adopted from Eisenthal and Bowden, 1974).

The direct linear plot has a few advantages over the other graphical methods: (a) it does not require additional calculation, and (b) it can be measured while the experiment is proceeding, so that an immediate visual idea can be obtained. Disadvantages include not coping with large amounts of data, and also, poor presentation of data.

3.6   Enzyme Inhibition

Substances which reduce the rate of an enzyme catalyzed reaction are called inhibitors. However, there are several substances which may cause a reduction in rate of an enzyme catalyzed reaction. Some of them, such as protein denaturant, are non-specific, but others exist which are specific for an enzyme. Those substances which act on a specific site of an enzyme and show specificity in binding are termed as inhibitors. There are several ways an inhibitor can inhibit the reaction and it is a good tool not only for therapeutic application, but it also provides much important information about how an enzyme works. There is a situation where the inhibitor makes the enzyme totally inactive (lower V_{max}) whereas in other cases it leads to incomplete inactivation, affecting either K_m or V_{max} or both. There can be both reversible inhibition and irreversible inhibition (or catalytic poisoning). Reversible inhibition can form noncovalent binding of the inhibitor. In irreversible inhibition, the molecule is covalently bound to the enzyme. Irreversible inhibitors that poison the enzyme are not suitable for further development for therapeutic purposes.

Reversible inhibition: All reversible inhibitors form noncovalent bonds with the enzyme but they differ in their mechanisms through which they decrease the activity of the enzyme and the way they affect the kinetics of the reaction. As mentioned, the reaction rate is often dependent on [ES], therefore reducing the enzyme concentration that leads to decreased reaction rates.

Reversible inhibitors are generally divided into the following categories: *competitive inhibitors*, *noncompetitive inhibitors* and *uncompetitive inhibitors* (Figures 3.11 and 3.12). There also are cases of mixed inhibition, a term that describes a process of inhibition which cannot be explained by any of the above categories individually.

3.6.1   Competitive Inhibition

When an enzyme comes within close proximity of the substance resembling the substrate, it accepts this molecule at the same site where its natural substrate binds to proceed with the reaction. If the enzyme is not able to undergo a catalytic step in the presence of such a molecule, it is said to be a competitive inhibition and the molecule is called competitive inhibitor. Usually, competitive inhibitors have a higher affinity and stronger binding than the natural substrate (Figures 3.11 and 3.12). Competitive inhibitors bind to the active site of an enzyme and stop its catalytic function.

$$\mathrm{E + S} \underset{k_{-1}}{\overset{k_1}{\rightleftharpoons}} \mathrm{ES} \xrightarrow{k_2} \mathrm{E + P}$$

$$\mathrm{+}$$

$$\mathrm{I}$$

$$k_{-3} \Big\Vert k_3$$

$$\mathrm{EI}$$

"I" stands for inhibitory molecule and the dissociation constant for inhibitor binding is given by K_I, defined as $K_I = [\mathrm{E}][\mathrm{I}]/[\mathrm{E}]$ where, [I] is the concentration of free inhibitor. So, the rate equation can be solved as

$$[\mathrm{E}]_t = [\mathrm{E}] + [\mathrm{ES}] + [\mathrm{EI}]$$

where,
$[\mathrm{E}]_t$ = concentration of total enzyme present
$[\mathrm{E}]$ = concentration of free enzyme
$[\mathrm{ES}]$ = concentration of enzyme–substrate complex
$[\mathrm{EI}]$ = concentration of enzyme–inhibitor complex

Therefore, the rate equation for competitive inhibition will be given by

$$v = \frac{V_{max}[S]}{K'_m + [S]} \qquad \qquad \text{(Eq. 3.34)}$$

where, $K'_m = K_m(1 + [I]/K_I)$, is also referred as $K_m{}^{app}$.

Implying that with an increase in [I], there is an increase in K_m which means lower affinity for the substrate (higher K_m = lower affinity). This makes sense as inhibitors compete for the same site for binding as the substrate. The maximum velocity remains unchanged and, for large [S] the value of v approaches V_{max}. This is similar to the absence of inhibition, and from Equation 3.28, $V_{max} = k_{cat}[E]_t$. High K_m implies that increasing the substrate concentration would outcompete the binding sites.

3.6.2   Noncompetitive Inhibition

This form of inhibition occurs when the inhibitor binds to the second site (allosteric sites) on the enzyme surface other than the active site in such a way that it distorts the enzyme so that the binding of the substrate will be inhibited. In this case, the inhibitor either binds to the free enzyme or the enzyme–substrate complex. However, binding to one does not necessarily interfere with the other, and either binding type, leads to no product formation. The noncompetitive inhibitor does not resemble the substrate and does not have any affinity to the active site. The inhibitor molecule does not interfere with the substrate molecule in any way but it completely stops the catalysis. Reaction of this form of inhibition is shown below:

$$[E]+[S] \xleftrightarrow{K_s} [E \cdot S] \xrightarrow{k_2} [E]+[P]$$

$$+ \qquad\qquad\qquad +$$

$$[I] \qquad\qquad\qquad [I]$$

$$\Updownarrow K_I \qquad\qquad\qquad \searrow K_I$$

$$[E \cdot I]+[S] \xleftrightarrow{K_s} [E \cdot S \cdot I]$$

The K_m is unaffected by the inhibitor, but the k_{cat} decreases with the increasing [I], and so, there is a change in V_{max}. For a high [S], we find

$$v = \frac{V'_{max}[S]}{K_m + [S]} \tag{Eq. 3.35}$$

where, V' is $Vmax \, / \left(1 + \dfrac{[I]}{Ki}\right)$ and referred to as V_{max}^{app}.

In Equation 3.35, $Vmax$ term is altered, referred as $Vmax^{app}$, by a term that includes the contribution from [I]. Equation also suggests that affinity for the substrate is unaltered, while the maximum reaction rate is changed.

3.6.3 Uncompetitive Inhibition

This form of inhibition takes place when an inhibitor of the enzyme binds only to the ES complex to inhibit enzyme from reacting with substrate to form product. In this inhibition the inhibitor does not interact with free enzyme. This is why, at least in principle, the mechanism is different from competitive inhibition. One can hypothesize that binding of the substrate to its enzyme leads to conformational changes which provide a binding site for the inhibitor. The enzyme–substrate–inhibitor complex does not produce any product. Reaction of this form of inhibition is shown below:

$$E + S \underset{k_{-1}}{\overset{k_1}{\rightleftharpoons}} ES \xrightarrow{k_2} E + P$$

$$+$$

$$I$$

$$k_{-3} \Updownarrow k_3$$

$$ESI$$

The rate equation is as follows

$$v = \frac{V'_{max}[S]}{K'_m + [S]} \tag{Eq. 3.36}$$

where, V' is $Vmax / \left(1 + \dfrac{[I]}{Ki}\right)$ and $Ki = k_3/k_{-3}$,

$K'm$ is $K_m / \left(1 + \dfrac{[I]}{Ki}\right)$

In this inhibition, as [S] increases to infinity, not all enzyme is converted to [ES]. This means that there is a finite amount of [ESI] complex even at infinite [S]. So, under these conditions, V' is less than V_{max} and K'_m also decreases, which makes sense because if inhibitor, I, binds to ES alone, and not E, it will shift the equilibrium of $E + S \rightleftarrows ES$ towards the right (Le Chatelier's principle) which decreases K'_m and appears as increased affinity of substrate to its enzyme.

Equation 3.36 suggests four important things: (i) that both V_{max} and K_m are affected by [I] and its dissociation constant, Ki; (ii) altering the inhibitor concentration will alter the V' and K'_m; (iii) with the decrease of maximum velocity, K_m also decreases, meaning the affinity for the substrate is increasing; and (iv) the impact of $\left(1 + \dfrac{[I]}{Ki}\right)$ is greater as this term is in the numerator, and so, the net result always decreases the reaction rate with increase of [I].

3.6.4 Mixed Inhibition

Mixed inhibition is a type of enzyme inhibition which can be seen as mixture of competitive and uncompetitive inhibition. In this sort of inhibition, the inhibitor may bind to the enzyme or [ES] complex but with greater affinity of one state or the other. It can be considered as a subtype of non-competitive inhibition. Notably, inhibitors that bind to the allosteric site are not all mixed inhibitors.

Mixed inhibition may result in either of the two situations mentioned below:

- An increase in K_m, which is reflected as the decreased affinity with substrate. Therefore, in this condition, the binding of inhibitor to the free enzyme is favorable thus **mimicking competitive binding**.
- Decrease in K_m, which means an increase in the affinity of enzyme with its substrate. In this situation, the binding of inhibitor to the ES complex is favorable thus **mimicking closely uncompetitive binding**.

In either case the inhibition decreases the apparent maximum enzyme reaction rate.

$$E + S \rightleftarrows ES \longrightarrow P$$

$$+I \Big\Uparrow K_{ic} \qquad K_{iu} \Big\Uparrow +I$$

$$EI \qquad\qquad ESI$$

In this case the V^{app} or $V' = \dfrac{V}{1 + i \,/\, Kiu}$ (Eq. 3.37)

$$K_m{}^{app} \; of \; K' = \dfrac{K_m\left(1 + \dfrac{[I]}{Kic}\right)}{1 + [I] \,/\, Kiu}$$ (Eq. 3.38)

$$\frac{V'}{K'} = \frac{\dfrac{V_{max}}{K_m}}{1 + \left[I\right] / Kic}$$ (Eq. 3.39)

where, $Kic = K_I = \dfrac{[E][I]}{[EI]}$ and $K_{iu} = K_I' = \dfrac{[ES][I]}{[ESI]}$

Questions to ponder over

1. Consider a situation where the concentration of inhibitor is less than that of the substrate. If the affinity for the substrate is higher for the active site, then what are the types of inhibition that the reaction follows? Is the enzyme inhibited a lot or a little? What happens to the product formation?
2. Prepare a protocol that could be tested experimentally whether an inhibitor was competitive or noncompetitive. *Hint*: Consider concentration effects.

Table 3.1 Comparison between different types of inhibition.

Inhibitor Type	Binding Site on Enzyme	Kinetic Effect
Competitive Inhibitor	At the active site of the enzyme. Inhibitor competes with the substrate and binding is dynamic. Reversible inhibition; can be reversed by increasing substrate concentration.	Unchanged V_{max}; increased K_m.
Noncompetitive Inhibitor	Inhibitor binds either the free enzyme or the enzyme-substrate complex at a site different from the active site. Binding of substrate to enzyme is unaltered. Irreversible inhibition.	Unaltered K_m; decreased V_{max}.
Uncompetitive Inhibitor	Inhibitor binds only to ES complexes at sites different from the active site. Modification of enzyme conformation upon substrate binding facilitates this. Irreversible inhibition.	Decreased V_{max}; decreased K_m.
Mixed inhibition	Inhibitor binds, both, to the free enzyme and enzyme substrate complex.	Both V_{max} and K_m are altered and depend on inhibitor concentration.

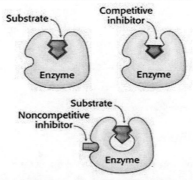

Fig. 3.11 Different modes of enzyme inhibition.

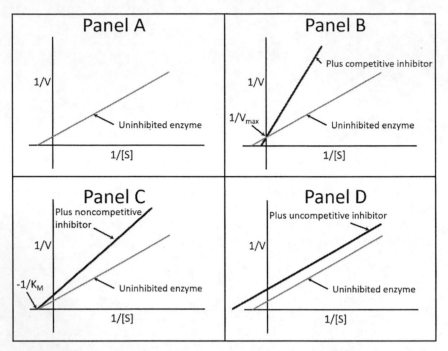

Fig. 3.12 Typical Lineweaver–Burk (L–B) plots of different inhibition modes. Panel A shows the L–B plot for a typical enzymatic reaction in the absence of its inhibitor. Panel B shows the L–B plot when an enzyme is inhibited by a competitive inhibitor. For competitive inhibition, the two straight lines cross at the y-axis indicating no change in V_{max}. Panel C shows the L–B plot when an enzyme is inhibited by a noncompetitive inhibitor. Both lines meet at the negative x-axis indicating no change in the affinity, K_m, of enzyme for its substrate. Panel D shows the L–B plots when an enzyme is inhibited by an uncompetitive inhibitor. The two lines are parallel to each other indicating that both V_{max} and K_m change.

3.6.5 Irreversible Inhibition

Here, the inhibitor binds to the enzyme covalently and makes it inactivate. Since the covalent bond is strong and requires considerable energy to be broken, the inhibition is termed as irreversible. Almost all irreversible reactions are toxic in nature. The extent of inhibition depends on the reaction rate constant. For the inhibitors to bind so selectively, they must bind very strongly with the active site. Many natural toxins are enzyme inhibitors and cannot be removed by physical techniques. The main function of the inhibitor is to reduce the availability of enzyme molecules for an enzymatic reaction. Binding with a hydroxyl group, or sulfhydryl or metal ions, at the active or allosteric site produce this type of inhibition.

3.7 Inhibitory Effect of Substrates

3.7.1 Non-productive Binding

Consider the example of α-chymotrypsin. Its natural substrate is ill-defined. An enzyme that can bind a macromolecule is also able to bind several molecules in many different ways. So, there may be a possibility where the binding is not productive, and leads to nonproductive enzyme–substrate complexes that do not form product/s.

$$A + E \leftrightarrow EA \rightarrow E + P$$

$$E + A \leftrightarrow AE \rightarrow \text{no product}$$

This binding follows the Michaelis–Menten equation, however V_{max} and K_m may be lower. Therefore, the ratio V_{max}/K_m is a better way for the determination of catalytic properties on an enzyme.

3.7.2 Substrate Inhibition

For some enzymes, it is possible that a second substrate molecule will bind to the enzyme–substrate complex. However, it will not happen at lower concentrations or closer to physiological value, but as concentration of substrate increases, it starts inhibiting the enzyme and affecting its kinetics (Figure 3.13).

$$A + E \leftrightarrow EA \rightarrow E + P$$

$$A + EA \leftrightarrow AEA \rightarrow \text{no product}$$

The rate of second equation is given by K_{si}, rate constant for substrate inhibition.

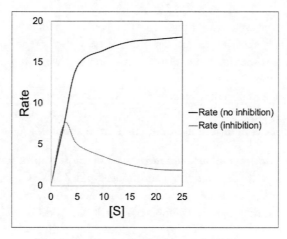

Fig. 3.13 Example of substrate inhibition.

Overall rate equation of substrate inhibition is given by

$$v = \frac{V_{max}\left[S\right]}{K_m + [S]^* \left(1 + \dfrac{[S]}{Ksi}\right)} \tag{Eq. 3.40}$$

Equation 3.40 is similar to the Michaelis–Menten equation for a two-step model. However, the term $[S]^2$ makes the rate approach zero rather than V_{max} when [S] is large. Also, K_m is not equal to [S] when v = $V_{max}/2$.

3.8   General Protocol for an Inhibition Experiment

In general, inhibition experiments have two major components: (a) design, which is preceded by (b) analysis. There are two main objectives of any inhibition experiment: identification of the type of inhibition and estimating the value of inhibition constants. And, as far as experimental design is concerned, there are four main aspects:

(a) *Choice of substrate concentration*: In an enzyme assay, the first step is to find conditions in which the experimental rate depends on the concentration of enzyme (slight variation in other conditions has very little effect), whereas in an investigation of the kinetic parameters of an enzyme one needs to be concerned about variation in other parameters. Therefore, in general, the conditions that are optimum for assaying an enzyme are unlikely to be appropriate for determination of its kinetic parameters.

Assuming an enzyme obeys the Michaelis–Menten mechanism, consideration of [S] will define K_m and V_{max} precisely. In Michaelis–Menten kinetics, v (rate) becomes V_{max} as [S] becomes very large. In principle, larger [S] will be better for precise measurement. But this is not always the case. Two reasons for this: (i) at high [S], many enzymes show substrate inhibition resulting in a rate that would not be expected from the K_m and V_{max} at low [S] and (ii) if the substrate is an ion it may be inappropriate to vary the ionic strength if excessively high [S] is used. Moreover, one must pay attention to the maximum [S] that can be used for an assay using absorbance measurement. However, this can be improved by using narrower path-length cuvette. Wider path-length cuvettes will be useful for assaying weakly absorbing solutions. Both these options require special modifications in the instrument and this should be one of the considerations while opting for one or the other option in an assay's conditions.

Notably, at high substrate concentration, the rate is largely dependent on V_{max} whereas at low [S] rate is dependent on V_{max}/K_m. In general, defining K_m requires accurate measurement of both V_{max} and V_{max}/K_m and substrate concentration should range from about 0.2 K_m to about 10 K_m.

(b) *Choice of pH, temperature, and other conditions*: The most appropriate condition for most mammalian enzyme assays are physiological conditions -- pH 7.5, 37°C, and ionic strength of 150 mM. However, one can deviate from this condition because many enzymes become denatured appreciably at 37°C, and are comparatively more stable at 25°C. Additionally, pH of reaction should be selected such that the reaction rate is largely unaffected by small changes in pH.

(c) *Use of replicate measurements*: At the end of any kinetic study there is always some discrepancy while fitting the data of every observation with the formulated equation. The discrepancy in the obtained parameters and equation should be dismissed by considering the experimental errors. One of the ways to minimize random errors is to include replicates of observations. If the replicate observations agree, within statistical limits, then the obtained parameters and equation would satisfy the precise enzyme kinetics. If, on the other hand, data are scattered in these replicates, then measured parameters and the equation may be rejected until the precise observations become available.

The disagreement between an experimentally observed and a fitted line may be either caused by experimental errors on the measurements or inadequacy of the theoretical model, or both. Another pertinent question would be how many repeats should be appropriate for a kinetic experiment. The answer will depend on several factors: (i) amount of work that is needed for each measurement,

(ii) stability of the enzyme or other reagents, (iii) determination and quantification of the experimental error, and (iv) experimental and other complexities related to analysis. First and foremost imperative, in the experimental parameters, is to include the number of different concentrations of substrate or inhibitor which should be appropriate to characterize the shape of the curve. In general, for a one substrate enzyme, there should be at least five substrate concentrations in the range of 0.5 K_m to 5 K_m. Whereas for two substrate enzymes one might require a minimum of 25 different combinations of concentrations of substrate and enzyme.

(d) *Effect of inhibitor on the kinetics*: Competitive inhibition decreases the value of V_{max}/K_m, and that is why at low concentration of substrate [S], the component which is involved in competitive inhibition will be more pronounced. Similarly, at high substrate concentration the component which is involved in uncompetitive inhibition is more pronounced. So, an inhibition experiment should be designed to include both high and low concentrations of substrate for complete characterization of inhibition kinetics. Note that there is no such requirement for using the same set of [I] values at each [S] value. Nonetheless, if several of the identical [S] and [I] values are used, it will produce a reasonable number of points on each line when one uses [S] or [I] as abscissa.

3.9 Applications of Enzyme Inhibition

The mechanism of enzyme inhibition is effective in various ways:

1. It provides insights into the mechanism of the catalytic activity of the enzyme.
2. Understanding it, allows controlling of the mechanism of the enzymatic activity in vivo
3. It helps in design of inhibitors for use in therapeutics.

3.10 Methodologies for Studying Catalytic Mechanism of the Enzyme

Among characteristics of any enzyme are their specificity, catalytic activity and regulating capacity, reflecting a 3D interaction of the enzymes with its substrates. A wide range of experimental strategies and techniques are required to develop a complete elucidation of the mechanism involved in the activity of the enzyme with the substrate and conversion of the substrates to its end products. These include:

X-ray crystallography: The diffraction patterns measured by X-ray can give the exact location of the amino acid in the proteins and details about substrate binding and reaction. The determination of amino acids are performed by growing a crystal in the presence and absence of substrate or inhibition or both. These crystals are analyzed by using X-ray crystallography technique. The 3D modeling facilitates in predicting the formation of products. This is the general approach which is being used in the development of theoretical molecules by the pharmaceutical industry.

Irreversible inhibitor and affinity label study: Irreversible inhibitors form covalent bonds with the enzyme's active or allosteric sites. Location of the binding site of the inhibitor in the enzyme facilitates study about the identity and possible interaction of specific amino acids with the inhibitor molecule at the binding site. To identify the binding location, inhibitor molecules are either tagged with a radioisotope or by using docking study or MD-simulation based drug design.

Kinetics: As just discussed in detail, this is based on the determination of K_m, k_{cat} and K_i values for a range of substrates and/or competitive inhibitors. These allow for correlation between the molecular structures of the active site and kinetic constants, and constructing the structure of the active site. Further information can be gathered by carefully examining the influence of pH and temperature on the kinetic parameters.

Isotope exchange: Reactions in which the natural isotope of an element is exchanged with its different isotopes can also provide information about kinetic parameters and effect of enzymatic reaction due to modification in stereoselectivity. Therefore, by following its isotopic exchange, we can examine the mechanistic model of the reaction.

Site directed mutagenesis: By mutating key amino acids, by site-directed mutagenesis, we can examine various enzymatic parameters, such as binding, catalysis, and kinetics.

3.11   Enzyme Activation

In enzymology, there are several disparate meanings of the term "enzyme activation." In general, an activator is a species that increases the activity of an enzyme, without any change in itself, during the reaction (similar to what are called catalysts).

There are various processes where the term "enzyme activation" has been used:

1. Some enzymes are secreted as inactivated precursors or zymogens. By partial proteolytic reaction, these precursors are converted into an active enzyme. This process of activation is termed as "zymogen activation." For example, pepsinogen is the zymogen and after activation it is converted into the active enzyme pepsin.
2. Several metabolic enzymes are activated by metabolic regulations, such as phosphorylation, from inactivated state to activated state. However, in general, such processes do not correspond to activation or inactivation of enzyme.
3. Many enzymes are activated by metal ions. In fact, these metal ions are not activators but instead they are co-factors and part of the substrate. For example, nearly all the ATP-dependent kinases are "activated" by Mg^{2+}. It's not because Mg^{2+} binds to the enzyme directly and activates it, the true substrate in $MgATP^{2-}$. Free Mg^{2+} is an inhibitor for several enzymes.

3.11.1   Specific Activation

This is a simplest type of activation. In this the free enzyme has no activity without a bound activator. Depicted below, the activator is represented as X.

$$\begin{array}{c} X \\ + \\ E \\ \Big\updownarrow K_{Sp} \\ S + EX \underset{K'_{-1}}{\overset{K'_1}{\rightleftharpoons}} ESX \xrightarrow{K'_2} EX + P \end{array}$$

The rate equation of this inhibition is similar to competitive inhibition and can be represented as:

$$v = \frac{V_{max}[S]}{K'_m\left(1 + \dfrac{Ksp}{x}\right) + [S]} \qquad \text{(Eq. 3.41)}$$

In which, $K'_m = (K'_{-1} + K'_2)/K'_1$ and x is the concentration of activator, X.

The mathematical difference between competitive inhibition and specific activation is the replacement of denominator $[I]/K_1$ in Equation 3.41 by K_{sp}/x. This makes sense as the rate will be zero in the absence of activator. Enzyme affinity for its substrate cannot be negligible. Therefore, it is practically not possible for an enzyme that cannot bind substrate in the absence of an activator. Moreover, the proton is one of the commonest activators and does not produce any steric effect.

3.11.2 Hyperbolic Activation and Inhibition

Realistically, activators behave in a more complex fashion than the mechanism just described in section 3.11.1. In practice, the activation process is better described as given below:

Some important points for consideration while analyzing this mechanism are:

(a) The activator-dissociation steps are not dead-end reactions. They are in the loop.
(b) This is not necessarily the mechanism of activation, as it could lead to inhibition if the EX complex is less reactive than the free enzyme, E.
(c) If $K_2 > K_2'$ then X inhibits at high substrate concentration.
(d) If $K_1K_2/(K_{-1} + K_2) > K_1'K_2'/(K_{-1}' + K_2')$, then X inhibits at low substrate concentration.

In this case, the plot of 1/V' or K_m'/V' versus inhibitor or reciprocal activator concentration, is a rectangular hyperbola, which is why it is called hyperbolic activation or hyperbolic inhibition. Hyperbolic effects are not very hard to recognize experimentally. Perform experiments with wide range of inhibitor and activator concentrations to get a sense of whether rate tends to be zero at high inhibitor concentration or low activator concentration. Deviation from linear behavior of the plot should be checked; if deviation is determined then it must be due to hyperbolic effects.

Questions

1. How does an enzyme speed up a chemical reaction?
2. Explain the differences in terms of K_m and V_{max} between competitive, noncompetitive and uncompetitive inhibition. Use a Lineweaver–Burk plot to describe each of the inhibition terms graphically.

3. Given enzyme A from species X with a K_m of 0.23 mM and enzyme B from species Y with a K_m of 1.33 mM; which one would have an apparent higher affinity for the substrate used to determine K_m?
4. Why is it important to study enzyme kinetics?
5. What are the general methodologies to study the structure and mechanism of enzymes?
6. What are inhibitors?
7. What happens when an enzyme is heated beyond its optimum temperature?
8. What type of inhibitor should be useful in trying in identifying the features of a substrate that are important for binding the substrate to the active site of an enzyme catalyzing a single-substrate reaction? Why? How would one use the inhibitor to obtain this information?
9. Why is initial velocity important in enzyme kinetics?
10. What can replace enzymes?

3.12   Proteomics

Proteins are quintessential biomolecules for life on this planet. They comprise of amino acids arranged according to defined templates. Proteomics refer to the study of the all the proteins in a cell, tissue, or organism under a defined set of conditions. It involves a large-scale study of proteins, their quantities, their structure, dynamics, and physiological role or functions. The analysis of any disease also targets the changes in protein profile of the cell, tissue, or organ. The process helps us design appropriate therapies to treat disease (almost every therapeutic drug which is being used today has a protein as a target). The term first appeared in 1997 and originated from the word proteome (protein and genome) conceived by Mark Wilkins in 1994. In other words, proteome is the entire database of proteins produced by living organisms. Proteomics relies on three basic technological platforms which include fractionation of complex protein and peptide mixtures, MS (Mass Spectrometry) to acquire the data of individual protein (see more discussion below), and finally bioinformatics to analyze.

Molecular biology suggests to us that the amino acid sequence can be obtained from the DNA sequence. However, this is not always true. Reasons for this: (a) in a given condition different sets of genes are expressed in different tissues even though the DNA in each cell is same. Apart from the house keeping genes (proteins that are common to all cells), some specific proteins unique to that tissue are expressed for very specialized function of that tissue. Additionally, single chain DNA sequences can be translated into multiple proteins using alternate splicing, variation in the translation "start" and "stop" sites, frameshifting and post-translational modifications.

These two arguments, suggest that protein content of the cell is more complex than the genome. For example, the human genome sequence suggests there may be 30,000–40,000 genes whereas the number of proteins could be as many as 200,000 or more. This is shattering to the dogma of one gene code for one protein. In view of this, there is a need for an understanding of the biological role of each and every protein in the cell individually. This led to development of the terminology proteomics.

Proteomics is a large-scale study of proteins in an organism, system or biological context. In biological entities, the concentration and number of proteins are not constant; they vary from cell to cell and change over time. Proteomics can provide sufficient information about the interaction, location, and involvement in biological processes of a protein of particular interest. Therefore, proteomics can be used to examine the following (Figure 3.14):

1. when and where proteins are expressed,
2. rates of protein production,
3. stability of protein (degradation and steady state abundance),
4. protein modification,
5. biological functions of proteins, and
6. involvement of proteins in metabolic pathways.

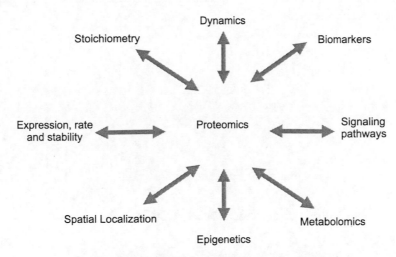

Fig. 3.14   Fields where proteomics can be used.

So, the main purpose of proteomics is to determine the identity and amount of every protein in a cell and examine their functions.

Proteomic study is a blend of conventional and modern techniques, which allow us to determine and analyze the total protein content of the cell. In general, there are two major steps involved: separation of proteins (using gel-based techniques) and analysis of proteins (using mass spectrometry).

3.12.1   2-D PAGE

The goal of 2-D electrophoresis is to separate all gene products present in a sample. It can differentiate gene expressions between the two different biological states of the cell. This has immense utility in finding the possible target for the disease. For example, we can compare the 2-D gel pattern for a diseased tissue/cell and compare it with that of a normal tissue/cell. If a particular protein is present (or absent) in the diseased tissue/cell, then by identifying (sequence and molecular characteristics) this protein, we can trace back to the gene. This will allow us to understand why the expression of this gene is more (or less, or without expression) in the diseased state. Finally, we can understand the mechanism of the disease. Similarly, we can compare the information from diseased tissue/cell with treated tissue/cell to examine the effect of drugs, changes in the protein expression of proteins in different stages of tissue development, changes due to external stimuli, and determine bacterial infection.

If performed in a favorable condition, 2-D gels can separate 5000 proteins. In the first dimension, isoelectric focusing (IEF) is performed and in the second dimension SDS-PAGE (Sodium Dodecyl

Sulphate – Polyacrylamide Gel Electrophoresis) is performed. First dimension separates protein based on their isoelectric point (pI) and second dimension separates them based on their size. It is not mandatory to have IEF first and SDS second, the reverse order may also be followed. But, there are two reasons for using the classical order: (a) it is better that the second separation should be the cheapest one (economical reason), and (b) it is much easier to stain SDS gels and resolutions are better than IEF ones. In a 2-D gel the proteins appear as spots on the gel rather than bands.

Although, the name 2-D electrophoresis suggests that it is a two-step process, it, in fact consists of five step as shown in Figure 3.15.

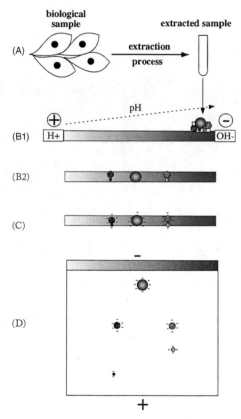

Fig. 3.15 Schematic representation of classical 2-D gel electrophoresis. First step is the extraction of proteins from the complex biological samples (A) which are then separated onto a pH gradient (B1), IEF strip, with anode and cathode on acidic and basic side, respectively. After IEF, proteins in the sample are separated based on their pI (B2). After separation, the strip is equilibrated in a SDS-containing buffer (C). Then the separated proteins on IEF strip is transferred to SDS gel by loading IEF strip on top of a SDS–PAGE gel, where proteins are further separated based on their molecular masses (D) (Reproduced with permission from Rabilloud and Lelong, 2011).

Step 1: Sample preparation

The main objective of sample preparation for this method is to maintain protein in its native state with unaltered charge. Therefore, avoid using any charged detergent, such as SDS, and use uncharged chemicals to extract proteins. A combination of chaotropes and detergents are generally used to achieve this. Chaotropes, such as urea, are excellent solubilizing and denaturing agents. However, chaotropes alone are not very efficient in solubilizing lipids, and under the condition of IEF (pH3.0 – 10.0), they are not able to keep proteins in solution. Therefore, electrically neutral detergents (over the pH range of IEF), such as CHAPS, and compatible with chaotropes should be used.

Another aspect in sample preparation is to break the protein–protein and protein–DNA ionic interactions. In most cases, protein denaturation should break protein–protein ionic interaction, whereas, protein–DNA ionic interactions are difficult to break. Generally two approaches are used to break protein–DNA interactions: (a) Dissolving the sample in a high pH buffer in the presence of a nucleic acid precipitant; the nucleic acid can then be degraded with trichloroacetic acid. (b) Using other interfering agents such as polysaccharides, polyphenols, and hydrophobic chemicals. Then, these agents should be eliminated using proper protocols. Another caveat in sample preparation would be dealing with protein modifications, such as carbamylation induced by the presence of urea or protease activity. Proper precautions should be applied to avoid these situations during sample preparation, such as using protease inhibitors and preparing the sample at 4°C.

Step 2: First separation (IEF)

This step is relatively straightforward and is described in Chapter 4. However, there are a few things which need careful attention. IEF is a steady-state technique. IEF strips are designed in such a way that they form a pH gradient and the sample can be introduced at any point on this gradient, but it is always preferable to apply the sample at the anodic side of the focusing gel, to avoid sample loss. Other factors that need attention are voltage profile, thiol ionization, and isoelectric precipitation (discussed in Chapter 4).

Step 3: Interfacing with the second separation

The purpose of this step is to coat the protein separated in IEF onto SDS, so that they can be run appropriately in the second dimension. Therefore, for this step IEF strip is equilibrated in a SDS-containing buffer. Using organic disulfides can simplify issues related to electroendosmosis (the motion of liquid under the influence of an applied potential across a porous material, capillary tube, membrane, microchannel, or any other fluid conduit).

Step 4: The second separation (SDS-PAGE)

Process of SDS is described in Chapter 4. However in IEF, the protein may not be truly precipitated, and it is possible that protein is in a somewhat solubilized form. So, it is preferable to start the SDS separation at low voltage, giving time to the SDS front to re-solubilize the proteins.

Step 5: Protein detection

This step is an important one, as (a) detection is required for further analysis, and (b) it helps the experimenter to identify a few spots of interest, which can be processed further for mass spectrometry to complete additional analysis. Important requirements for the protein detection are sample homogeneity, compatibility with steps involved (especially mass spectrometry), sensitivity, and linearity. There are three in-gel detection methods: detection with organic dyes, silver staining, and fluorescence. Detection with organic dyes, such as Coomassie blue, is the most popular one with moderate sensitivity (10–47 ng); have good linearity, homogeneity and excellent compatibility with mass spectrometry. Conversely, silver staining sensitivity is very good (0.5–1.2 ng) but less linearity and homogeneity, and less compatibility with mass spectrometry. Best alternative for protein detection is the fluorescence detection method which offers good sensitivity (1–2 ng), excellent linearity and compatibility with mass spectrometry. Immunodetection is the preferred choice for detection because of several reasons: (a) multiple options of conjugated secondary antibodies (radioisotopes, fluorescent or chemiluminescent), (b) signals are comparatively stable, and (c) stripping and re-probing allows using the same blot with different primary antibodies. Using various types of labeled antibodies, pico-gram sensitivity can be achieved.

An important point to note here is that the image analysis of 2-D gel-based proteomics requires multiple comparison of several reproducible gels; it is not based on just comparison of one IEF and a single subsequent SDS-PAGE gel. Also, careful design of experiment and proper statistical consideration are needed to avoid false positive results. The complexity of 2-D gel and data under consideration is daunting. Fortunately, several commercial 2-D gel electrophoresis softwares, compatible with available operating systems, are available. Together all these steps can provide both quantitative and qualitative information from gel pattern and comparison of two-different 2-D gels. They are also able to create a database and compare the data from the available 2-D electrophoresis databases, such as SWISS-2D PAGE (maintained at Geneva University Hospital, (http://au.expasy.org/ch2d/).

Flicker is one of the interesting programs to compare 2-D gel patterns (http:/open2dprot. sourceforge.net/Flicker). In this program, the majority of spots appear as fixed spots when comparing the two gels. Spots that appear on one gel and not on the other will be seen as flashing spots.

2-D electrophoresis is hampered by some limitations, such as low abundancy of identified proteins, detecting low and high mass proteins, difficulties associated with membrane proteins and proteins with extreme isoelectric points.

3.12.2 Mass-fingerprinting

Proteomics using mass-spectrometry involve two methodologies: (a) peptide mass mapping (or PMF) and (b) peptide sequencing (Figure 3.16). Peptide mass-fingerprinting is an analytical technique used in proteomics, which can be combined with 2-D gel electrophoresis to identify a unknown protein. PMF involves an identification and quantification of protein spots from 2-D gel followed by in situ protein protease digestion of protein. The absolute mass of the peptides can be accurately analyzed by a mass spectrometer, such as MALDI-TOF (Matrix-assisted Laser Desorption Ionization – Time of Flight) or ESI-TOF (Electro Spray Ionization – Time of Flight). Both ion sources have their own pros and cons. ESI requires more of the peptide sample than MALDI. However, for a few peptides MALDI is better, but for identifying large number of peptides ESI provides better results. MALDI-TOF is preferred in PMF analysis because of two reasons: (a) MALDI-TOF has wide sequence coverage, and (b) can analyze rapidly a large number of samples, at the same time.

The observed accurate mass values provide a "fingerprint." This set of masses or fingerprint, obtained from the digestion of protein provides highly diagnostic information for the subjected protein. This set of masses, are termed "fingerprint", because no two proteins have the same set of peptide masses. This peptide fingerprint can be compared to a predicted list (using protease digestion of peptides and available databases such as the Mascot or Protein Prospector). With a sufficient number of peptide masses a match is usually found. In general, for better confidence of identification 5 or more accurate masses are required, while 3 or 4 might yield a more ambiguous match. When one has a significant number of matches, the protein is identified with greater confidence.

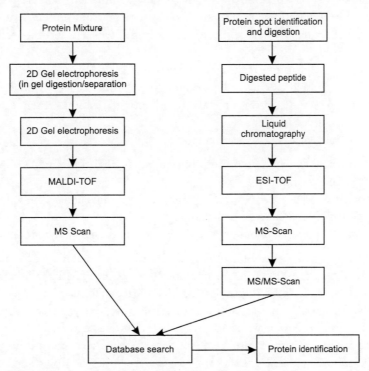

Fig. 3.16 Schematics of two approaches for mass spectrometric based proteomic analysis: peptide mass mapping (or PMF) and peptide sequencing.

Peptide sequencing is done through the production of ions followed by fragmentation of ions by tandem MS (or by sequential MS experiments using an ion trap). Inside the mass spectrometer, gas molecules are made to collide with other gas molecules causing fragmentation of peptide bonds. The usual result of this process is to form two types of fragments: the n-terminus fragment, known as b-ions, and c-terminus fragments, known as y-ions (Figure 3.17).

As mentioned earlier, MALDI-TOF and ESI-TOF are the two common approaches for peptide fingerprinting and sequencing. Schematics for them are provided below (Figure 3.17).

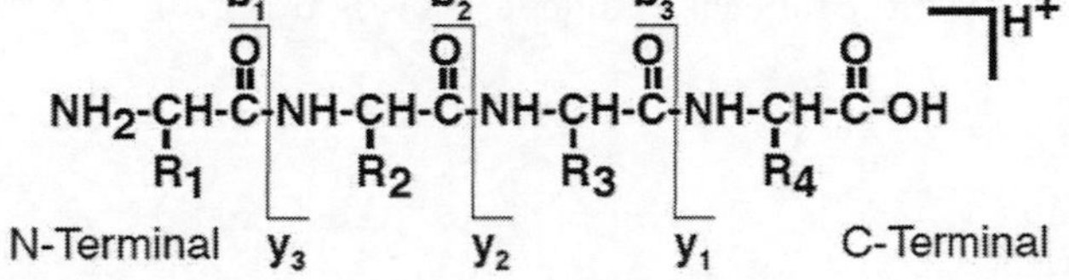

Fig. 3.17 A schematic diagram of fragmentation creating two fragments: N-terminal b-ions and C-terminal y-ions.

3.13   Mass Spectrometry

3.13.1   Introduction

Mass spectrometry (MS) is an immensely valuable technique, which is based on the principle that different gaseous ions (released from the sample under examination) will have differing mass-to-charge ratios. The applications of mass spectrometry range from protein structure, function, modification, global protein dynamics, proteomics, drug discovery, clinical testing, genomics, environment, and geology.

Mass spectrometry is a sensitive technique that was developed almost 100 years ago to measure elemental atomic weight and the natural abundance of specific isotopes. Initially MS was used in the biological samples to detect trace metals. In recent years, MS has extended applications in sequencing oligonucleotides and peptides.

The essential features of all mass spectrometers are:

- **The ion source:** Production of ions in the gas phase. A small amount of sample is ionized to cations by loss of electrons.
- **The mass analyzer:** The ions are sorted by using electric and magnetic field. Different masses are separated based on their mass and charge.
- **The detector:** The separated ions are then measured, and each analyte is detected.

The development of two ionization techniques: electrospray ionization (ESI) and atmospheric pressure chemical ionization (APCI), has revolutionized the utility of MS. Additionally, techniques like matrix-assisted laser desorption/ionization (MALDI) have enabled accurate mass determination of high-molecular-mass compounds as well as low-molecular mass molecules and expanded its utility to the biological molecules. New isotopic tagging added additional features for the quantification of target molecule both in relative and absolute quantities. All these developments have led to analysis of the samples in solid, liquid, and gas states.

Any material that is ionizable and when its ions can exist in gas phase can be investigated by MS. So in chemistry laboratories, well developed but simple MS or LC-MS (Liquid Chromatography-MS) find a wide range of application. However, for biomolecules, MS investigation of protein, nucleic acids and oligosaccharides require quadrupole ion trap mass analyzers. The aim of this section is to provide an overview of mass spectrometry and its efficacy in the analysis of biological samples. It will briefly cover the types of instrumentation, their main use, advantages/disadvantages, and their particular applications. Data analysis and sample preparation will also be covered.

Essential components

All mass spectrometers have the following components (Figure. 3.18):

(a) A vacuum system
(b) A sample system
(c) An ion source
(d) A mass filter/analyzer
(e) A detector

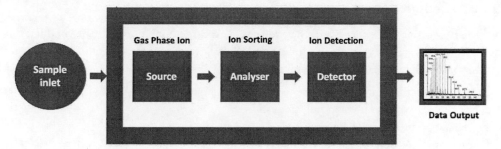

Fig. 3.18 Basic components of mass spectrometers. Sample inlet could be either direct probe or chromatographic system outlet. Source, analyzer and detector are placed under vacuum. Data output system consist of spectrum, computer and printer.

3.13.1.1 *Principles*

The first step of mass spectroscopic analysis is conversion of molecules into gas phase ions.

$$M + e^- \longrightarrow M^{\cdot+} + 2e^-$$

$M^{\cdot+}$ ions are called molecular ions. Ions that normally undergo fragmentation, are radical cations which break up into either even ions and radicals or odd ions and also neutral molecules. Each ion derived from a molecular ion can undergo further fragmentation on applying enough collision energy. All these ions are separated and detected based on their mass-to-charge ratio. A mass spectrum is a plot of relative abundance (number of ions, ion counts or relative intensity are other ways of representation) versus m/z.

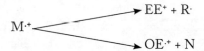

$EE^+, R^{\cdot}, OE^{\cdot+}$, and N represent an even ion, a radical, an odd ion, and neutral molecule, respectively.

The most intense peak is called the base peak and is arbitrarily assigned the relative abundance of 100%, being the base peak (Figure 3.19). The other peaks are given as percentages of the base peak.

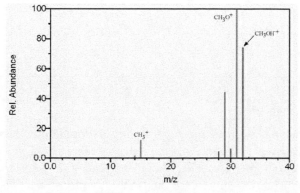

Fig. 3.19 Mass spectrum of methanol. CH_3OH^+ is the molecular ion and CH_3O^+ and CH_3^+ are other fragments.

3.13.1.2 *Vacuum System*

Ions are very reactive and short-lived; their formation and manipulation must be conducted in a vacuum. Operating under vacuum minimizes collisions between ions and air molecules. In mass spectrometery, a high level of vacuum assists in the following ways:

- By providing an adequate mean free path for the analyte ions
- By providing collision free ion trajectories
- By reducing ion-molecular reactions
- By reducing collisions of ions and air molecules
- By reducing background interference
- Facilitating target ions to reach the detectors

To get the required vacuum, the mass spectrometers have turbomolecular pumps, diffusion pumps, and rotary vane pumps. The required mean free path of the instrument is dictated by the distance travelled by analyte ions between the ion source and the detector.

According to the kinetic theory of gases, the mean free path L (in m) is given by

$$L = kT/\sqrt{2}\,p\sigma$$

> ### Pressure units
>
> **The official SI unit is the pascal.**
> 1 pascal (Pa) = 1 newton (N) per m^2
> 1 bar = 10^6 dyn cm^{-2} = 10^5 Pa
> 1 millibar (mbar) = 10^{-3} bar = 10^2 Pa
> 1 microbar (µbar) = 10^{-6} bar = 10^{-1} Pa
> 1 nanobar (nbar) = 10^{-9} bar = 10^{-4} Pa
> 1 atmosphere (atm) = 1.013 bar = 101 308 Pa
> 1 torr = 1 mmHg = 1.333 mbar = 133.3 Pa
> 1 psi = 1 pound per square inch = 0.07 atm

where, k is the Boltzmann constant, T is the temperature (in K), p is the pressure (in Pa) and σ is the collision cross-section (in m^2) = πd^2, where d is the sum of the radii of the stationary molecule.

The mean free path dictates the pressure required within the instrument. Mean free path and required pressure for various analyzer types are presented in the table below (Table 3.2).

Table 3.2 Mean free path and required pressure for various analyzer types.

Analyzer	Pressure (torr)	Mean Free Path
FTMS	$<10^{-8}$	5 km
Magnetic Sector	$<10^{-6}$	50 m
TOF	$<10^{-6}$	50 m
Quadrupole	$<10^{-4}$	50 cm
Ion Trap	$<10^{-4}$	50 cm

3.13.1.3 *Sample System*

Samples can be introduced to the mass spectrometer directly through a solid probe, or in the case of mixtures, by a chromatography device (e.g., gas chromatography, liquid chromatography, capillary electrophoresis). The selection of a sample inlet depends upon the sample matrix. Introduction of sample depends on the nature of sample. Gases and samples with high vapor pressure are introduced into the source directly. Liquids and solids are usually heated to increase their vapor pressure. If the analyte is thermally stable or if it does not have sufficient vapor pressure, then the sample must be directly ionized from the condensed phase. Different sample introduction systems are as follows:

Direct vapor inlet: It is the simplest sample introduction method which works well for gases, liquid, or solid with a high vapor pressure.

Gas chromatography: One of the most common techniques to introduce the samples into a mass spectrometer. Complex mixtures are routinely separated by gas chromatography and identified using mass spectrometer. Several different interface designs are used to connect these two instruments.

Liquid chromatography: This kind of inlet is used to introduce thermally labile compounds not easily separated by gas chromatography.

Direct insertion probe: This is used to introduce low vapor pressure liquids and solids into the mass spectrometer. The sample is loaded into a short capillary tube at the end of a heated sleeve. This sleeve is then inserted through a vacuum lock, so the sample is inside the source region. After the probe is positioned, the temperature of the capillary tube is increased to vaporize the sample. This probe is used at higher temperatures than are possible with a direct vapor inlet.

Direct ionization of sample: Unfortunately, some compounds either decompose when heated or have no significant vapor pressure. These samples may be introduced to the mass spectrometer by direct ionization from the condensed phase. These direct ionization techniques are used for liquid chromatography/mass spectrometry, glow discharge mass spectrometry, fast atom bombardment and laser ablation.

Direct infusion: This is the simplest form of mass spectrometry and involves pumping the analyte sample directly into the mass spectrometer. This method is compatible with mass spectrometers equipped with ESI to acquire molecular masses of the samples and their respective fragmentation pattern for qualitative analysis. The sample is injected using a syringe and a syringe pump facilitates the regular flow of liquid. This method is generally used for samples that are pure and not a complex matrix. It is most crucial that samples be free of contaminants as they may interfere with the measurements. Direct infusion is typically used for identification of small molecules or small proteins.

3.13.1.4 *Ion Source (Ionization)*

Ionization methods are mainly divided into two categories: (a) classical methods which include electron impact (EI) and fast atom bombardment (FAB), and (b) modern methods which include atmospheric pressure chemical ionization (APCI), electro-spray ionization (ESI), matrix assisted laser desorption ionization (MALDI) and other derivative methods. EI is mainly used in GC-MS, whereas APCI is more compatible with liquid chromatography (LC). FAB was popular earlier, but the technological development of ESI coupled with MALDI eliminated the use of FAB mainly because the former technique is more sensitive. In addition, MALDI along with ESI is very useful for the measurement of large molecular weight samples. ESI is also very compatible with LC.

(a) Electron Impact ionization (EI): EI is done by volatilizing a sample directly in the source that is contained in a vacuum system. A stream of electrons from a heated filament, bombard the gas phase ions of the sample. The most commonly used biased voltage is - 70 eV. Interaction of electrons with the analyte, results in either the loss (to produce a cation) or the capture of an electron (to produce an anion) (Figure 3.20). The disadvantage of this technique is the necessity for the analyte to be in vapor state which limits its applicability to biological molecules. However, this technique is useful in the analysis of metabolites, pollutants, and pharmaceutical compounds.

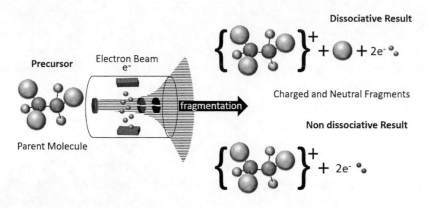

Fig. 3.20   Electron impact ionization interface.

In this technique, ionization results out of the loss of an electron which creates a molecule with a single unpaired electron. Therefore, this species is cation as well as radical and represented as $M^{\cdot+}$, where (·) stands for for radical and (+) sign indicates cation. Similarly, a negatively charge radical when formed is represented as $M^{\cdot-}$. Such radical ions are termed as parent ions, molecular ions or precursor ions. These molecular ions are very unstable and further disintegrate into a number of smaller fragment ions. When the precursor ion fragments, one of the fragments carries a charge and other the unpaired electron, i.e. it splits into a radical and an ion. The radical produced in the fragmentation process is a neutral species and does not take part in the mass spectrometry and is pumped away by the vacuum system. Only the charged species are directed towards the mass analyzer. It is customary to use dot outside the abbreviated bracket sign and IUPAC recommends use of the following notation: $M^{+\cdot}$ or $M^{-\cdot}$. While all possible bond breakages can occur, the distribution depends on the thermodynamic stability of the product formed. This whole process gives rise to several daughter ions, which will be recorded in the mass spectrum.

(b) Fast Atom Bombardment (FAB): This technique was very popular in the 80's and early 90's and revolutionized MS for biologists. In this technique the ions formed have low internal energy and very little fragmentation. This had an advantage for the biologists because they did not require prior derivatization of biomolecules in solution. In this technique, the sample is mixed with a relatively involatile and viscous matix, such as glycerol, nitro glycerol, 3 nitro-benzoic acid, and m-nitro benzoyl alcohol. This sample is placed in the source and bombarded in a vacuum with a beam of neutral atoms of high velocity, typically, Ar, He or Xe. Later developments included the use of cesium ions (Cs^{+}) and these were called liquid secondary ion mass spectrometers (LSIMS) or secondary ion mass spectrometers (SIMS). Pseudo molecular ions are formed in the process either by gaining a proton $[M + H]^{+}$ or loss of proton $[M - H]^{-}$. Other charge adducts can also be formed, such as $[M + Na]^{+}$, $[M+ K]^{+}$ and $[M+NH_{4}]^{+}$.

(c) Electrospray ionization (ESI): This is a soft ionization technique and very useful for biomolecules, such as protein and DNA. The process involves production of ions by forcing a liquid stream through a needle or capillary into a ionization source. A potential difference exists between the outlet of the sample stream and the inlet. Because of the applied voltage liquid inside the needle tries to retain more and more charge and becomes unstable. At the tip of needle, the droplet can assume a conical shape referred to as the *Taylor cone* which results in a fine jet with tiny and highly charged droplets. These charged droplets move in the space between the needle tip and the cone, causing solvent evaporation to occur, in turn causing these droplets to become smaller and smaller. The desolvation process is further assisted by the flow of carrier gas. As the solvent evaporation occurs, the droplets shrink until the point where the surface tension can no longer sustain the charge, known as the Rayleigh limit. At this point a Coulombic explosion occurs and the droplet is ripped apart producing even smaller droplets. The whole process is repeated until the ion passes through the cone to the vacuum region of the mass analyzer.

Both ESI negative- and positive-ion mass spectrometry can be used, and the principle of detection is essentially the same. However, positive-ion MS is more common.

(d) Chemical Ionization: Chemical ionization is a soft ionization technique that produces ions with little excess energy and yields a spectrum with less fragmentation. In chemical ionization the source is enclosed in a small cell with openings for the electron beam, the reagent gas and the sample. The reagent gas is added to this cell at approximately 10 Pa (0.1 torr) pressure. This is higher than the 10^{-3} Pa (10^{-5} torr) pressure typical for a mass spectrometer source. At 10^{-3} Pa the mean free path between collisions is approximately 2 meters and ion–molecule reactions are unlikely. In the CI source, however, the mean free path between collisions is only 10^{-4} meters and analyte molecules undergo many collisions with the reagent gas. The reagent gas in the CI source is ionized with an electron beam to produce a cloud of ions.

When analyte molecules (M) are introduced to a source region with this cloud of ions, the reagent gas ions donate a proton to the analyte molecule and produce MH^+ ions. The energetics of the proton transfer is controlled by using different reagent gases. The most common reagent gases are methane, isobutane, and ammonia. Methane is the strongest proton donor commonly used with a proton affinity (PA) of 5.7 eV. For softer ionization, isobutane (PA 8.5 eV) and ammonia (PA 9.0 eV) are frequently used. Acid base chemistry is frequently used to describe the chemical ionization reactions. The reagent gas must be a strong enough Brønsted acid to transfer a proton to the analyte. Fragmentation is minimized in CI by reducing the amount of excess energy produced by the reaction. Because the adduct ions have little excess energy and are relatively stable, CI is very useful for molecular mass determination.

The concentration of sample is usually around 1 – 10 pmol mm^{-3}. Typical solvents are 50/50 acetonitrile (or methanol/H_2O with 1% acetic acid or 0.1% formic acid, ammonium acetate, ammonium hydroxide or 0.02% trifluoroacetic acid. At basic pH, the carboxylic acid side chains as well as stronger anions such as phosphate and sulphate groups will be ionized.

(e) Atmospheric Pressure Chemical Ionization (APCI): Atmospheric pressure chemical ionization (APCI) is an ionization method, softer than standard chemical ionization. It is usually coupled with high performance liquid chromatography (HPLC) as it can work with higher flow rates and is used in mass spectrometry which utilizes ions in gaseous phase at atmospheric pressure. Since the ions are in the gaseous phase and not in liquid solution, the solvent need not be polar. This is an advantage of using APCI over ESI as it can ionize nonpolar or less polar molecules. Hence, APCI has been used in trace analysis of steroids, pesticides, drug metabolites pharmacology, and many such applications.

The APCI is composed of three parts as shown in Figure 3.21: a nebulizer probe which can be heated under pressure, an ionization region which is equipped with a corona discharge needle, and an ion-transfer region for an average (intermediate) pressure. The sample is dissolved in a suitable solvent and is introduced from a direct inlet probe or a LC column where the sample elutes and enters a pneumatic nebulizer. The nebulizer has a temperature of 350–500°C and with the flow of nitrogen gas the sample is converted into an aerosol. The sample aerosol in the solvent with the gas stream enters into the ionization region under atmospheric pressure, where the gaseous sample (A) and solvent (B) molecules are ionized at corona discharge. At this point, a highly charged electrode produces an electric field due to the applied potential of 2–3 kV resulting in fragmenting into radical cations through the removal of electrons from a neutral molecule. Since the solvent molecules are present in excess, they undergo the ionization in a similar way.

$$A + e^- \rightarrow A^{+\bullet} + 2e^-$$

$$B + e^- \rightarrow B^{+\bullet} + 2e^-$$

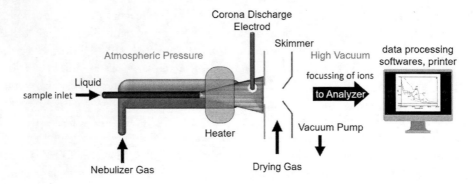

Fig. 3.21   The interface of APCI.

Due to the collisions between the ions and molecules, charge transfer takes place from an ion to other neutral molecules. The collision between solvent radial cation with a sample molecule can also result in a direct charge transfer to form a radical cation sample ion.

$$B^{+\bullet} + A \rightarrow A^{+\bullet} + B$$

Alternatively, a radical solvent cation can collide with a neutral solvent molecule resulting in abstraction of a hydrogen atom from the molecule. This resulting ionized solvent can further ionize the neutral sample molecules via proton transfer:

$$B^{+\bullet} + B \rightarrow [B+H]^+ + B[-H]$$

$$[B+H]^+ + A \rightarrow [A+H]^+ + B$$

The resulting sample ions, ($A^{+\bullet}$ or $[A+H]^+$) now pass through a skimmer into the ion-transfer region where they are transported into a mass analyzer for detection.

APCI utilizes high temperature and since the sample must be converted into gaseous phase, it is very important for the sample to be stable and volatile. Therefore, this method of ionization cannot be applied to analytes that are unstable or non-volatile and hence cannot be used for samples with molecular weight greater than 1500 Da.

(f) Matrix Assisted Laser Desorption/Ionization (MALDI): MALDI is a soft ionization technique in mass spectrometry in which the sample is ionized with minimal fragmentation using a laser energy absorbing matrix consisting of crystalized molecules. This method is similar in principle to electro-spray ionization (ESI) such that both techniques ionize large molecules in gaseous phase with minimal fragmentation. MALDI typically produces far fewer multi-charged ions when compared with ESI. It has been widely used in the analysis of fragile macromolecules like DNA, proteins, carbohydrates, polymers and such.

MALDI is conducted in three-steps as follows:

1. *Preparation of matrix solution*: The sample is mixed with a suitable matrix material which consists of crystallized molecules and applied to the metal plate. The commonly used matrix material is sinapinic acid, α-cyano-4-hydroxycinnamic acid, and 2,5-dihydroxybenzoic acid (DHB).
2. *Ablation and desorption*: A pulsed laser is used to irradiate the sample (in matrix) which triggers ablation and desorption of the sample and matrix material.
3. *Ionization*: The last step is ionization, where the sample molecules are ionized by protonation or deprotonation in the hot plume of the ablated gases and accelerated to mass analyzer for analysis.

Table 3.3   Summary of different ion sources.

Ion Source	Applications	Advantages	Disadvantages
EI	Pollutants, drug metabolites, organic molecules	High ionization efficiency and sensitivity	Analyte in vapor state only
FAB	Proteins, peptides, polar antibiotics, nucleotides	No derivatization of samples, thermally unstable, high sensitivity, low sample size	Cannot separate mixture of different volatility
ESI	Organometallics, bio-macromolecules, proteins and peptides	High molecular weight samples, multiple ionization modes, improved sensitivity and accuracy	Ion signal fluctuations
CI	Pesticides and organic compounds	Reduced fragmentation, lower energy than ESI	Cannot be used for thermally unstable and non-volatile samples, expensive
APCI	Steroids, pesticides, drug metabolites pharmacology	Accommodate higher flow rates, no signal overlap and improved resolution	Cannot be used for thermally unstable and non-volatile samples, molecular weight < 1500 Da
MALDI	Microbial identification	Rapid, better accuracy, fewer charged ions minimizing spectral complexity	Low analytical sensitivity

3.13.1.5 *Mass Analyzer*

A mass analyzer is an important component of the mass spectrometer and plays an important role in separating ions. The ions that are released from the ion source are sorted and separated based on their mass to charge ratio. General types of mass analyzers are as follows:

(a) Magnetic sector mass analyzer: An ion's mass to charge ratio is proportional to the degree of deflection when beamed through a magnetic field. Ions are accelerated in magnetic sector mass analyzer so that they have the same kinetic energy. All the ions are accelerated into a focused beam followed by deflection by the magnetic field according to the masses of ions. The lighter the ions, more is the deflection. The extent to which deflection occurs depends on the number of positive charges. The ions with the same degree of deflection will follow the same trajectory path.

(b) Time of flight (TOF): Time of flight measurements are used to determine an ion's mass to charge ratio as they travel through the flight tube. An electric field of known voltage is applied for acceleration of ions. Ions with equal charge will have the same kinetic energy. The ions separate based on velocity. The ions with higher mass have lower velocity than the ions with the lower mass. An increase in the charge will result in increased velocity. The time taken by an ion to reach the detector is measured. The time taken is inversely proportional to the velocity and hence is dependent on mass to charge ratio. A time of flight analyzer consists of four components: a pulsed ion source, an accelerating grid, a field-free flight tube, and a detector. The ion source needs to be pulsed so that ions with different m/z do not arrive at the detector at the same time. The ions with higher mass do not migrate at their ideal velocities. To overcome this problem, the end of the flight tube is equipped with a reflection assembly (reflectron) which consists of a series of ring electrodes with high voltage that causes reflection of ions in the opposite direction. For the ions of same m/z value, faster ions travel a greater distance than the slower ones in the reflectron. This results in the slow and fast ions of the same m/z value reaching the detector at the same time, making the bandwidth of output signal narrower .

Tandem time-of-flight (TOF/TOF) method employs two time-of-flight spectrometers back to back. TOF/TOF operates in MS mode to record full spectrum of the parent ions, also known as precursor ions. When operating in a tandem (MS/MS) mode, the laser energy is elevated considerably above the threshold of MALDI. The first TOF mass spectrometer uses a velocity filter and isolates precursor ions of the target and the second TOF-MS analyzes the fragment ions.

(c) Quadrupole: As the name suggests, quadrupoles consist of four parallel metal rods, the opposite pairs of which are connected together electrically. To one pair of rods is applied a radio frequency (RF) voltage, while the other pair is given a direct current (DC) voltage. At a selected DC and RF, only the ions of a particular m/z show a stable trajectory and can reach the detector, while other ions with unstable trajectories do not, because the amplitude of their oscillation becomes infinite. By changing the DC and RF ratio in steps for given intervals of time, ions with different m/z values can be transmitted to the detector in sequence.

3.13.1.6 *Applications*

The major application of mass spectrometry is for qualitative analysis. It has however, expanded its scope for quantitative analysis with tandem quadrupole mass spectrometry that offers greater reliability and performance.

Drug development

Mass spectrometry is frequently used to confirm the molecular mass and structure elucidation. Hence, it is widely used in drug development. Its ability to identify small molecules speeds up the process of generating, testing, and validating a drug discovery starting from a vast array of products with potential application. The technique is used for peptide mapping, bio affinity screening, purity analysis, presence of metabolites in the samples, quality control, in vivo drug screening, and much more.

Tandem mass spectrometry is extensively used in the analysis of natural food such as anthocyanins and flavonoid determination from blueberries. Similar analysis can open the path towards novel drug discovery based on health benefits of food, through analysis of secondary metabolites.

Pharmacokinetics

Pharmacokinetic study is very crucial and plays an important role in understanding drug absorption and time required for the drug to dissipate from body organs and hepatic blood flow. MS analyzers are useful in these studies because they have shorter analysis times, couple with higher sensitivity and specificity. Tandem MS-MS can help detect the metabolites through examination of fragmentation patterns as it can be programmed to fragment specific ions.

MS and Proteomics

Mass spectrometry is used in proteomics as a method for qualitative and quantitative analysis of the components of a complex biological sample like blood serum that contains thousands of proteins. The analysis of protein can be done in three ways: top down proteomics in which an intact protein is introduced into the mass analyzer, bottom-up proteomics in which the protein is digested into smaller peptides and subsequently introduced into the mass analyzer, and shotgun proteomics in which proteins in a mixture are digested and then processed for analysis. The process is depicted in Figure 3.22.

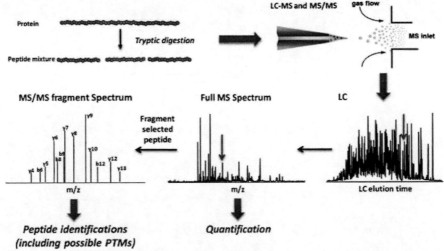

Fig. 3.22 Process of application of LC-MS/MS in proteomics (Adopted from Xie et al., 2011).

3.13.1.7 *Identification and Sequence Determination of Peptides and Proteins*

For structure determination, the first step is to conduct fragmentation of sample molecules and produce stable ions. For producing stable ions and subsequent fragmentation as well, the most common method is collision-induced dissociation (CID). Therefore, CID with tandem mass spectrometry (MS/MS) is an important technique for the sequence determination of peptides and proteins. In CID, ions obtain high kinetic energy and collide with neutral molecules. Some of the kinetic energy is converted into internal energy which leads to bond breakage and fragmentation of molecular ions into smaller pieces. The tandem mass spectra can then be obtained by sector, reflection TOF, triple quadrupole, MALDI-TOF PSD (post source decay). The major difference in all these techniques is in the kinetic energy of the ions, which ranges from a few electron volts (ev) to several kilo electron volts. Recently developed techniques, such as electron capture dissociation (ECD), electron transfer dissociation (ETD), and infrared multiphoton dissociation (IRMPD) have also been in use in place of CID.

For protein sequencing, mass spectrometry is performed in positive ion mode. The type of fragmentation employed depends on amino acid composition and sequence, amount of internal energy, ion activation method, and other unspecific fragmentation of bonds. However, there are a few types of fragmentation of peptides which normally can be seen in peptide mass spectrum:

(1) The first type of ions are derived from the cleavage of one or two bonds in the peptide chains such as Cα-C, C-N, N-Cα or C-O bonds, which will then create six different ions. The first set of ions are formed when positive charge is on the N- terminal and labeled as **a**, **b** and **c** (Figure 3.23). The other set of ions, created when the positive charge is on C-terminal side, are labeled as **x**, **y** and **z** (also Figure 3.23).

Mass of a – ions = [N] + [M] -CHO

Mass of b – ions = [N] + [M] - H

Mass of c – ions = [N] + [M] + NH_2

Mass of x – ions = [C] + [M] + CO-H

Mass of y – ions = [C] + [M] + H

Mass of z – ions = [C] + [M] – NH_2

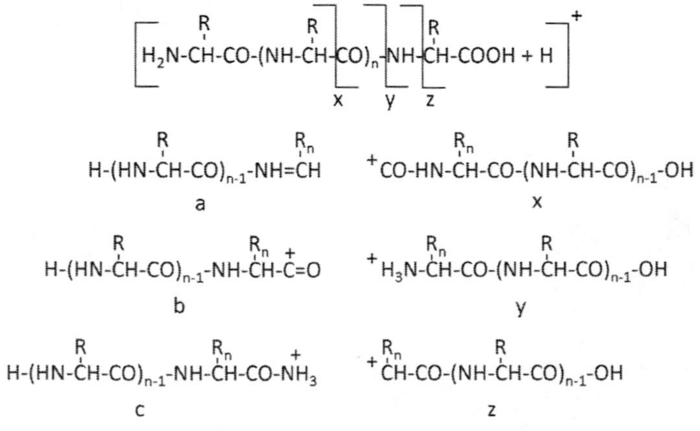

Fig. 3.23 Fragmentation of peptide: a, b, c, x, y, and z – ions.

where, [N] is the molecular mass of the neutral N-terminal group, [C] is the molecular mass of the neutral C-terminal group, and [M] is molecular mass of the neutral *amino acid residues*. Other ions are a-NH_3, a - H_2O, b-NH_3, b-H_2O, y-NH_3, and y-H_2O and represented as a*, a°, b*, b°, y* and b°, respectively.

The "a" ions are often used as a diagnostic for "b" ions, such as "a-b" spectra. The a-b pair is separated by 28 u in terms of atomic mass units.

(2) The second type of ions, are derived from the cleavage of the amino acid lateral chain. In addition to the ions described earlier, **d**, **v** and **w** are three other types of ions which can be observed in high-energy mass spectra (Figure 3.24); where,

Mass of d – ions = mass of a ion – partial side chain

Mass of v – ions = mass of y ion – complete side chain

Mass of w – ions = mass of z ion - partial side chain

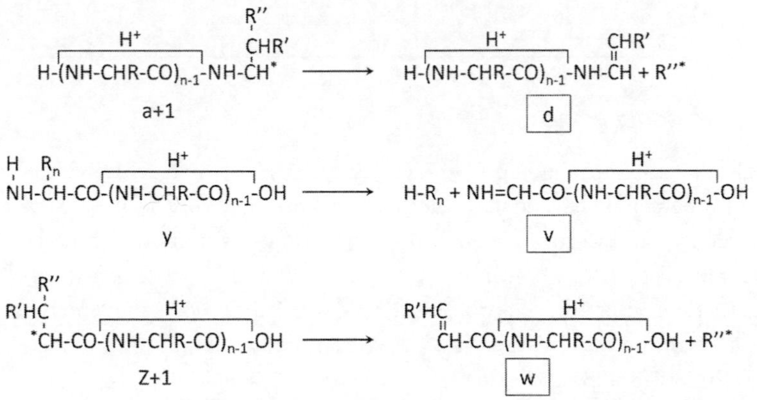

Fig. 3.24 Fragmentation into d, v, and w – ions.

The fragments are represented by "d", "v" or "w" according to the position of the positive charge. For d ions, positive charge is on the N-terminal and for w ions positive charge is on the C-terminal. These ions are created by cleavage of the bond between the β and γ carbon atoms of the side chain of the amino acids. They are useful in distinguishing between the isomers leucine and isoleucine. Amino acids, such as histidine, phenylalanine tryptophan and tyrosine, which have an aromatic group attached to the b-carbon atom do not display these fragments because of very low traces. V-type fragments result from the complete loss of the side chain. Amount of fractionation depends on the localization of the positive charge. If the positive charge is carried on the N-terminal side, it will increase the "a" and "d" fragments and outnumber "b" and "y" fragments. Similarly, if the positive charge is on the C-terminal side, it will increase the "v" and "w" fragments.

(3) Two other types of ions can also be formed due to cleavage of internal bonds in the peptide chain: immonium ions and internal fragments. Immonium ions result from multiple cleavage of the peptide chains and appear in the low mass part of the spectrum (Figure 3.25 and Table 3.4).

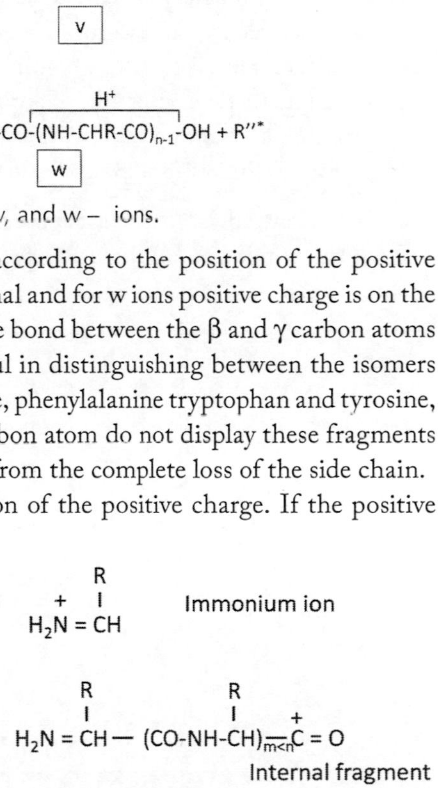

Fig. 3.25 Fragments derived from double cleavage of peptide main chain.

Table 3.4   Masses of most often found immonium ions.

Amino Acid	One Letter Symbol	Characteristic Mass in amu (u)
Proline	P	70
Valine	V	72
Leucine	L	86
Isoleucine	I	86
Methionine	M	104
Histidine	H	110
Phenylalanine	F	120
Tyrosine	Y	136
Tryptophan	W	159

Rules for de novo sequencing

The main goal of *de novo* sequencing is to identify the peaks which will give the mass difference between two fragment ions to calculate the mass of amino acid residue. For example, the mass difference between y1 and y2 ions is equal to 104 atomic mass units which is the mass of residue serine, S. Such a process can be continued until all the residues are determined. A few rules that are useful for the determination of amino acid residues and de novo sequencing are given below. Somatostatin, a 14 amino acid peptide, is used as example to explain the fragmentation of b and y ions (Figures 3.26, 3.27, 3.28, and 3.29).

(a) It is always advisable to start at the high mass end of the spectrum. The base peak is determined at the outset and all the other peaks show up conveniently as lower percentages, making it easier to start sequencing.

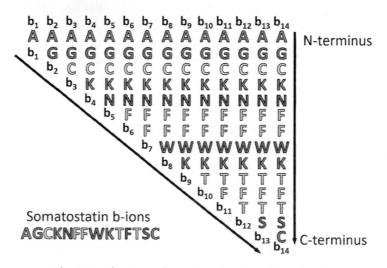

Fig. 3.26   b – ions of somatostatin. [See color plates]

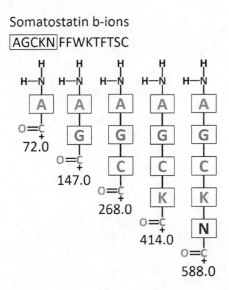

Fig. 3.27   Formation of b – ions. [See color plates]

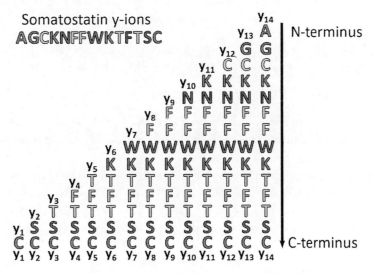

Fig. 3.28   y – ions of somatostatin. [See color plates]

(b) Once you know the mass of a *b* or *y* ion the corresponding mass of *b* or *y* molecules can be calculated as follows:

$y = (M + H)^{1+} - b \text{ ion} + 1$

$b = (M + H)^{1+} - y \text{ ion} + 1$

(c) *b*-ion intensity will drop when the next residue is proline (P), and similarly drop further (progressing to) glycine (G), histidine (H), lysine (K) and arginine (R).

(d) Take the example of CSGIPILQKN. This may display PILQKN, PILQN, PILQ, etc., due to internal fragmentation. Therefore, if the P of H residues in the sequence, internal fragmentation can occur. This can be detected by the intensity of y ions which will be the most prominent

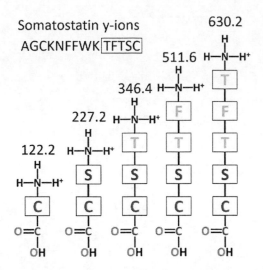

Fig. 3.29 Formation of y – ions of somatostatin. [See color plates]

peak in the spectrum. However, in case of proline in the sequence, it is possible that *b* and *y* ions or *y* and *b* ions may swap their intensity. Sometimes, this phenomena may also occur when basic residues such as H, K or R are present in the sequence.

(e) If *y* and *b* - ion fragments contain the amino acid residues arginine (R), lysine (K), glutamine (Q), and asparagine (N), the original molecule may appear to lose NH_3 (-17 atomic mass units). When cleavage happens before or after arginine (R) the loss of -17 mass units is more prominent than the corresponding *y* or *b* ion.

(f) If *y* and *b* - ion fragments contain the amino acid residues serine (S), threonine (T), and glutamic acid (E) the original molecule may appear to lose water, -18 atomic mass units. *Note*: E must be at the N-terminus of the fragment.

(g) The ion series can die out, when encountering aspartic acid (D) in a sequence.

(h) Presence of immonium ions can provide clues about the amino acid composition of a peptide.

(i) In case of isobaric masses, q-TOF mass spectrometer is often capable of higher mass accuracy and resolution. Lower mass accuracy can be dealt through conducting additionals reaction, such as acetylation, to shift the mass.

(j) Tables 3.5, 3.6, and 3.7 will be useful for determining fragmentation of peptide.

Table 3.5 Common amino acids and their monomeric mass units.

Amino Acid	Symbol	Monomeric Mass Units
Glycine (Gly)	G	57.02146
Alanine (Ala)	A	71.037114
Serine (Ser)	S	87.032029
Proline (Pro)	P	97.052764
Valine (Val)	W	99.068414

Contd.

Table 3.5 *contd.*

Amino Acid	Symbol	Monomeric Mass Units
Threonine (Thr)	T	101.04768
Cystine (Cys)	C	103.00919
Leucine (Leu)	L	113.08406
Isoleucine (Ile)	I	113.08406
Asparagine (Asn)	N	114.04293
Aspartic Acid (Asp)	D	115.02694
Glutamine (Gln)	Q	128.05858
Lysine (Lys)	K	128.09496
Glutamic Acid (Glu)	E	129.04250
Methionine (Met)	M	131.04048
Histidine (His)	H	137.05891
Phenylalanine (Phe)	F	147.06841
Arginine (Arg)	R	156.10111
Tyrosine (Tyr)	Y	163.06333
Tryptophan (trp)	W	186.07931

Table 3.6 List of common conflicting masses encountered in the mass spectrometry of peptides and proteins.

Amino Acids (symbol)	Monomeric mass		Mass in amu (u)	Difference in Mass
V	99.068414	Acetyl-Gly	99.032034	0.03638
L	113.08406	Isoleucine	113.08406	0
L	113.08406	Acetyl-Ala	113.047684	0.036376
N	114.04293	Gly - Gly	114.04298	0.000002
Q	128.05858	Lys	128.09496	0.03638
Q	128.05858	Gly - Ala	128.058578	0.0000002
K	128.09496	Gly - Ala	128.058578	0.036382
E	129.04259	Acetyl - Ser	129.042599	0.000009
F	147.06841	Met sulfoxide	147.0354	0.033
R	156.10111	Val - Gly	156. 089878	0.011232
R	156.10111	Acetyl - Asn	156.0535	0.04761
Y	163.06333	Met Sulfone	163.0303	0.033
W	186.07931	Ala – Asp	186.064054	0.015256
W	186.07931	Ser – Val	186.100443	0.021133
W	186.07931	Gly – Glu	186.064054	0.015256

Table 3.7 Important chemicals that are used for fragmentation of peptide chains for mass spectrometry. X is any amino acid residue.

Reagent	Cleavage Site
Cyanogen bromide	Met – X
Hydroxylamine	Asn – Gly
Formic Acid	Asp – Pro
Phenyl isothiocyanate (Edman's)	Terminal amino group of peptide
2-Nitro-5-thiocyanobenzoate	X – Cys
Trypsin	Arg – X, Lys – X
Chymotrypsin	Tyr – X, Trp – X, Phe – X
Endoprotease V8	Glu – X, Asp – Y
Endoprotease Asp-N	X – Asp, X – Cys

In sequence determination, the following need careful attention:

(a) Incorrect assignment of b and y – ions must be checked for and corrected.
(b) It is possible some fragments are missing.
(c) Existence of other fragment ion type other than what has been described earlier.
(d) Existence of conflicting masses.
(e) The post-translational modifications on the residues may cause mass ambiguity.

General Protocol for De Novo Sequencing of Protein or Peptide

Example: Tryptic peptides. In this case look for the arginine (mass unit: 175) and lysine (mass unit: 147).

1. Identifying lysine and arginine will provide clues about C – terminal residue. Calculate the b ions by using the following formula.

   for Arginine $(M + H)^{1+} - 18 - 156$ = penultimate b ion
   for Lysine $(M + H)^{1+} - 18 - 128$ = penultimate b ion
   (General formula: protonated peptide - 18 - AA residue mass = penultimate b ion)

   To identify b – ion look for an ion at – 28 mass unit (– CHO, as given above). Also, loss of water and ammonia at –18 atomic mass unist and – 17 atomic mass units, respectively, will provide further pointers for such assignments. After determination of b – ion, find the corresponding y – ion by using

   $$y = (M + H)^{1+} - b + 1$$

   Or alternatively, use the following formulae if the y – ions are already identified:

   $$(M + H)^{1+} - y_1 + 1 = \text{penultimate b} - \text{ion.}$$

   Such exercises help in enhancing accuracy in assignments.
   This works for the low end of the spectrum, while ion trap instruments do not provide determination at the low ends of spectrum. Therefore both methods of calculation need to be conducted to confirm the peak.

2. Now look for the next b – ion and corresponding y – ion. It is possible you will not find a – ion every time. Continue finding b – ions till it is not possible to go any further to construct b – ion series.

   Meanwhile, continue calculating the corresponding y – ion series.
3. It is not always directly possible to get the b – ions accurately. Therefore, use the formula given below to calculate the y – ion first and derive the b – ion from it.

   $(M + H)^{1+}$ – AA = penultimate **y** ion

   The y – ion should be found between amino acids of 57 to 186 atomic mass units. Once a y – ion is found, then find the corresponding b – ion by calculating using the following formula,

   $b = (M + H)^{1+} - y + 1$

   After this follow the same protocol as in the case of b – ion series, and so on.
4. Carefully observe the data generated on isobaric residues, immonium ions and other relevant parameters.

References

Angel, T. E., Aryal, U. K., Hengel, et al. (2012). Mass spectrometry-based proteomics: existing capabilities and future directions. *Chemical Society Reviews*, 41(10), 3912–3928.

Bruins, A. P. (1991). Mass spectrometry with ion sources operating at atmospheric pressure. *Mass Spectrometry Reviews*, 10(1), 53–77.

Carmical, J. and Brown, S. (2016). The impact of phospholipids and phospholipid removal on bioanalytical method performance. *Biomedical Chromatography*, 30(5), 710–720.

Clarke, W., Molinaro, R. J., Bachmann, L. M., et al. (2014). Liquid chromatography-mass spectrometry methods; approved guideline. *Clinical and Laboratory Standards Institute (CLSI): C62-A*, 34(16), 1–62.

Cornish-Bowden, A. (2013). *Fundamentals of Enzyme Kinetics*. New Jersey: John Wiley & Sons.

Deng, G., Gu, R. F., Marmor, S., Fisher, S. L., Jahic, H. and Sanyal, G. (2004). Development of an LC–MS based enzyme activity assay for MurC: application to evaluation of inhibitors and kinetic analysis. *Journal of Pharmaceutical and Biomedical Analysis*, 35(4), 817–828.

Hoffman, E. D. and Stroobant, V. (2007). *Mass Spectrometry: Principles and Applications*. West Sussex: Wiley.

Gika, H. G., Theodoridis, G. A., Plumb, R. S. and Wilson, I. D. (2014). Current practice of liquid chromatography–mass spectrometry in metabolomics and metabonomics. *Journal of Pharmaceutical and Biomedical Analysis*, 87, 12–25.

Grace, M. H., Xiong, J., Esposito, D., Ehlenfeldt, M. and Lila, M. A. (2019). Simultaneous LC-MS quantification of anthocyanins and non-anthocyanin phenolics from blueberries with widely divergent profiles and biological activities. *Food Chemistry*, 277, 336–346.

Hardouin, J. (2007). Protein sequence information by matrix-assisted laser desorption/ionization in-source decay mass spectrometry. *Mass Spectrometry Reviews*, 26(5), 672–682.

Hwang, S. I., Lundgren, D. H., Mayya, V., et al. (2006). Systematic characterization of nuclear proteome during apoptosis: a quantitative proteomic study by differential extraction and stable isotope labeling. *Molecular & Cellular Proteomics*, 5(6), 1131–1145.

Jorge, T. F., Rodrigues, J. A., Caldana, C., et al. (2016). Mass spectrometry-based plant metabolomics: Metabolite responses to abiotic stress. *Mass Spectrometry Reviews*, 35(5), 620–649.

Lee, M. S. and Kerns, E. H. (1999). LC/MS applications in drug development. *Mass Spectrometry Reviews*, 18(3-4), 187–279.

Majors, R. E. (2012). Supported liquid extraction: the best-kept secret in sample preparation. *LC GC North America*, 30(8).

Mathews, K. C., Van Holde, K. E. and Ahern K. G. (2003) *Biochemistry* 3rd ed. Singapore: Pearson Education. pp 360–411.

Mørtz, E., O'Connor, P. B., Roepstorff, P., et al. (1996). Sequence tag identification of intact proteins by matching tanden mass spectral data against sequence data bases. *Proceedings of the National Academy of Sciences*, 93(16), 8264–8267.

Niessen, Wilfried. (2006). *Liquid Chromatography-Mass Spectrometry*. Boca Raton: CRC Press.

Polson, C., Sarkar, P., Incledon, B., Raguvaran, V. and Grant, R. (2003). Optimization of protein precipitation based upon effectiveness of protein removal and ionization effect in liquid chromatography–tandem mass spectrometry. *Journal of Chromatography B*, 785(2), 263–275.

Scientific Working Group for Forensic Toxicology. (2013). Scientific Working Group for Forensic Toxicology (SWGTOX) standard practices for method validation in forensic toxicology. *Journal of Analytical Toxicology*, 37(7), 452–474.

Segel, I. H. (1976). *Biochemical Calculations* 2nd ed. New York: John Wiley & Sons. pp. 214–272.

Stenesh, J. (1984). *Experimental Biochemistry* 1st ed. New Jersey: Prentice Hall. pp. 167–171.

Sudhakar, P., Latha, P. and Reddy, P. V. (2016). *Phenotyping Crop Plants for Physiological and Biochemical Traits*. Cambridge, Massachusetts: Academic Press.

Wysocki, V. H., Resing, K. A., Zhang, Q. and Cheng, G. (2005). Mass spectrometry of peptides and proteins. *Methods*, 35(3), 211–222.

Xie, F., Liu, T., Qian, W. J., Petyuk, V. A. and Smith, R. D. (2011). Liquid chromatography-mass spectrometry-based quantitative proteomics. *The Journal of Biological Chemistry*, 286(29), 25443–25449.

Zhang, J. H., Roddy, T. P., Ho, P. I., et al. (2010). Assay development and screening of human DGAT1 inhibitors with an LC/MS-based assay: application of mass spectrometry for large-scale primary screening. *Journal of Biomolecular Screening*, 15(6), 695–702.

4

Bioanalytical Techniques

4.1 Introduction

Protein Science is the study of protein molecules by researchers from varied fields of science, including chemistry, physics, mathematics, and biology. The primary interest of such research is on the structure, function, design, and possible applications of protein molecules. Proteins are considered a part of family called biological macromolecules and before broaching their molecular structure, clarity about the definition of molecule is essential. Defining a molecule in biochemistry is a little different than in general chemistry. In general chemistry, a molecule normally comprises of two or more atoms bonded covalently in specific stoichiometry and defined geometry. For example, ethane, C_2H_6 has well defined stoichiometry and defined geometry. But this is not the case with the chiral molecule or cis-trans isomers of biochemistry.

In biochemistry, molecules are considered as components which may or may not be bonded together covalently in all parts. Local and non-local interactions play important roles in their structures. For example in a protein molecule there are several weak interactions taking place in the functional structure of that protein, apart from covalent bonds. Also in a complex protein, non-covalent interactions play roles in the very assembling of the constituent molecules. Take the case of apoptosomes and proteosomes. The geometry of biological molecules are unique 3-D arrangements of its components. There are various levels of structural organization of such biological macromolecules. These levels of complexity, in them, are described below:

Four degrees of structure

(a) Monomers are simple building blocks of macromolecules; and include sugars, amino acids and nucleotides.
(b) Primary structure (1°) is the linear rearrangement of residues in the covalently linked polymers.
(c) Secondary structure (2°) is a local regular structure, such as a-helix, b-sheets.
(d) Tertiary structure (3°) is a global 3-D fold or topology, such as native structure of protein.
(e) Quaternary structure (4°) is spatial arrangement of multiple distinct polymers, such as hemoglobin and proteosomes.

Biochemists devoted considerable effort over a very long time, employing a variety of biochemical techniques in order to understand the relationship between structure and function of biomolecules.

The current focus in life sciences is on learning more about proteomes with emphasis on the study of individual structures of biomolecules in order to understand their role in cellular functions. The tens of thousands of biomolecules encountered in living cells are mainly in two general groups. The first group characterized by high molecular weight, such as protein and DNA, is generally unstable in extreme chemical conditions (by either losing their structure or degradation into building blocks). The second group consists of low molecular weight molecules, which are more robust chemically, such as lipids, and fatty acids. Both these groups display wide ranging disparity in terms of water solubility, chemical composition, and reactivity.

4.1.1 Requirements for Structure and Function of Biomolecules and Affecting Factors

Biomolecules share certain common attributes as regards their structures and functions. The first and most obvious one is that these molecules are produced and degraded inside the cell under mild and regulated environment: of pH, temperature, polarity, and pressure. There are two effects as a result of variation in these chemical conditions. Structural effects take place often accompanied by irreversible changes in the molecule (protein denaturation, hydrolysis of covalent bonds). Functional effects are more subtle and may be reversible (protonation/deprotonation, partial unfolding). Techniques described in Tables 4.1 and 4.2 are some of the available ways to monitor how environmental changes affect structural/ functional attributes of biomolecules.

Table 4.1 Important physical attributes of biomolecules and connected biophysical techniques to study them.

Physical Attributes	Biophysical Techniques
Mass	MS, electrophoresis, gel filtrations, light scattering
Volume/density	Gel filtration, centrifugation, light scattering, spectroscopy
Charge	Ion-exchange chromatography, IEF, MS
Shape	Centrifugation, crystallization, electrophoresis, light scattering, spectroscopy
Energy	Spectroscopy, calorimetry

Table 4.2 Important chemical attributes of biomolecules and connected biophysical techniques to study them.

Chemical Attributes	Biophysical Techniques
Composition	MS, spectroscopy, chemical reactions
Molecular structure	Crystallization, spectroscopy
Covalent bonds	Bioinformatics, MS
Noncovalent bonds	Electrophoresis, chromatography
Native/Denatured structure	Spectroscopy
Complex formation/ interactions	Chromatography, spectroscopy, crystallography

4.2   Hydrodynamic Methods

There is no doubt about the importance of water as a biological solvent. Most of the interactions of biomolecules occur due to the presence of water molecules. Their structures and functions are greatly influenced by flow interaction arising from their hydrodynamic properties. These properties arise from various physical interactions that occur between molecules and water/solvent molecules. Centrifugation is the main technique for exploiting hydrodynamic properties to study biomolecules.

The solution is always more viscous than the solvent (alone) and primarily depends on the concentration, shape, and mass of the molecule. The molecular effect of viscosity is due to intermolecular interactions within the solution (Van der Waals, hydrogen bonds, electrostatic interactions, and such), and partly on the overall size and shape of solute and solvent molecules. By definition, viscosity is the friction of a stationary surface with flowing fluid. If the fluid is moving at *velocity v* in a container, then that part of this fluid around the center of the container is moving at this velocity **v**, while the velocity of fluid next to the stationary surface is close to zero. The next layer has a slightly higher velocity, and so on, giving rise to a velocity gradient, until **v** is achieved in the center. Newton demonstrated that the shear force, f, between layers of liquid is proportional to both the areas of the layers and the velocity gradient between them, thus

$$f \propto A. \, dy/dx \qquad \text{(Eq. 4.1)}$$

$$f = \eta . A . dy/dx \qquad \text{(Eq. 4.2)}$$

where, η is constant of proportionality known as viscosity.

Viscosity measurements are performed by measuring the time taken for a solution of volume **V**, of a particle, dissolved in solvent of viscosity η_0 to flow through a narrow capillary tube of radius r and length L, under hydrostatic pressure. The most popular instrument is the Ostwald Viscometer (Figure 4.1). The viscosity of a sample solution, η, is given by

$$\eta = \pi . h . g . \rho . r^4 . t/8Lv \qquad \text{(Eq. 4.3)}$$

where, h is the average liquid height, g the gravitational constant, t is time taken by solution of volume **V** to flow through the capillary and ρ is the density of the solution.

Since viscosity measurements of the solvent alone (η_0) and of various concentration of the particle (η) are carried out under identical experimental conditions

$$\eta/\eta_0 = t.\rho/t_0.\rho_0 \qquad \text{(Eq. 4.4)}$$

Thus, prior knowledge of the density of the solutions is required in this method.

Establishing the relationship between viscosity, η, and molecular mass and shape is complex. Generally the larger the molecule and more extended its shape, the greater is the

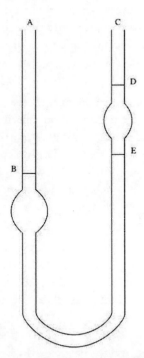

Fig. 4.1   Ostwald viscometer. Solution is added at opening A till the meniscus of B. Suction is applied so that solution reaches point D. The time required for meniscus of solution at D to reach the meniscus at point E is measured.

value of η. An important factor in overall shape is the axial ratio, i.e., the ratio of longest to shortest axis of the molecules.

Fibrous molecules have larger axial ratios than globular molecules of the same mass and therefore produce more viscous solutions. For double-stranded DNA the relationship between mass and η has been empirically determined as

$$\log(\eta + 5) = 0.665.\ \log M - 2.863 \qquad \text{(Eq. 4.5)}$$

While for random coil proteins of n residues dissolved in 6N guanidinium hydrochloride it is.

$$\eta = 0.716.\ n^{0.66} \qquad \text{(Eq. 4.6)}$$

The change in viscosity can be used to follow the processes.

4.2.1 Sedimentation

When particles are forced through a solution they resist movement. The quantum of resistance depends on specific properties of the particles and those of the solvent. A commonly used sedimentation technique is centrifugation. This can not only be used to separate complex mixtures but is a very valuable tool for determining mass, shape, or density of particles.

As a particle passes through the solvent it experiences a resistance due to a frictional force F, in this case centrifugal force, operating in the opposite direction

$$F = f.\ v \qquad \text{(Eq. 4.7)}$$

where, f a frictional coefficient depends on the shape and mass of the particle and the viscosity of the solvent, and v is the velocity of the particle.

At the beginning of centrifugation, the particle accelerates through the solvent, until the frictional force (constantly increasing with increase in velocity) balances with the centrifugal force being applied and so halts this acceleration. At this point, a constant velocity called sedimentation velocity is achieved. The sedimentation velocity is given by

$$v_{sed} = m_0.\ (1 - Y.\ \rho).\ \omega^2.\ r\ /\ f \qquad \text{(Eq. 4.8)}$$

where, m_o is the mass of the particle, Y is the partial specific volume, ρ is the density of solvent, ω is the angular velocity of rotation, r is the radius, and f is the frictional coefficient (depends on the mass and shape of the particle, and viscosity of the solvent).

Sedimentation velocity depends on the shape of particle, but for a perfect sphere

$$v_{sed} = d^2.\ [\rho_p - \rho_m].\ \omega^2.\ r\ /\ 18\eta \qquad \text{(Eq. 4.9)}$$

where, d is the particle diameter, ρ_p and ρ_m are the density of particle and solvent, respectively, and η is the viscosity of solvent.

It is difficult to determine v_{sed}, ρ, and f accurately so a useful measure of differential behavior of different particle in a centrifugal field is provided by the sedimentation coefficient, s:

$$s = v_{sed}/\omega^2.\ r = m_0.\ (1 - Y.\ \rho)/f \qquad \text{(Eq. 4.10)}$$

Since both $m_0.(1-Y.\rho)$ and f are inherent properties of the particle and solvent, respectively, s is a constant for any given particle/solvent. The spread of values observed in biomolecules range from 1×10^{-13} s for a protein to 10000×10^{-13} s for intercellular organelles. A more widely used notation is provided by Svedberg, S, with $1S = 1 \times 10^{-13}$s. Examples: cytochrome c (1S), ribosomes (~70S), tobacco mosaic virus (~400S) or lysosomes (10000S). Although there is no linear relationship between sedimentation coefficient and molecular mass, nonetheless it is useful as indicator of relative size.

Sedimentation or centrifugation is performed in a device called centrifuge. Generally, for biological samples a high speed centrifuge is used. These centrifuges include a rotor chamber into which the sample is inserted. Rotors are mainly of two kinds: fixed angle rotors and swinging bucket rotors. Because rotor design varies between manufacturers and radial distance can also differ widely, it is often convenient to express centrifugal force as a value relative to that of the Earth's gravitational field called the relative centrifugal force, g:

$$g = 1.119 \times 10^{-5}.(rpm)^2.r \qquad \text{(Eq. 4.11)}$$

The most common centrifuge is the bench top centrifuge, which can provide up to 6000 g. While low volume bench-top centrifuges (minifuge) can achieve relative centrifugal force up to 12,000 g, ultracentrifuges can deliver relative centrifugal forces of 150,000 g.

4.2.2 Use of Sedimentation or Centrifugation Techniques

(a) Fractionation of subcellular organelles

Individual subcellular organelles of eukaryotic cells may be regarded as individual types of particles with characteristic ranges of mass and density. Centrifugation of cell homogenates, therefore, allows preparation of highly-purified fractions enriched in one or other cell compartment such as the nucleus, endoplasmic reticulum or mitochondria in a process called subcellular fractionation (Figure 4.2).

(b) Density gradient centrifugation

Sedimentation velocity depends on solvent and particle density. This dependence can be used to create a density gradient to achieve separation of different particles from complex biological samples. This is achieved by establishing a density gradient between a region of high density at the bottom and a region of low density at the top. The density

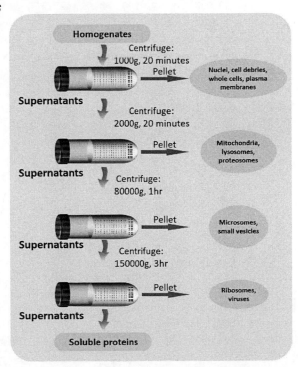

Fig. 4.2 Subcellular fractionation.

gradient can be established either before particle centrifugation (zonal centrifugation) or during centrifugation (isopycnic centrifugation).

The zonal centrifugation experiment involves creation of a density gradient before centrifugation by mixing high and low density solutions of materials such as sucrose and glycerol. This gradient is created in a centrifuge tube prior to centrifugation and the sample is then layered on top. As velocity gradually decreases along the gradient, particles begin to sediment out. Because different particles have different densities, they sediment out at different rates and separate out at different points from the sample mixture.

In isopycnic centrifugation, the metal salt CsCl is used because it is highly dense (1.8 g/ml). A solution of CsCl is mixed with the sample and then centrifuged forming a CsCl density gradient from low density, at the top of the centrifuged tube, to high density, at the bottom. Sample particles in the region of highest density at the bottom of the tube are less dense than the surrounding medium. Therefore they tend to float towards the top of the tube to a region of lower density. Conversely, some of the same types of particle in the region of lowest density at the top of the tube will sediment towards the bottom of the tube. Eventually each type of particle gets concentrated in a narrow band specific to its isopycnic density. Material such as ficoll and percol are particularly useful for separation of individual organelles or cell types by density gradient centrifugation since they do not subject particles of the sample to high osmotic pressure or shear forces.

(c) Analytical Ultracentrifugation

It is also possible to combine analysis with the process of sedimentation and to learn about many physical properties of particles from analysis of their dynamic behavior under centrifugal forces. This is known as analytical ultracentrifugation and it offers the advantage of making it possible to study the behavior of bio-macromolecules under a wide range of solvent conditions.

4.3   Biocalorimetry

Biological samples can be extremely heat sensitive and function in a narrow range of temperatures. Heat is an important factor in depicting chemical equations in terms of thermodynamic parameters. Analysis of such thermodynamic parameters helps us understand the flow of energy within the system. One of the popular instruments to measure the flow of heat is the calorimeter. Biocalorimetry is the term for using calorimetric measurement to study the interactions and properties of biomolecules and there are three important methods to study it.

(a) Iso-thermal Calorimetry

Biocalorimetry allows direct measurements of enthalpy changes. Iso-thermal calorimetry (ITC) is be used to directly measure changes in enthalpy (ΔH) associated with processes such as ligand binding and complex formation.

A typical experiment involves measurement of enthalpy (heat) change as a function of addition of small quantities of a reagent (ligand) to the calorimetry cells containing other components (enzyme) of the system under investigation. At the beginning of the experiment, there is a large excess of enzyme compared to the ligand. This allows ΔH tobe individually measured (because it is correspondingly large as well). As aliquots of reagents are progressively added, ΔH values drop because of dilution of enzyme–ligand interactions. The ΔH is a measure of total enthalpy change which includes heat associated with the process of enzyme–ligand interactions, conformational changes, ionization of polar groups or changes in interaction with the solvents.

ITCs provide a useful method for studying binding processes such as those involving a protein (P) and ligand (L)

$$P + L \leftrightarrow PL$$

It allows estimation of, both, a binding (K_b) and a dissociation (K_d)constant

$$K_b = [PL]/[P][L] \qquad\qquad\qquad\qquad\qquad\qquad (Eq.\ 4.12)$$

and $\qquad\qquad\qquad K_d = [P][L]/[PL] \qquad\qquad\qquad\qquad\qquad\qquad (Eq.\ 4.13)$

K_d is related to Gibbs Free Energy or ΔG by

$$\Delta G = - RT \ln K_d \qquad\qquad\qquad\qquad\qquad\qquad (Eq.\ 4.14)$$

Further, ΔG is related to ΔH and ΔS

$$\Delta G = \Delta H - T\Delta S \qquad\qquad\qquad\qquad\qquad\qquad (Eq.\ 4.15)$$

So even if two ligands have similar values of K_d but quite different ΔH and ΔS values, ITC allows direct determination of ΔH; and therefore, helps identify detail differences in binding thermodynamics.

As mentioned, ITC measures the heat absorbed or released in any chemical reaction. A solution of the biomolecule under investigation is first placed in the sample cell and ligand solution in a similar buffer solution is placed in syringe (Figure 4.3A). When the ligand solution is injected into the cell, the ITC instrument detects heat that is released or absorbed as a result of interaction. Injections are performed repeatedly, and result in peaks that become smaller as the biomolecule solution becomes saturated. Eventually the peak sizes remain constant and represent only the heat of dilution (Figure 4.3B). Once titration is completed, the individual peaks are integrated by the instrument software and finally presented in the form of a Wiseman plot (Figure 4.3C). An appropriate binding model is chosen and the isotherm is fitted to yield the binding enthalpy, ΔH, the K_d, and the stoichiometry, n. From such data, Gibb's free energy, ΔG, and entropy, ΔS, are calculated.

ITC can also be used to determine the heat capacity. By definition heat capacity, or Cp, is the quantity of heat which will change the temperature of exactly 1 g of substance by 1°C. For low molecular mass reagents, Cp of reactants and products are not significantly different. However, for large molecules such as proteins, there may be significant changes due to change in conformation, exposure of hydrophobic residues and denaturation; Cp can vary. For example, when temperature is raised the rigidity is reduced in proteins, leading to large increase in Cp of the denatured state versus the native state. The variation in Cp due to enthalpy and entropy at two different temperatures T_1 and T_2 is given by the following equation:

$$\Delta Cp = \Delta H_{T2} - \Delta H_{T1}/(T_2 - T_1) = \Delta S_{T2} - \Delta S_{T1} / \ln (T_2/T_1) \qquad (Eq.\ 4.16)$$

Plot of ΔH versus temperature gives a slope corresponding to ΔCp.

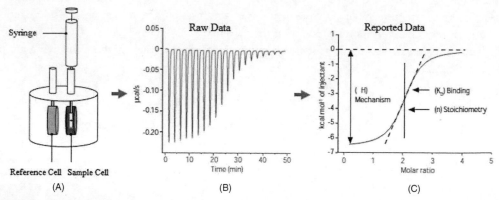

Fig. 4.3 Isothermal calorimetry. (A) A model of ITC instrument, (B) Raw data of titration, and (C) Wiseman plot.

(b) Differential Scanning Calorimetry (DSC)

DSC is another method of biocalorimetry experimentation that involves measurement of changes in Cp as a function of change in temperature. This technique is especially sensitive to phase changes in biopolymers arising during phenomenon such as protein–protein binding, protein unfolding, and ligand binding. A typical DSC signal is shown in Figure 4.4. The area under the curve is the ΔH which is a function of the melting temperature (T_m) and ΔCp. These thermodynamic parameters ideally should show no dependence on either scan rate or sample concentration. In general, any process involving a temperature-induced change of phase in a bio-macromolecule is amenable to study by DSC. It is possible to vary the experimental conditions used such as pH, ion strength, or including denaturing and stabilizing molecules (Figure 4.5). Moreover, comparison of mutant and wild type protein allows estimation of the contribution of a single amino acid. This technique can be used on DNA, polysaccharides, and other biopolymers.

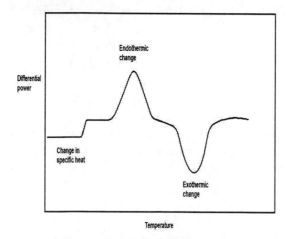

Fig. 4.4 Typical DSC thermogram.

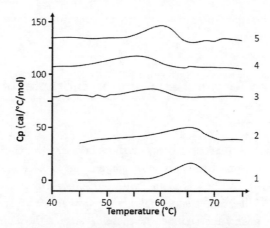

Fig. 4.5 DSC heating curves for the thermal denaturation of GLUT-1. *Curve 1*, no addition; *curve 2*, in the presence of 0.4 M NaCl; *curve 3*, in the presence of 4.8 mM ATP and 0.4 M NaCl; *curve 4*, in the presence of 4.8 mM ATP; *curve 5*, in the presence of 4.8 mM ATP and 500 mM D-glucose (Adopted from Epand et al., 2001, Protein Science, 10, 1363).

(c) Determination of thermodynamic parameters by non-calorimetric means

Heat content of a biomolecular system is largely defined by two factors:

1. The exponential effect of temperature as described by Arrhenius equation

$$k = Ae^{-Ea/RT} \qquad \text{(Eq. 4.17)}$$

This basically means that rates of reaction increase exponentially with temperature.

2. The conformational changes of biomolecules are associated with temperature fluctuation.

If we determine the rate of any reaction at different temperatures, then plot ln k versus 1/T should produce a straight line with slope −Ea/R (Arrhenius plot; Figure 4.6).

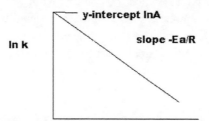

Fig. 4.6 Arrhenius plot.

For any chemical reaction the equilibrium constant, K_{eq}, is simply the ratio of concentration of product and concentration of reactant. These values are related to enthalpy changes of the reaction by the van't Hoff equation:

$$d(\ln K_{eq})/dT = \Delta H/RT^2 \qquad \text{(Eq. 4.18)}$$

van't Hoff and Arrhenius equations provide means for determination of useful parameters without using any calorimetric methods.

4.4   Spectroscopic Techniques Used on Biomolecules

4.4.1   Basis and Purpose

The fundamental basis of molecular spectroscopy is the energy involved in the formation of chemical bonds between two atoms. Upon bond formation some energy is lost, stabilizing the bond. That lower energy of the molecule can be augmented with light, resulting in a higher energy state or in the breaking of the bond. The former is generally referred to as spectroscopy whereas the latter is considered to be photochemistry as it changes the chemical state of the molecule. Photochemistry is used to modify molecules, create reactions with other compounds, and understand the mechanism of action in biological systems. Spectroscopy, on the other hand, is extensively used to examine the structure–function relationship, test purity, develop detection methods, and assay chemical reactions.

To understand the chemical nature of molecular spectroscopy, one needs to establish familiarity with basic concepts of molecular orbital theory. According to this theory, molecular orbitals (MO) are linear combinations of atomic orbitals (LCAO). LCAO implies that the MOs are results of addition and subtraction of atomic orbitals, which result in bonding and antibonding orbitals. Thus the number of MOs, continue to remain equal to the number of AOs that were originally involved in forming the MOs.

4.4.2   Sigma (s) and Pi (p) Orbitals and Bonds

s MOs are formed through two overlapping atomic orbitals along an internuclear axis and are cylindrical in symmetry. Consider two hydrogen atoms combining to form a hydrogen molecule. The linear combination of atomic orbitals of Atom A ($1s_A$) and Atom B ($1s_B$) yields two MOs as shown in Figure 4.7. The s orbital is called the bonding MO, which is formed by the addition of two 1s atomic orbitals. The antibonding MO, s*, is also formed by the same atomic orbitals but with a combination of orbitals in opposite (negative) symmetry. The process is also referred to as subtraction of the two atomic orbitals, in contrast to addition ($1s_A + 1s_B$) of orbitals in s MO. The symbols of g (gerade) and u (ungerade) stand for wavefunctions which are symmetric and asymmetric, respectively, with reference to the center of the molecule.

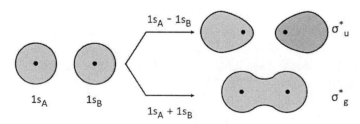

Fig. 4.7   Schematics of *s bonding* and antibonding molecular orbital formation from a pair of 1s orbitals (A and B). Solid points represent the positions of nuclei in the atomic orbitals.

The s_g molecular orbital, if occupied, is in a low energy state as a stable MO. The s^*_u MO, formed from negative overlap of the two atomic orbitals in a molecule, is an unstable state. In a ground state hydrogen (H_2) molecule, s_g MO is occupied by a pair of electrons. Similar to s and s orbital overlap, it is also possible to form MOs by overlapping between s and p atomic orbitals, and p and p orbitals, as shown in Figure 4.8.

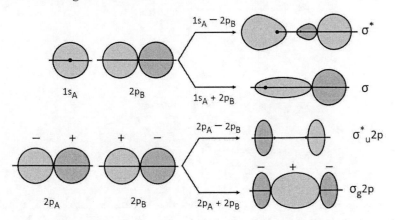

Fig. 4.8 Schematics of *s bonding* and antibonding molecular orbital formation from a pair of *s* and *p* orbitals or a pair of *p* orbitals (A and B). Solid points represent the positions of nuclei in the *s* atomic orbitals, and nodal points represent positions of nuclei in *p* orbitals.

In contrast to the s MOs where the s and/or p atomic orbitals overlap head on against each other, when the p orbitals combine by overlapping laterally, a p bonding MO and a p* antibonding MO is formed (Figure 4.9).

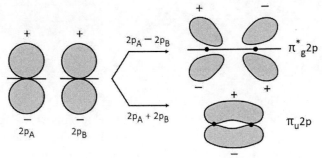

Fig. 4.9 Schematics of π *bonding* and antibonding molecular orbital formation from a pair of *p* orbitals (A and B).

In most biological systems both s and p bonds are involved. Thus both s and p bonds are formed from the linear combinations of 2s and 2p orbitals. Figure 4.10 summarizes the MOs of the homonuclear diatomic molecules (such as N_2) along with their energies. This diagram provides a fundamental concept for MO energy levels. Energies of bonding and antibonding MOs depend upon several factors, including types of atoms involved, geometric orientation of bonds, and the nature of surrounding atoms.

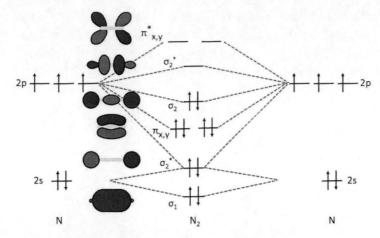

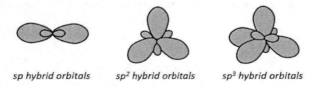

Fig. 4.10 Schematics of *s* and *p* *bonding* and antibonding molecular orbital formation from a pair of *s* and *s* orbitals, or a pair of *p* orbitals (A and B).

Biological systems are generally polyatomic molecules, having single, double, and tipple bonds. Such bonds involve the concept of *hybrid orbitals*. A linear combination of one 1s orbital and one p orbital forms two equivalent sp hybrid orbitals. A linear combination of one s orbital and two or three p orbitals form three equivalent sp² hybrid orbitals or four sp³ hybrid orbitals, respectively. A pair of sp orbitals has a linear structure. The sp² orbitals form a triangular planar. A set of sp³ hybrid orbitals has a structure of tetrahedron. Figure 4.11 shows the geometries of the hybrid orbitals.

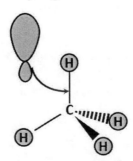

sp hybrid orbitals   *sp² hybrid orbitals*   *sp³ hybrid orbitals*

Fig. 4.11   Hybrid orbitals.

Overlap of hybrid orbitals of a given atom and atomic orbitals of other atoms form sMOs. For example, in CH_4 the 2s orbital and three 2p orbitals of C form four sp³ hybrid orbitals each of which is occupied by one electron. Thus, a CH_4 molecule consists of four s bonds each of which is formed by overlapping a sp³ hybrid orbital with hydrogen 1s orbital as in shown in Figure 4.12.

Fig. 4.12   *sp³* hybrid orbitals on C atom form an *s* bond each with 4 H 1*s* orbital in methane (CH_4).

A double bond consists of a s bond and a p bond. A triple bond consists of a s bond and two p bonds (Figure 4.13).

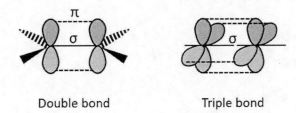

Double bond   **Triple bond**

Fig. 4.13 Double and triple bonds involving **s** and **p** bonds. The solid line represents **s** bond between 2 **p** orbitals, and the dotted lines represent the formation of **p** bonds from the overlapping of pairs of **p** orbitals.

Non-bonding (n) orbitals are the atomic orbitals in an atom which do not form molecular orbitals. For example, in a carbonyl (>C=O) group, the 2s orbital and two of the 2p orbitals in the O form three sp^2 hybrid orbitals. Two of these orbitals are filled and the third one which is occupied by one electron overlaps with a C sp^2 orbital to form a s bond (Figure 4.14). The remaining 2p orbital on O combines with one on C atom to form a p bond. The two filled sp^2 orbitals on the O atom are non-bonding.

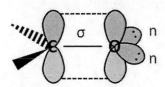

Fig. 4.14 Depiction of **s, p,** and **n** orbitals in a carboxy (>C = O) group. Groups which consist of **s, p,** and **n** orbitals are common in biological molecules. Examples are pyridine, pyrimidines, purines, nicotine, and flavins.

4.4.3 Benzene and Aromatic Molecular Stabilities

The most widely used example of electron delocalization is benzene which provides the basic concept of aromatic molecules. The six 2p orbitals around the Carbon atom overlap to give six p orbitals that spread all around the benzene ring. According to the Huckle approximation, the molecular orbitals and their relative energies are presented in Figure 4.15.

The above approximation does not take into account electron repulsion. If electron repulsion is considered, the degenerate states split and a new pattern of energy levels emerge. Thus the lowest energy excitation (arrows in Figure 4.15) absorbs different wavelengths of radiation.

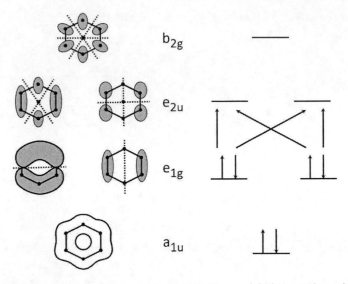

Fig. 4.15 The **p** molecular orbitals of benzene (top view). The nodal planes (where the electron density is zero) perpendicular to the molecular plane are represented by dash lines. a, e and b are eigen functions of different point groups which are assigned into gerade (g) and ungerade (u) groups.

4.4.4 Molecular Structure and Transitions

Electronic transitions are from the highest occupied molecular orbital (HOMO) to the lowest unoccupied molecular orbital (LUMO) in linear compounds. Energy induced transitions occur when the transition dipole integral is non-zero. Light induced transitions in linear compounds occur at higher wavelengths (l) compared to cyclic compounds, as the HOMO electron in cyclic compounds can go to higher unoccupied orbitals, making the transitions at lower l. Electrons in linear compounds can be considered as particles in a box in one dimension and those in cyclic compounds as particles in a box of two dimensions.

4.4.4.1 *Conjugated p Electron System*

The p bond system in double bonded atoms provides a test system for structure-spectroscopy relationships. Consider the following structures

$$>C=C< \quad \text{vs.} \quad >C=C-C=C< \quad \text{vs.} \quad >C=C-C=C-C=C<$$
$$\text{2 p electrons} \qquad \text{4 p electrons} \qquad \text{6 p electrons}$$

The conjugated double bonds provide a system of delocalized p electrons, leading to decrease in the energy difference between HOMO and LUMO with increase in the number of double bonds. This is because y functions for a particle in a box have increasingly higher levels of energy in the ground state. For such a phenomenon to occur the molecule ought to possess a conjugated bonding system, where the orbitals overlap, where the electrons behave like particles in a box, free to move in one dimension along the x-axis corresponding to the conjugated bonds.

It is possible to calculate the energy of transition between HOMO and LUMO by considering the following:

$$En = n^2h^2/8mL^2 \qquad \text{(Eq. 4.19)}$$

where, L is the length of the conjugated p bond system.

In order to determine the longest wavelength of transition, the energy levels of the LUMO and HOMO, the energy difference (ΔE) between the HOMO and LUMO is calculated, which is difficult. However, absolute energy levels are needed for the estimation of ΔE.

For a polyene with k double bonds

$$n = k \text{ for HOMO}$$

and $\qquad\qquad\qquad\qquad N = k{+}1 \text{ for the LUMO}$

$$\Delta E = E_{k+1} - E_k = (k + 1)^2h^2/8m_eL^2 - k^2h^2/8m_eL^2$$

$$= (2k + 1)h^2/8mL^2 \qquad \text{(Eq. 4.20)}$$

where, h, the Planck's constant, and m_e, the mass of an electron are constants.

Knowing $\qquad\qquad\qquad \Delta E = hv = hc/\lambda \qquad\qquad\qquad$ (Eq. 4.21)

where, c = speed of light
λ = wavelength

$$\text{or}$$

$$\lambda = hc/\Delta E \qquad \text{(Eq. 4.22)}$$

Substituting with Equation 4.20,

$$\lambda = hc \times 8\ m_eL^2/h^2\ (2k + 1) = 8m_eL^2c/2k + 1 \qquad \text{(Eq. 4.23)}$$

4.4.4.2 *Molecular Features and Electronic Transitions*

Equation 4.23 allows calculation of λ for an electronic transition to the first approximation. However, one needs to know the value of L, which is the bond length of delocalized electrons, although it may not be the added value of single and double bonds. In fact, the bond length is determined by spectral characteristics. This feature is particularly helpful in determining if the molecule is non-linear, such as semi-cyclic (carotene, phytochrome) or cyclic (such as heme or chlorophyll) (Figures 4.16 to 4.18).

The spectral properties of cyclic compounds with conjugated p electrons are influenced by electron movement in circles, leading to angular momentum associated with such movement. This angular momentum gives rise to an angular momentum quantum number, which determines feasibility of the transitions. The concept can be understood with the following description of four types of quantum numbers:

1. Principal quantum number, n, that represents the electronic transitions from ground to excited states. "n" is always a positive integer, i.e., 1, 2, 3, and so on.
2. Azimuthal or angular momentum quantum number, l, where l = n-1. So this can be 0, 1, 2, and so on.

3. Orientation quantum number or magnetic quantum number, m_l, with integrs from -l to +l. This is associated with different orientations of the vector representing the angular momentum.

4. Spin quantum number, s measure of angular momentum due to the spin of the electron (+1/2 or -1/2).

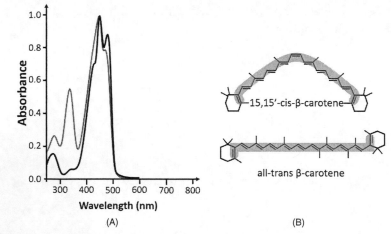

Fig. 4.16 Electronic absorption spectra of β-carotene (A) in linear (blue) all trans and 15,15-cis (red) structure forms (B) (Adopted from Fiedor et al., 2016). [See color plates]

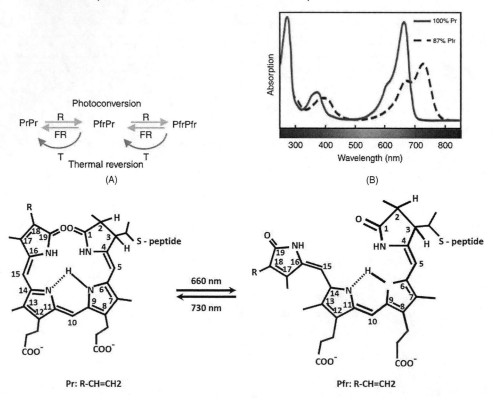

Fig. 4.17 Pr (red light absorbing) and Pfr (far-red light absorbing) forms of phytochrome (A) showing spectral shift (B) showing in part the trans and cis forms of the tetrapyrrolic chromophore (C) (Adopted from Legris et al., 2019).

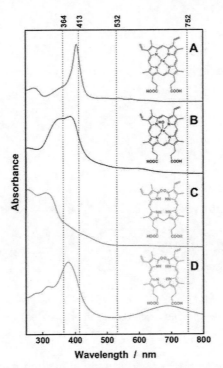

Fig. 4.18 Absorption spectra of hemoglobin (A), hematin (B), bilirubin (C), and biliverdin (D), along with the chromophore structures, respectively. The simplified heme structure represents the chromophoric unit of hemoglobin. The applied laser excitation wavelengths $\lambda_{exc.}$ = 364 nm, $\lambda_{exc.}$ = 413 nm, $\lambda_{exc.}$ = 532 nm, and $\lambda_{xc.}$ = 752 nm are depicted as vertical dashed lines. These can be carefully tuned into the electronic absorption bands of the individual chromophores and strongly resonating Raman enhancements can be achieved for the vibrational modes that are coupled to these electronic transitions (Adopted from Yan et al., 2016).

According to the selection rule of transitions, a transition resulting in a large change in the linear or angular momentum is momentum forbidden.

Oscillator strength, f, of a transition = $p_s \times p_o \times p_p \times p_m \times f_a$, where p_s, p_o, p_p, and p_m represent the probability of transitions due to electron spin, orbital symmetry, parity, and momentum, respectively. f_a is the oscillator strength of a fully allowed transition. Here we are concerned with the momentum factor for transition, the selection rule for which states that any transition resulting in a large change in the linear or angular momentum is momentum forbidden, meaning the transition will be weak. Momentum probability of transitions (pm) ranges between 10^{-1} and 10^{-3}.

As an example, one could consider compounds containing aromatic rings as a chromophore having an aromatic ring, containing 6 p electrons, naphthalene with 10 p electrons, and porphyrins with 18 conjugated p electrons to follow the 4n+2 aromatic ring rule. It is to be noted that the p electrons in conjugated double bonds be in an aromatic ring, thus the porphyrin ring with 20 conjugated p electrons does not display the same characteristics as the 18 p electrons which are part of the aromatic ring.

To begin with, take the case of benzene, an aromatic compound with 6 p electrons, following the 4n+2 rule.

n = 2
l = n − 1 = 2 − 1 = 1
m_e = −1 to + 1; −1, 0, +1

The electronic structure of benzene can be represented as follows (in Figure 4.19):

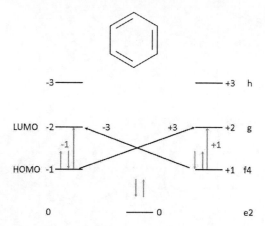

Fig. 4.19 Structure of benzene (left) and its electronic energy states (right) showing transitions between HOMO and LUMO orbitals.

Because of the degenerate nature of the orientation quantum number, l, the transitions could be from -1 or 1 ground states (HOMO) to -2 and +2 excited states (LUMO) resulting in orbital angular quantum number changes (Δq) of ±1 and ±3.

As a general rule, if transitions from q = me to q = me+1, then

$$\Delta q = \pm 1 \quad \text{or} \quad \pm(2me + 1) \qquad \text{(Eq. 4.24)}$$

For porphyrins with 18 p electrons in an aromatic ring, the electronic structure will be as follows, showing the Δq for HOMO-LUMO transition as ±9 (Figure 4.20).

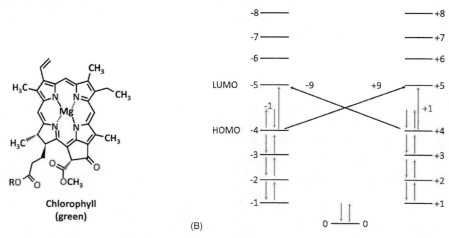

Fig. 4.20 Structure of chlorophyll, a porphyrin (A) and its electronic energy states (B) showing transitions between HOMO and LUMO orbitals.

Each of the HOMO-LUMO transitions with $\Delta q = \pm 1$ and $\Delta q = \pm(2m_e+1)$ is doubly degenerate and this holds true for a perfect circle. However, these real aromatic rings are not perfect circles, leading to the polarization of the transitions along "a" and "b" axes as shown below for benzene.

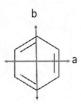

+1 transitions are referred to as B state, which is less stable because of higher energy $\pm(2m_e+1)$ transitions are referred to as L state, which is most stable, with lower energy.

The higher energy band (< l) is polarized along the short axis, whereas the lower energy (>l) b band is polarized along the longer axis. For the naphthalene molecule which is much less symmetrical, the degeneracy in the energy of the states is more pronounced. In Figure 4.21, energy states of HOMO-LUMO transition of 10 p electron system ($\Delta q = \pm 1$ and ± 5) are shown, with a pronounced split in the degenerate energy levels of the S1 excited state.

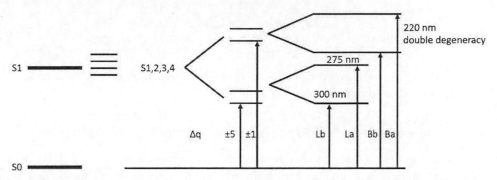

Fig. 4.21 Ground and excited states of naphthalene, showing excited state degeneracy and B and L transitions corresponding to two different angular momentum quantum number changes (Dq as ± 1 and ± 5).

The resulting sub-levels are denoted as *a* and *b*, depending on the orientation of the new nodal plane introduced into the electronic wave function. For the "a" state, the nodal planes are situated in such a manner, that the electron density is located at the **atoms**, while the effective charges go to the **bonds** for the "b" state. This is illustrated in Figure 4.22 for the states of naphthalene. According to Hund's third rule, the *L* states are energetically, always lower than the *B* states (from Band. C., https://thedelocalizedchemist.com/indole/).

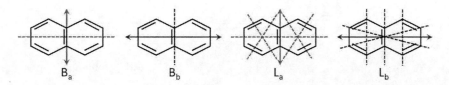

Fig. 4.22 Transition dipole orientation and electron density distribution for naphthalene n=2 and Δq as +1 and +5). +1 or the B-states and 5 for the L-states. Δq also corresponds to the number of nodal planes. At these planes (dashed lines) there is no electron density. Hence, the electrons are pushed more to the atoms for the "a" states and to the bonds for the "b" states. The resulting orientation of the transition dipole moment is indicated by the arrows (from Band. C., https://thedelocalizedchemist.com/indole/).

Absorption spectra of benzene, naphthalene, and anthracene with increasing number of delocalized aromatic p electrons are shown in Figure 4.23.

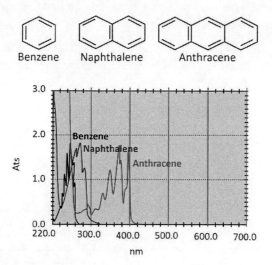

Fig. 4.23   Structure and absorption spectra of benzene, naphthalene, and anthracene, showing transitions corresponding to degenerate energy states.

4.4.4.3   *Structure and Optical Properties of Biological Chromophores*

Such transition degeneracies are more clearly resolved in porphyrins, which consist of tetrapyrroles. Chlorophylls are the best representative of such spectra (Figure 4.24), showing clear ± 1 and ± 9 values for ΔQ (with 18 aromatic p electrons, as per Figure 4.20) transitions which are traditionally labeled as B_{xy} and Q_{xy}, instead of B_{ab} and L_{ab} (Figure 4.21).

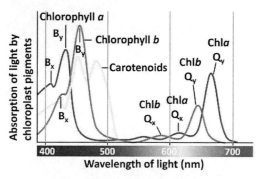

Fig. 4.24   The absorption bands of Chlorophyll a, Chlorophyll b, and Carotenoids, showing transition bands (Adopted from Dingle, 2014).

Another interesting example of a tetrapyrrolic protein is Phytochrome, a blue-green chromoprotein that regulates plant growth and physiology. It is a 124 kDa sized protein that contains tetrapyrrolic chromophore that undergoes photoconversion. Upon red light absorption (660 nm), the red light absorbing (Pr) form of phytochrome convert into a far-red light absorbing Pfr form, which maximally absorbs at 730 nm (Figure 4.25). Upon absorption of 730 nm the Pfr form converts into the Pr form. This photo-transformation is critical for the photomorphogenic responses. The band around 280 nm is due to the aromatic amino acid groups of the protein.

Fig. 4.25 UV-Vis absorption spectra of phytochrome in its Pr (solid line) and Pfr (broken line) forms. The spectral peak below 300 nm is due to protein aromatic amino acid residues, while the remaining spectral features are due to the tetrapyrrolic chromophore.

Spectroscopic techniques allow examination of the molecular mechanism of action involved in not only the photo-transformation but also the mechanism involved in the mediation of molecular events following the photo-transformation. This photo-transformation involves two molecular events – in one of which, the tetrapyrrolic chromophore in the Pr form of the phytochrome that exists in a circular form, when photo-transformed to the Pfr form, becomes isomerized at the C15-C16 double bond to give a 15-E isomer (Figure 4.26).

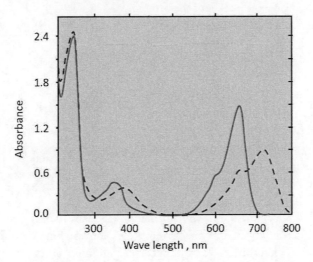

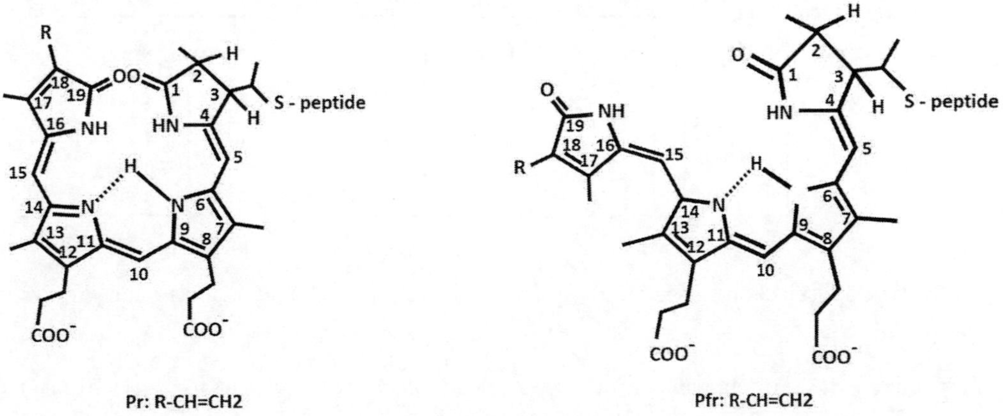

Fig. 4.26 Tetrapyrrolic chromophore structure and conformation in the Pr and Pfr forms of chromophore.

The second molecular event concerns the phytochrome chromophore that exists in a semi-circular conformation in both the Pr and Pfr forms, although with differing configurations. The chromophore in the Pr form sits in a hydrophobic pocket of the protein. In the Pfr form, the chromophore interacts with the N-terminus polypeptide segment of about 6 kDa size while emerging out of the pocket, in a relatively more exposed state (Figure 4.27).

This example of phytochrome chromophore, or porphyrins, in general, provides a system to demonstrate how the spectral characteristics of linear and cyclic compounds differ by way of the electronic transitions that are reflected in spectral characteristics. Energy levels of the spectral transitions are shown in Figure 4.28 for Chlorophyll "a" (Chl a), and Pr and Pfr forms

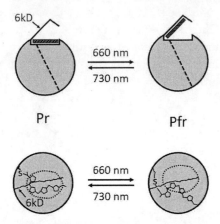

Fig. 4.27 A model for photo-transformation of phytochrome, exhibiting the topography of its tetrapyrrolic chromophore.

of the phytochrome. Based on the photo-transformation mechanism of the phytochrome, it is clear that when the aromatic ring formed by the tetrapyrroles converts into a semi-circular shape, the low energy transitions get red shifted, as would be expected in linear molecules. Furthermore, the chromophore spectral characteristics are also determined by the surrounding environment provided by the protein moiety, which appears to change in the Pr and Pfr forms, as indicated in Figure 4.27. Chlorophyll "a", being the more compliant with a circular structure due to the presence of coordinating metal in the middle of the ring, shows well resolved B and Q transitions.

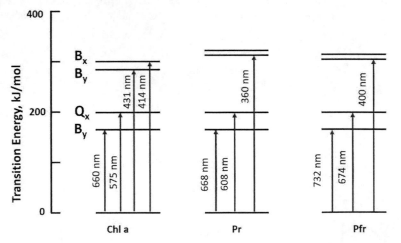

Fig. 4.28 Levels of electronic spectral transitions of chlorophyll "a" (Chl a), and Pr and Pfr forms of phytochrome.

Electromagnetic radiation spans a wide range of electromagnetic frequencies in the electromagnetic spectrum. Depending upon its energy content (wavelength), energy from different parts of the electromagnetic spectrum may interact with biomolecules in different ways. This section describes some of the experimental techniques and the possible applications that should come about from studying interactions of biomolecules and electromagnetic radiation.

The human eye only detects a comparatively narrow part of the electromagnetic spectrum. The precise nature of the interaction of these different types of electromagnetic radiation with matter differs depending on wavelength, and hence we need different approaches to measure these interactions. Absorption of light energy from electromagnetic spectrum elevates electrons from their ground state to an excited state. Excited state electron return to ground state only by losing energy. This transition is only possible between allowed energy levels. The phenomenon of transition of energy level is not only confined to electrons. Chemical bonds can also vibrate and rotate and give rise to similar quantized energy levels. However, the gap in these (vibrational and rotational) energy levels is small and needs higher wavelength radiation to generate a spectrum.

4.4.5 Ultraviolet/Visible Absorption Spectroscopy

If light in the ultraviolet/visible part of spectrum is passed through a sample in solution, light energy may be absorbed. Molecules (or parts of molecules) capable of absorbing light are called chromophores. This is the principle employed in *absorption spectroscopy*. Each chemical structure absorbs light of different frequencies (Table 4.3).

The absorption phenomenon may be quantified by the Beer–Lambert Law:

$$\log(I_0/I) = \varepsilon.c.l$$

where,

I_0 is the intensity of incident light,
I is the intensity of transmitted light,
c is the molar concentration,
l is the length of the light path, and
ε is molar extinction coefficient.

$\text{Log}(I_0/I)$ then, is the absorbance (A) at a particular wavelength. A plot of A or ε versus frequency or wavelength is known as an absorption spectrum. Wavelength corresponding to maximum absorption is called λmax. When light is absorbed, the absorbance value increases. In theory, the parameter is linear, but practically, it is not possible to measure absorbance accurately above 3.0. The accuracy of quantification decreases with high concentration and for most linear measurement obtained below absorbance 1.0. Schematics of the instrumentation of an UV spectrophotometer are shown in Figure 4.29.

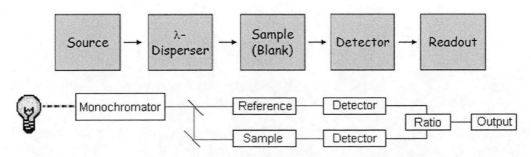

Fig. 4.29 UV spectroscopy. Schematic of an UV spectrometer.

The absorption spectrum of a chromophore not only depends upon its chemical structure, the environment in which these chromophore is placed also plays a major role. The most important environmental factors affecting absorption spectra are pH, solvent polarity, and orientation of molecule. These effects are especially important in the study of biomolecules and may acts as a reporter of microenvironment within these molecules.

For example, protonation/deprotonation effects in protein result from change in pH or oxidation/ reduction and affect electronic environment of chromophores. This often results in dramatic differences between the absorption spectra of protonated and deprotonated forms (Figure 4.30). Solvent polarity also affects the absorption spectrum. Dimethylsulfoxide, dioxane, ethylene glycol, glycerol, and sucrose are some of the alternatives of water. Absorbance spectra in these solvents give a slightly different spectrum compared to water and thus can be used to monitor such changes in the microenvironment of biomolecules. Orientation effects are a spectroscopic consequence of the relative geometry of neighboring chromophore molecules. A good example is hyperchromicity of nucleic acids. A solution of free nucleotides has a higher A_{260} than an identical concentration of single-stranded polynucleotide. Double-stranded nucleic acids in turn have a lower absorbance at this wavelength than single-stranded polynucleotides. For this reason, absorbance measurements are useful in monitoring assembly or denaturation of nucleotides in vitro. An absorption characteristic of some common biomolecules is shown in Table 4.3.

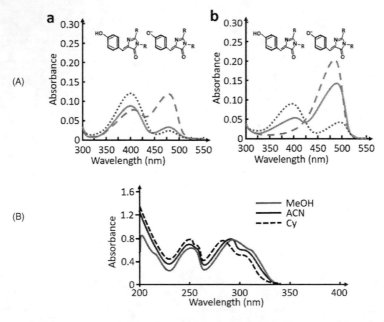

Fig. 4.30 (A) Absorbance spectra of unbound *(gray, solid line)*, minimizer-bound *(gray, dashed line)* or enhancer-bound *(black, dotted line)* wt GFP (a) or eGFP (b). The absorption at 395 nm corresponds to the protonated chromophore and absorption at 475 nm to the anionic chromophore. Both enhancer and minimizer affected the absorption of deprotonated form (Kirchoffer et al., 2010, Nature Structural and Molecular Biology, 17, 133–138). (B) Absorbance spectra of Flavones in methanol (red), acetonitrile (ACN, blue), and cyclohexane (Cy, black). Both hydrogen bond donating ability and non-specific dipolar interaction can affect absorption spectra (Sancho et al., 2011). [See color plates]

Absorption spectra of biomolecules are routinely utilized for examining physiological states, effects of environmental factors, yield, and much more. Spectral changes are also utilized for monitoring biochemical reactions, such as for dehydrogenases and glutathione-S-transferases.

Table 4.3 Wavelength maxima and molar extinction coefficients of representative chromophores.

Common Chromophores	Symbol	λ_{max} (nm)
Amine	$-NH_2$	195
Ethylene	$-C=C-$	190
Carbonyl group	$C=O$	270–285
Pyrrole		324
Porphyrin		405
Heme		413
Carotenoids		450 and 480
Melanin		335

Contd.

Table 4.3 *contd.*

Common Chromophores	Symbol	λ_{max} (nm)
Tryptophan		280 and 219
Tyrosine		274
Phenylalanine		257
Adenosine		260
DNA		260
RNA		260

Questions to ponder over

Please consider the following questions while evaluating these spectra.

1. How does a solvent affect spectral properties (band positions, spectral shape and intensity)?
2. How could two entirely different classes of biochemical compounds absorb light in the spectral region?
3. Why would spectral shapes of two compounds absorbing in the same spectral region be different?
4. Why does substitution of groups in a chemical structure (as a result of chemical or biochemical reaction) alter spectral properties?
5. What is the relationship between demo-experiments and fundamental quantum chemical principles, as discussed in a biological spectroscopy course?

Another way in which absorption spectra may be presented is as *derivative* spectra. This involves plotting the rate of change of absorbance dAλ as a function of λ (Figure 4.31). It is particularly useful for high-resolution comparison of spectra.

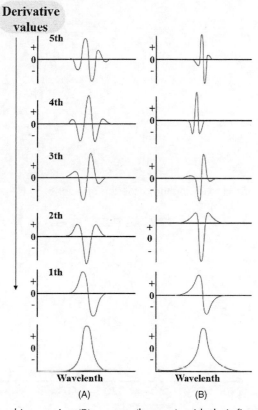

Fig. 4.31 Gaussian (A) and Lorentzian (B) spectra (bottom), with their first to fifth *derivative spectra*.

Box 4.1 Assignment 1

(A) Glutathione-S-transferase catalyzes a reaction between glutathione (GSH) and dichlorobenzene (CDNB) and glutathione (GSH, a tripeptide. 8-Methoxypsoralen (8-MOP) is a competitive inhibitor of this reaction.

Spectral recordings of CDNB, CDNB-SG conjugate, NADH and anthocyanins under different conditions are shown below

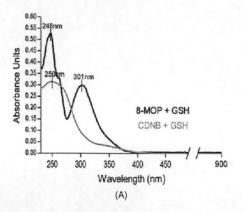

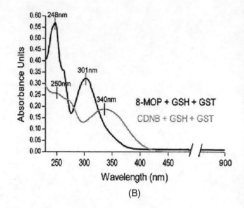

(A)   (B)

(B) Spectral change in NADH following the oxidation of alcohol by NAD+

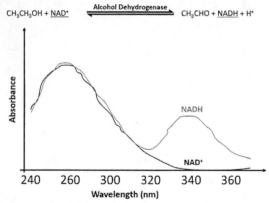

(C) Spectral changes in anthocyanin with solvent pH changes

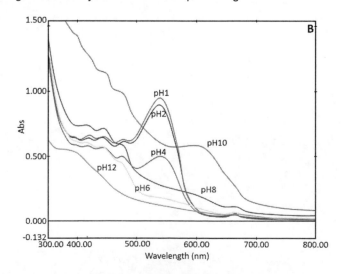

Box 4.2   Demonstration/Hands-on Experiment 4.1

DNA Denaturation Monitored by UV Absorption and Derivative Spectroscopy

Purpose

To understand how to use UV spectroscopy of DNA to demonstrate hypochromism; and estimate thermodynamic parameters of DNA denaturation.

Principles

Nucleic acids, ribonucleic acid (RNA) and deoxyribonucleic acid (DNA), consist of purines (adenine, guanine) and pyrimidines (cytosine, thymine, uracil), which have several conjugated π bonds. The presence of oxygen and nitrogen provide non-bonding orbitals. Both π–$\pi*$ and n-$\pi*$ electronic transitions readily occur in the UV region, leading to an absorption band around 260 nm.

The band at 260 nm is a broad band consisting of several molecular transitions, including those representing different orientation of the transition dipole with the purine and pyrimidine rings. These electronic transitions, particularly under different environmental conditions, could play a significant role in causing mis-pairing and biases leading to mutations in the genetic material.

Near neighbor stacking of chromophores (bases), occurs in the helical polynucleotides resulting in significant hypochromism in a double-stranded DNA helix. The magnitude of the chromophore–chromophore interactions determines the degree of hypochromism. This feature is exploited to study denaturation and renaturation of the DNA helix, usually with temperature mediated melting of DNA molecules.

The basic principle in this set of experiments involves resolution of spectral bands corresponding to different transition of DNA bases with the fourth derivative of an UV absorption spectrum of a DNA preparation (plasmid isolated from E. coli). Electronic transitions of the bases in 230–330 nm region, are sensitive to denaturation of the DNA, and changes can be monitored by comparing 4th derivative spectra of DNA before and after temperature-induced melting.

The phenomenon of hypochromism is used to follow denaturation of DNA by monitoring change in absorbance at 260 nm as a function of heating (temperature). T_m (melting temperature) of DNA depends on factors like GC content, buffer pH, salt concentrations, and coiling and supercoiling of the DNA.

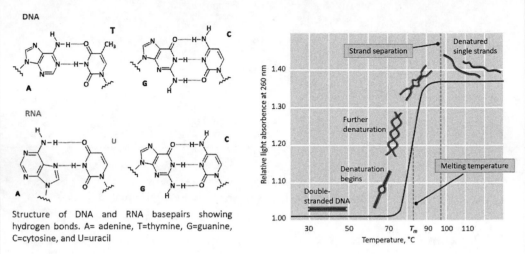

Structure of DNA and RNA basepairs showing hydrogen bonds. A= adenine, T=thymine, G=guanine, C=cytosine, and U=uracil

Fig. 4.32   Absorbance change in DNA at 260 nm as it is heated to melting point.

Temperature dependent denaturation of DNA can be followed by monitoring absorbance at 260 nm, and a plot of temperature and relative absorbance, plotted in Figure 4.32 shows different states of the DNA structure during the melting process. The curve can be plotted as absorbance at 260 versus. T (K), and the curve labeled as shown in Figure 4.33.

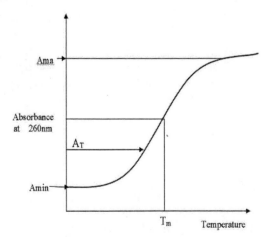

Fig. 4.33   DNA denaturation curve showing absorbance change at 260 nm as a function of temperature.

Fraction denatured DNA at any temperature, T, can be calculated by the following equation:

$$F_d = (A_T - A_{min})/(A_{max} - A_{min})$$

Equilibrium constant, K, can be calculated at any temperature, T, as

$$K = F_d/(1 - F_d)$$

With K available in this way, one can use the $\Delta G° = -RT \ln K$ relationship to calculate the Gibbs Free Energy.

Using relationship, $\Delta G° = \Delta H° - T\Delta S°$

One can write, $-RT \ln K = \Delta H° - T\Delta S°$

Or $\ln K = -\Delta H°/R \, (1/T) + \Delta S°/R$ (van't Hoff equation)

Plotting ln K versus 1/T gives a slope (Figure 4.34) which is $-\Delta H°/R$, and a y-intercept as $\Delta S°/R$. Using an R value of 1.987 cal·K^{-1}mole^{-1}, one can calculate enthalpy and entropy values for the melting of the DNA.

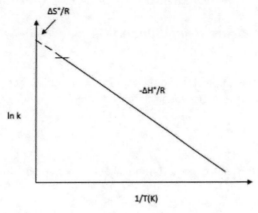

Fig. 4.34   van't Hoff plot of DNA denaturation.

Experimental procedure

The experiment involves recording absorption spectra of DNA, provided, under native (physiological pH and room temperature) and denatured conditions. Students are expected to record their own data and carry out calculations.

Experimental plans

1. Approximately 18 ug/ml DNA solution is prepared in water. One may have time to do this recording in another buffer as well with salt and higher pH. Ask questions regarding the selection of conditions.

2. A brief introduction to the instrument, sample compartment, special needs, computer software, would be useful. Be prepared to take notes on how to start the instrument, how to record data, and special care to be exercised and reasons for such – concentration, cuvette sizes, etc.

3. The UV/Vis spectrometer will be used to record reference and sample spectra at room temperature. We will also show you how to process the data, and transform the absorption spectrum into a 4th derivative spectrum.

4. You will record the spectrum of DNA at about 100°C. What do you expect to happen to the DNA and why? Would that be visible in spectral changes?

5. Record absorbance at different temperatures, between 25 and 100°C, and collate the data into F_d and $1-F_d$ forms to calculate K at every temperature. Also calculate melting temperature, T_m, which is the temperature at which $F_d = (1-F_d)$.

6. Using the van't Hoff equation, plot (as described above). Please calculate Gibbs Free Energy, enthalpy and entropy of DNA denaturation. You will need to write a brief report (2–3 pages) on the demonstration/hands-on, giving background, results obtained, and explanations of your observations.

Box 4.3   Demonstration/Hands-on Experiment 4.2

Estimation of Tyr Exposure Using Second Derivative UV Spectroscopy

Purpose

Develop understanding of the use of UV spectroscopy on proteins to resolve electronic transition bands corresponding to Tyr and Trp absorption, and calculate the degree of Tyr exposure in a protein.

Principles

The basic principle in this set of experiments would involve resolution of spectral bands corresponding to Tyr and Trp residues in the second derivative of UV absorption spectrum of a protein. Electronic transitions of Tyr residues in the 280–185 nm region are sensitive to Tyr exposure to polar environments. In contrast, Trp electronic transitions are virtually insensitive. This contrast in solvent sensitivity of Tyr and Trp residues is exploited to determine the degree of Tyr exposure by taking a ratio of *a* (an arithmetic sum of the negative $d^2A/d\lambda^2$ at 285 nm and a positive $d^2A/d\lambda^2$ at 289 nm) and *b* (an arithmetic sum of the negative $d^2A/d\lambda^2$ at 291 nm and the positive $d^2A/d\lambda^2$ at 295 nm), shown in Figure 4.35 below. The *a/b* ratio is estimated for the protein in a normal buffer (corresponding to physiological pH and salt conditions) and in a condition that will denature the protein (6 M guanidine.HCl). Comparison of the a/b ratio in native protein folding and denatured conditions allows the estimation of Tyr exposure under normal physiological conditions.

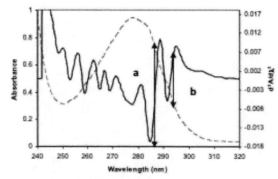

Fig. 4.35   Absorption (---) and second derivative (—) spectra of a protein dissolved in 10 mM sodium phosphate buffer, pH 6.0 at 25°C.

Experimental procedure

The experiment will involve recording the absorption spectra of a protein, lysozyme, under native (physiological pH and room temperature) and denatured conditions. You are expected to get the opportunity to record your own data and carry out calculations.

Experimental plans

1. 2 mg/ml lysozyme is prepared in phosphate buffered saline (PBS). Pay attention to the type of buffer, pH, and concentration of the lysozyme solution. Ask questions about the selection of conditions.
2. A brief introduction to the instrument, sample compartment, special needs, computer software, and related issues should be sought. Be prepared to take notes on how to start the instrument, how to record data, and reasons for special care – concentration, cuvette sizes, etc.
3. The UV/Vis spectrometer will be used to record reference and sample spectra at room temperature. We will also show you how to process the data, and transform the absorption spectrum into a second derivative spectrum.
4. The spectra of lysozyme dissolved PBS and in 6 M guanidine hydrochloride (HCl) will be recorded. What do you expect to happen to the protein in guanidine- HCl, and why? Would that be visible in spectral changes?
5. You will be able to record your own spectra for lysozyme in PBS and 6 M guanidine.HCl, using 2 mg/ml stock solution of lysozyme and 8 M stock solution of guanidine.HCl. You will obtain second derivative spectra, display the peaks, obtain peak tables to note down the values of peaks and troughs at appropriate wavelengths for calculating "a" and "b" to obtain a/b ratios of the protein in PBS and 6 M guanidine.HCl.
6. For estimation of the degree of Tyr exposure, **a**, use the following equation:

$$\alpha = (\gamma_v - \gamma_\alpha)/(\gamma_\upsilon - \gamma_\alpha)$$

where γ_n is the a/b ratio of the protein in native folding and γ_u is the a/b ratio under denatured condition. α is a correction factor calculated on the basis of Tyr and Trp ratio for a given protein according to the following equation (Ragone et al., 1984).

$$\gamma_u = (Ax + B)/Cx + 1$$

where A, B, and C are constants -0.18, 0.64, and -0.04, respectively (Table 1 in Ragone et al., 1984), and the **x** is Tyr/Trp ratio of the protein. For lysozyme, this ratio is 1.0.
7. You can record spectra of another protein of your interest under native and denatured conditions with known x value. You will be able to get the second derivative spectra and the peak and trough values of this protein so that you can calculate the Tyr exposure of this protein as well. You will need to submit a brief report (2–3 pages) on the hands-on experiment, giving background, results, and explanations for your observations.

4.4.6 Fluorescence Spectroscopy

When a chromophore absorbs light, then it has to lose its excess energy to return to a ground state; as heat, or nonradiative transition, or radiative transition. When it loses a portion of its energy as radiative transition this is released as in the form of light emission. This phenomenon is called fluorescence and such chromophores are called fluorophores (Table 4.4). Emitted light energy is always of higher wavelength than that which was absorbed (Figure 4.36). The schematics of fluorescence based instrumentation are shown in Figure 4.37.

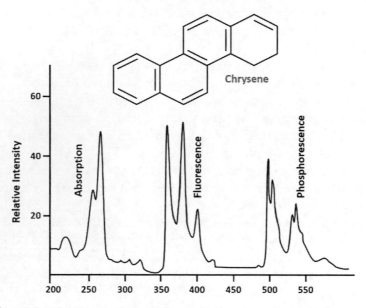

Fig. 4.36   Absorbance, fluorescence, and phosphorescence of chrysene.

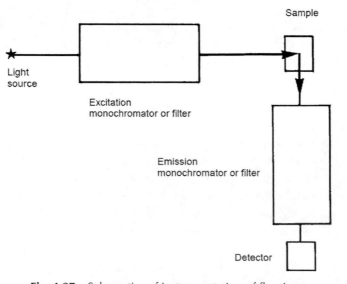

Fig. 4.37   Schematics of instrumentation of fluorimeter.

Table 4.4 Chemical structures of some compounds and their exhibition of fluorescence and chemiluminescence.

Structure	Use
NH2 Tyrosine CH—CH2— —OH COOH	Intrinsic fluorescence (protiens)
NH2 CH—CH2— COOH Tryptophan	Intrinsic fluorescence (protiens)
O⁻ H O=S=ON— 1-Anilino-8-naphthalene sulphonate (ANS)	Extrinsic fluorescence (protiens)
OH— O O COOH Fluorescein	Extrinsic fluorescence (protiens)
NH2 NH2 Ethidium bromide =N+B⁻ C2H5	Extrinsic fluorescence (DNA)
CH3—N—CH3 CH3 Acridine orange	Extrinsic fluorescence (DNA)
NH2 O NH NH Luminol O	Chemiluminescent substrate (peroxidase)
Luciferin N N COOH S S	Chemiluminescent substrate (firely inciferase)

Life times of excited states are usually very short (0.5 ns to 10 ns). However, it can be longer too. The latter case can arise as a consequence of a phenomenon called electron spin. In most atoms, the pair of electrons in single orbitals are oriented in opposite directions as a result of the Pauli Exclusion Principle. However, if electrons are placed in a higher energy orbital, then their spin can be oriented in either in the same (parallel), or opposite (antiparallel), orientation. When placed in a magnetic field, this atom can have three distinct energy levels which may be designated -1, 0, +1, and this state is a triplet state. When this molecule returns to the ground state, a radiative triplet-singlet transition occurs which is a much slower process than fluorescence and is called phosphorescence. Radiation emitted as a result of this transition is at an even longer wavelength than radiation emitted during fluorescence because the lowest-energy triplet state typically has only slightly higher energy than the lowest-energy singlet state (Figure 5.37).

Another phenomenon resulting from radiative transition is chemiluminescence. It occurs when molecules are promoted to excited state as a result of a chemical reaction, which then return to ground state with the emission of light. For example, the level of ATP may be quantified as follows:

$$\text{Luciferin} + \text{ATP} + O_2 \xrightarrow{\text{Firefly Luciferase}} \text{Oxyluciferin} + \text{AMP} + \text{pyrophosphate} + CO_2 + \text{light}$$

Both chemiluminescence and fluorescence need different types of instrumental arrangements if they are to be investigated. Only a portion of the light energy originally absorbed is emitted as radiation. Absorbed energy is lost in vibrational transition, internal quenching and external quenching. Internal quenching is due to some intrinsic structural rearrangement and external quenching is due to interaction of the excited molecule with some other molecule present in the sample. All forms of quenching result in nonradiative loss of energy. Acrylamide, iodide, and ascorbic acid are examples of external quencher.

External quenching is a complex process. This is possible by two mechanisms: dynamic quenching and static quenching. Dynamic quenching involves collision between the two molecules with the fluorophore losing energy as kinetic energy. Static quenching involves a more long-lasting formation of a complex between fluorophore and quencher, referred to as dark complex. It is often difficult to distinguish between two kinds of quenching but the Stern–Volmer relationship helps in differentiating these.

$$F_0/F = 1 + k_3 \cdot [q].T$$

where, $F_0 = k_1/(k_1 + k_2)$ is the fluorescence intensity in the absence of external quencher; $F = k_1/(k_1 + k_2 + k_3)$. [q] is the fluorescence intensity in the presence of external quencher; k_1, k_2, and k_3 are rate constants for fluorescence, internal quenching, and external quenching, respectively. [q] is concentration of quencher and $T = 1/(k_1 + k_2)$ is the excited state lifetime. Product of k_3 and lifetime is defined as the dynamic Stern–Volmer constant.

$$K_{sv} = k_3.T$$

A plot of F_0/F plotted against the function of concentration of external quencher [q] is called Stern–Volmer plot. By analyzing SV plot one can distinguish between dynamic quenching and static quenching.

A major difference between dynamic quenching and static quenching is the fact that temperature affects the two processes in an opposite way. Dynamic quenching depends upon collision between excited fluorophore and quencher and results in decrease in excited state lifetime, T, so temperature increase will increase dynamic quenching. Static quenching is due to complex formation between fluorophore and quencher. Complex formation is less at higher temperature and results in decrease in quenching.

Box 4.4   Assignment 1 Fluorescence Spectroscopy

The fluorescent behavior of phenanthrene is examined below (Figure 4.38):

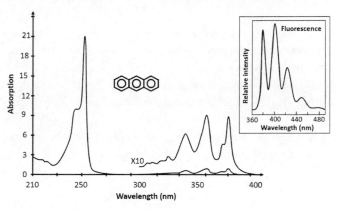

Fig. 4.38   Spectrum of phenanthrene.

(a) Select an optimum wavelength of excitation for recording a proper fluorescence spectrum. Provide a brief justification for your selection.
(b) Select an optimum emission wavelength of emission for recording a proper excitation spectrum. Provide a brief justification for your selection.
(c) Assume using a Xenon arc lamp as a light source in your spectrofluorometer, and plot approximately the uncorrected excitation spectrum of phenanthrene. Briefly explain your spectrum.
(d) What approximate bandpass will be needed to resolve spectral features of phenanthrene fluorescence spectrum? Provide a basis for your approximation.
(e) Calculate the size of slit width needed to obtain the bandpass you suggested in (d). Assume linear reciprocal dispersion of the monochromator in your spectrofluorometer as 1.6 nm/mm.

Box 4.5   Demonstration Experiment 4.4: Introduction to Fluorescence Excitation and Emission Spectra

Description

Fluorescence spectroscopy is one of the most sensitive and selective techniques for analysis of chromophores. Fluorescence excitation and emission spectra are of fundamental importance to utilizing fluorescence phenomenon for a variety of chemical and biochemical processes, including identification of emitting species, verification of purity, detection of artifacts, estimation of binding, molecular distance determination, effects of solvent polarity, etc. Excitation and emission spectra generally follow certain "Basic Rules" as outlined below.

Goal

To familiarize the student with a fluorimeter operated in steady state mode, to introduce the concept and strategic skills in recording excitation and emission spectra, and to illustrate the Basic Rules.

Introduction

This set of experiment involves recording of excitation and emission spectra and realization of the Basic Rules. The reasons for the Basic Rules can be understood from classroom discussions and in the textbook. These rules are:
1. The fluorescence emission occurs at longer wavelength (lower energy) than the excitation.
2. The shape of the emission spectrum does not change when the excitation wavelength is changed.
3. For a single emitting species, the excitation spectrum is the same as the absorption spectrum.
4. In many cases, the emission spectrum is a mirror image of the absorption/excitation spectrum.

Safety Issues

High voltages are produced by the detector and lamp power supplies. Ordinarily, students will have no need to have access to this circuitry. The fluorescent dyes used in this experiment are not known to be toxic under experimental circumstances. However, do not get them on your skin and cloth, as they are difficult to wash.

This experiment involves recording the emission and excitation spectra of fluorescein in aqueous solutions.

Materials

Samples (in 1 cm fluorescence cuvettes)

  1A: 1 µM fluorescein in 50 mM Na HCO_3 buffer, pH 9.5.
  1B: 50 mM Na HCO_3 buffer, pH 9.5.
  1C: 1 µM fluorescein, 5 mM anilinonaphthalenesulfonate (ANS) in 50 mM Na HCO_3 buffer, pH 9.5.
  1D: 1 µM fluorescein; with glycogen as scatterer, in 50 mM Na HCO3 buffer, pH 9.5.
  1E: Scatterer (glycogen) in 50 mM Na HCO_3 buffer, pH 9.5.
  1F: 100 pM fluorescein in 50 mM Na HCO_3 buffer, pH 9.5.

Operation of spectrofluorometers: see instructor sheets.

Procedures

Recording an Emission Spectrum – Rules 1 and 2.
1. Obtain Samples 1A and 1B from the instructor. Sample 1A is 1 µM fluorescein in 50 mM Na HCO_3 buffer, pH 9.5. Sample 1B is the same buffer without the fluorescein. Sample 1B is a "blank" or "control" sample.

2. After setting up the instrument, as described in the attached sheets, open the excitation shutter and verify that the emission shutter is closed. Set the excitation wavelength to 460 nm, and after opening the excitation shutter, note the color of the exciting light.

3. Insert a cuvette containing Sample 1A. In a darkened room, observe the sample fluorescence by eye. What color is it? Note how the apparent intensity does not change when you look at it from different angles; fluorescence is usually emitted isotropically.

4. Set the emission wavelength to 550 nm (see attached sheets), and set the excitation and emission band passes to 1 (students using fluorometer will set excitation bandpass to 1 and emission bandpass to 4). Open the emission shutter, and adjust the PMT voltage and slits to obtain optimum signal.

5. Once a suitable signal level is achieved, set the emission wavelength range to 500 to 700 nm, and record the emission spectrum. Where is the peak of emission? (Basic Rule 1).

6. Replace the Sample 1A in the cuvette with the Sample 1B (Note, you will need to wash the cuvette with nitric acid before putting Sample 1B in the cuvette). Record the emission spectrum under the same conditions as above. In case of same conditions, use the same instrument settings and gain. There are several reasons to do this (e.g. potential artifacts); do you know them?

7. Change the excitation wavelength to 440 nm, and reinsert the cuvette containing Sample 1A. Record its emission spectrum, and compare it to the one you recorded with excitation at 460 nm. How do they differ? (Basic Rule 2).

Rules 3 and 4 – Excitation Spectra

1. With Sample 1A still in place, change the emission wavelength to 550 nm, and set the excitation range to 310 to 510 nm. Measure the excitation spectrum and compare it to the absorption spectrum (provided by the instructor). How do they compare? Note the units.

2. Replace Sample 1A with Sample 1C in the cuvette (this contains 1 mM fluorescein and 5 mM nonfluorescent dye, ANS). Record its excitation spectrum. Compare with the excitation spectrum of the Sample 1A, and the absorption spectrum of Sample 1C (provided by the instructor). Why do they differ? (Basic Rule 3).

3. Plot the excitation and emission spectra of Sample 1A on the same sheet. How do they differ? (Basic Rule 4).

4.4.7   Use of Fluorescence

(a) In Binding Studies

Binding of ligands to proteins frequently cause changes to their three-dimensional structure. If this structural change has an effect on the environment of an intrinsic or extrinsic fluorophore, this can result in measurable changes in the fluorescence spectrum. Some extrinsic fluorophores such as 1-anilino 8-naphthalene sulphonate (ANS) are only strongly fluorescent when bound to proteins. ANS is binding to hydrophobic pockets on the protein. (Figure 4.39).

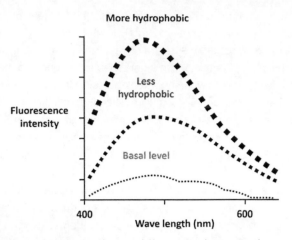

Fig. 4.39   Differential ANS binding to different conformational states of protein.

(b) Protein Folding Studies

Fluorescence is one of the main spectroscopic techniques used in the study of protein folding. Tryptophan is normally buried in the interior hydrophobic core of the protein. When protein unfolds, it exposes its core and tryptophan comes into contact with water and may be able to interact with quenching environment (Figure 4.40). Five main experimental parameters can be observed: (1) The fluorescence intensity may increase or decrease, (2) Fluorescence lifetime may decrease as a result of dynamic quenching, (3) The radiation emitted from an unfolded protein is usually lower in energy and therefore of longer wavelength, (4) The fluorophore rotational movement is less constrained in its unfolded state than in a folded state. So polarization can be affected by this process, (5) an external quencher can quench the fluorescence of tryptophan.

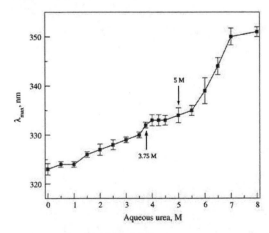

Fig. 4.40   Fluorescence maximum for BoNT/A LC in aqueous urea solution as a function of urea concentration. Samples were excited at $\lambda == 295$ nm and the wavelength corresponding to the maximum of fluorescence intensity were recorded for each concentration of urea. The profile of λmax shows a small plateau around 3.75–5.0M concentration of urea. This graph indicates that at 0M urea, protein is in a folded conformation, and at 8M urea it takes on an unfolded conformation.

Since a fluorophore has characteristic λmax values in both its absorbance and emission spectra, it is possible to conduct an experiment in which the emission λmax of one fluorophore (A) overlaps with the absorbance λmax of a second fluorophore (B). In this case it is possible that emission energy from one fluorophore will be absorbed by another fluorophore. This phenomenon is called Fluorescence Resonance Energy Transfer or FRET (Figure 4.41). FRET is strongly dependent on distance, R, between the fluorophore, especially in the range 10–80A. Efficiency of FRET is given by

$$E = R_0^6/(R_0^6 + R^6) \text{ or } 1 - (F_{da}/F_d) \quad \text{or} \quad 1 - (T_{da}/T_d)$$

where, R is the distance between donor and acceptor molecules, and R_0 is a constant related to the donar acceptor pair which can be calculated from their absorption and emission spectra. F_{da} and F_d are fluorescence intensities of donor in presence or absence of acceptor, respectively. Similarly, T_{da} and T_d are fluorescence lifetimes of donor in presence or absence of acceptor, respectively. Once the value of E is determined, R can be calculated.

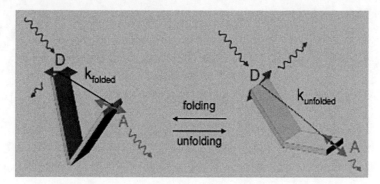

Fig. 4.41   Schematic representation of FRET analysis.

Box 4.6   Fluorescence Energy Transfer and Fluorescence Anisotropy

Description

Most fluorophores are hydrophobic in nature and some of them can bind to hydrophobic regions of a macromolecule such as protein. Such binding leads to drastic change in the microenvironment of the fluorophore compared to its aqueous solution. Environmental change could result in enhancement of fluorescence and in shift of the wavelength of maximum emission. Binding of fluorophores to proteins or other macromolecules allows estimation of energy transfer between intrinsic and extrinsic fluorophores, and determination of size, shape, and motions of the macromolecule.

Goal

The goal of this experiment is to observe the extent of energy transfer between Trp residues of bovine serum albumin (BSA), and to estimate rotational correlation time of BSA by monitoring ANS (aninlinonaphthalenesulfonate) anisotropy.

Samples

1. ANS in H_2O
2. H_2O as reference
3. BSA in H_2O
4. ANS + HSA in H_2O

Procedures

1. Based on previous two demonstrations, select excitation wavelength (340 nm) to measure ANS fluorescence spectrum between 400 and 500 nm.
2. Record the fluorescence spectrum of free and BSA bound ANS under identical instrumental settings.
3. The fluorescence lifetime of ANS bound to BSA is estimated as 9 ns. Estimate fluorescence lifetime of ANS in water. (Hint: $\tau \propto I_f$).
4. Record Trp emission spectra of BSA and BSA bound to ANS under identical conditions using identical concentrations of BSA. For Trp fluorescence, excitation at 295 nm and emission between 310 and 410 nm.
5. Measure steady state anisotropy of ANS bound to BSA (excitation 320 nm and emission by using 345 nm cut-off filter) by first determining $G = I_{HV}/I_{HH}$ at the emission wavelength of ANS, and then by determining I_{VV} and I_{VH}.

$$r = (I_{VV}-GI_{VH})/(I_{VV}+2GI_{VV})$$

6. Calculate rotational correlation time (θ) using the following equation:

$$r_0/r = 1 + \tau/\theta$$

    where, r_0 is limiting anisotropy (no rotation; assume value of 0.4), r is steady state anisotropy, τ is fluorescence lifetime (9 ns), and θ is the rotational correlation time

7. Using the relationship

$$\theta = \eta M (v + h)/RT$$

    where, η is viscosity of solution (0.01 Poise; 1 P = 1 dyne.s.cm^{-2}), M is molecular weight (g/mole, v is specific volume of the protein (assume 0.73 cm^3/g), h is hydration (d_wxV_w, where, d_w is hydration, typically 0.2g H_2O/gram protein, and V_w is specific volume of water, 1 cm^3/g, R is gas constant (8.314 x 10^7 ergs mol^{-1}K^{-1}; 1 erg = 1 dyne x cm), and T is absolute temperature (K). Calculate the molecular weight of BSA.

Safety Issues

High voltages are produced by the detector and lamp power supplies. Ordinarily, students will have no need to have access to this circuitry. The fluorescent dyes used in this experiment are not known to be toxic under experimental circumstances. However, do not get them on your skin and cloth, as they are difficult to wash away.

(c) Application of Fluorescence in Cell Biology

Due to high sensitivity, fluorescence has wide range of application in cellular microscopy. It allows the detection and visualization of specific cellular organelles and surface of individual cells. Combined with immunostaining these techniques can be used for more specific visualization (Figure 4.42).

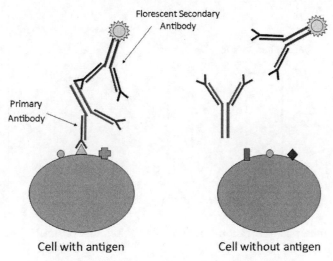

Fig. 4.42 Immunofluorescence microscopy.

4.5 Circular Dichroism (CD)

Light passing through a chromophore solution may interact with the sample in two main ways. The light may be refracted or absorbed. If the light is plane polarized and the sample is optically active then each enantiomer may interact differently with the left and right circularly polarized light. ORD (optical rotatory dispersion) arises from the fact that there is difference in refractive index of left and right polarized light. So, an ORD spectrum is a plot of Δn (difference in refractive index) versus wavelength (λ). Whereas, CD is absorption phenomenon in which left and right components of light are absorbed differently because of differences in molar extinction coefficient. So, plot of ΔA or $\Delta \varepsilon$ against wavelength (λ) is CD spectrum. Both CD and ORD spectra provide evidence of chirality of the sample leading to very useful techniques for chiral biopolymers such as proteins and nucleic acids.

Circular dichroism (CD) is basically the differential absorption of left- and right-handed circularly polarized light (Figure 4.44). This difference is expressed as absorption of ellipticity (θ).

Therefore,

$$\Delta A = A_L - A_R \quad \text{or} \quad \theta = \tan^{-1}(b/a) \quad \text{or} \quad 32.98\,\Delta A,$$

where, "b" and "a" describe the rotation of polarized light.

The data is normalized by scaling to molar concentrations of either the whole molecule or the repeating unit of a polymer. The Mean Residue Weight (MRW) for the peptide bond is calculated from $MRW = M/(N - 1)$, where M_{is} the molecular mass of the polypeptide chain (in Da), and N is the number of amino acids in the chain; the number of peptide bonds is N-1. For most proteins the MRW is 110±5 Da. The mean residue ellipticity at wavelength is

$$[\theta]_{MRW, \lambda} = MRW \times \theta_\lambda / 10 \times d \times c$$

where, θ_λ is the observed ellipticity (degrees) at wavelength λ, d is the path length (cm), and c is the concentration (g/ml).

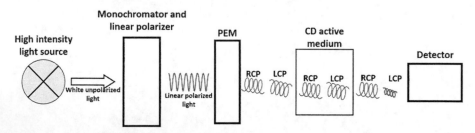

Fig. 4.43 Schematic representation of instrumentation for circular dichroism spectroscopy. RCP: Right Circularly Polarized Light, LCP: Left Circularly Polarized Light, while PEM stands for Photo Elastic Modulator.

If we know the molar concentration (m) of a solute, the molar ellipticity at wavelength k ([θ] molar λ) is given by:

$$[\theta]_{molar, \lambda} = 100 \times \theta_\lambda / m \times d$$

where, θ_λ and d have the same meaning as referred to earlier.

The size of signals in the far UV is a good way to check on the various experimental parameters and calibration of the instrument. Thus, a hypothetical protein which is 100% α-helix has a mean residue ellipticity at 222 nm of about -30,000 deg cm^2 dmol^{-1} ($\Delta\varepsilon$ = -9 M^{-1} cm^{-1}). Clearly the observed value for a real protein cannot be greater than this. For near UV CD, the mean residue ellipticities for the aromatic amino acid side chains of proteins should generally be less than 200 deg cm^2 dmol^{-1} ($\Delta\varepsilon$ less than 0.06 M^{-1} cm^{-1}).

4.5.1 Spectral Characteristics

(a) Near-UV Spectra of Proteins

Near-UV CD bands from individual residues in a protein may be either positive or negative and may vary dramatically in intensity. Knowledge of the position and intensity of CD bands expected for a particular chromophore is helpful in understanding the observed near-UV CD spectrum of a protein and the principal characteristics of the four chromophores are therefore summarized below:

- Phenylalanine has a sharp fine structure in the range 255–270 nm with peaks generally observed at wavelengths close to 262 and 268 nm.
- Tyrosine generally has a maximum in the range 275–282 nm, possibly with a red shifted shoulder (~6 nm) .

- Tryptophan often shows fine structure above 280 nm in the form of two ^{1}Lb bands (one at 288 to 293, and one some 7 nm towards the blue end; though both with the same sign) and a ^{1}La band (around 265 nm) with little fine structure.
- Cystine CD begins at long wavelength (> 320 nm) and shows one or two broad peaks above 240 nm; the long wavelength peak is frequently negative.

(b) Far-UV Spectra of Proteins

Far-UV CD spectra of proteins depend upon secondary structure content and just simple inspection of a spectrum will generally reveal information about the structural class of the protein. The characteristic features of the spectra of different protein classes may be summarized as follows (Table 4.5, Figure 4.45):

- All-α proteins show an intense negative band with two peaks (at 208 and 222 nm) and a strong positive band (at 191–193 nm). The intensities of these bands reflect alpha-helical content. $\Delta\varepsilon$mrw values for a totally helical protein would be of the order of -11 $M^{-1}cm^{-1}$ (at 208 and 222 nm) and +21 $M^{-1}cm^{-1}$ (at 191–193 nm).
- The spectra of regular all-β proteins are significantly weaker than those of all-α proteins. These spectra usually have a negative band (at 210–225 nm, $\Delta\varepsilon$mrw -1 to -3.5 $M^{-1}cm^{-1}$) and a stronger positive band (at 190–200 nm, $\Delta\varepsilon$mrw2 to 6 $M^{-1}cm^{-1}$).
- Unordered peptides and denatured proteins have a strong negative band (at 195–200 nm, $\Delta\varepsilon$mrw -4 to -8 $M^{-1}cm^{-1}$) and a much weaker band (which can be either positive or negative) between 215 and 230 nm ($\Delta\varepsilon$mrw +0.5 to -2.5 $M^{-1}cm^{-1}$).
- $\alpha+\beta$ and α/β proteins almost always have spectra dominated by the α-helical component and therefore often show bands at 222, 208 and 190–195 nm. In some cases there may be a single broad minimum between 210 and 220 nm because of overlapping α-helical and β-sheet contributions.

Table 4.5 Protein secondary structure elements and their maxima and minima in CD spectroscopy.

Secondary Structure	Electron Transition	Position of Minima or Maxima
α-helix	π to π* (positive)	190–195 nm
	π to π*	208 nm
	n to π*	222 nm
β-sheets	π to π*	195–200 nm
	n to π*	215–220 nm
Random coils	π to π*	~ 200 nm
	n to π*	220 nm

(c) Thermodynamics of unfolding

The thermodynamics of unfolding can be investigated by either (i) measuring the ellipticity at a single wavelength (usually 222 nm), and (ii) measuring ellipticity at single wavelength with respect to temperature. Additionally, free energy of folding and binding constants can be obtained by measuring CD as a function of denaturants, osmolytes or ligands, and determination of kinetic parameters can be done by measuring CD as a function of time.

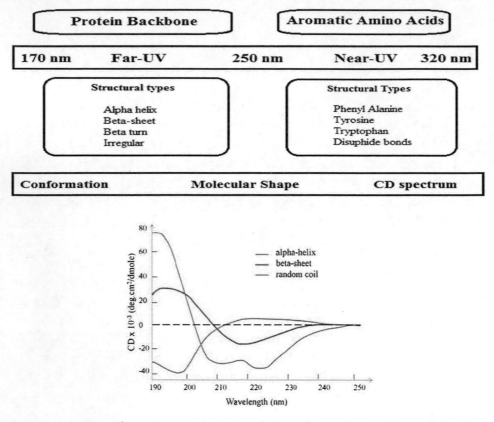

Fig. 4.44 Protein secondary structure elements and their CD spectrum (with permission from Wei et al., 2014).

Characterization of unfolding is done by following the change in ellipticity at a single wavelength as a function of temperature. In the simplest case, a molecule undergoes an unfolding transition between two states: folded, F, and unfolded, U. At a given temperature, the constant of folding, K, can be defined as:

$$K = [F]/[U]$$

Now, for defining thermodynamic parameters, we need to first define the free energy of folding, which can be given by

$$\Delta G = -RT \ln K$$

where, R is the Gas constant = 1.98 cal/mol and T is the absolute temperature (Kelvin).

The fraction folded at any temperature is α.

$$\alpha = [F]/([F] + [U])$$

$$\alpha = (\theta t - \theta u)/(\theta_F - \theta u)$$

where, θt is the observed ellipticity at any temperature, θ_F is the ellipticity of the fully folded form, and θu is the ellipticity of the unfolded form.

Now, along with all the above equations one can determine the melting temperature of the protein where $\alpha = 0.5$, and other thermodynamics parameters.

There are many different ways to analyze CD data. Analysis is mainly performed to estimate the percentage of secondary structure elements present in the data analysis; and, is done by using software. Some useful softwares are CDPro (lamar.colstate.edu/~sreeram/CDPro/ListPro.htm), Circular Dichroism at UMDNJ (www2.umdnj.edu/cdrwjweb), CONTIN (s-provencher.com/index. shtml), and DICROPROT (dicroprot-pbil.ibcp.fr). The algorithms of all these methods are based on the assumption that the CD spectrum of a protein can be represented by a linear combination of the spectra of its secondary structural components, plus a noise term. The noise is generated from aromatic chromophores and prosthetic groups.

$$\theta_\lambda = \Sigma \varepsilon_i S_{\lambda i} + \text{noise}$$

where, θ_λ is the CD of the protein as a function of wavelength; ε_i is the fraction of each secondary structure i; and $S_{\lambda i}$ is the ellipticity at each wavelength of each ith secondary structural element. The sum of all secondary structural elements should be equal to 1, and their fractional contribution must be greater than or equal to zero. Mainly, two methods are used to evaluate the protein conformation. In the first method, polypeptides with defined composition of known conformations are used as standards. Structures of these polypeptides are determined by X-ray scattering of films or by IR in solution. The second method uses spectra of proteins which are characterized by X-ray crystallography as standards. For analysis of unknown protein spectra, the methods may be any of least-square analysis, ridge regression, singular value decomposition (SVD), the self-consistent method, or neural network analysis.

All these methods and software programs are useful for the determination of α-helical content of globular proteins. However, K2D and CONTIN provide more accurate results for fibrous proteins such as collagen or coiled-coil proteins.

Although CD spectroscopy generally provides only low-resolution structural information, it does have two major advantages. First, it is extremely sensitive to changes in conformation, whatever their origin, and second, an extremely wide range of solvent conditions is accessible to study with relatively small amounts of material. The principal applications of CD spectroscopy in the study of biomolecules are:

(a) The estimation of protein secondary structure content from far-UV CD spectra.
(b) The detection of conformational changes in proteins and nucleic acids brought about by changes in pH, salt concentration, and added co-solvents (simple alcohols, trifluoroethanol, etc.) and the structural analysis of recombinant native proteins and their mutants.
(c) Monitoring protein or nucleic acid unfolding brought about by changes in temperature or by the addition of chemical denaturants (such as urea and guanidine hydrochloride; Figure 4.45).
(d) Monitoring protein–ligand, protein–nucleic acid, and protein–protein interactions.
(e) Studying (in favorable cases) the kinetics of macromolecule–macromolecule, macromolecule–ligand interactions (particularly slow dissociation processes), and the kinetics of protein folding reactions.

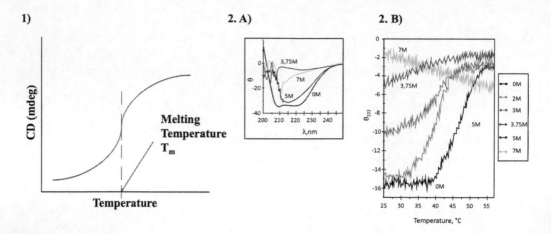

Fig. 4.45 Denaturation of a protein as measured by CD spectroscopy. Melting temperature (Tm) is dented by inflection point of the S-plot. 2(A) CD plot of Botulinum Toxin endopeptidase domain (BoNT/A LC) with respect to different concentration of urea. 2(B) Thermal denaturation of BoNT/A LC in (BoNT/A LC) in different concentrationss of urea.

Questions to ponder over

1. Why is it important to purge a CD spectrophotometer with nitrogen prior to measurement of CD spectra?
2. What is circular dichroism?
3. What is circular dichroism used for?
4. Different components used in CD spectrophotometer and their use?

Box 4.7   Thermodynamic Parameters of Protein Denaturation Monitored by CD Spectral Analysis

Experiment

Creating a record of the CD spectra of a protein under native (physiological pH and room temperature) and in denatured condition (at high temperature of 90–100°C).

Experimental plans

1. Prepare the protein solution in a buffer. Pay attention to the type of buffer, its pH and concentration in the protein solution. Check if the buffer used is the same as the one used for dissolving the protein. Also, check out the concentration of the protein being used for CD recordings.

2. Familiarize yourself with the instrument, sample compartment, special needs, computer software, etc. Be prepared to take notes on how to start the instrument, how to record data, and reasons for special needs – nitrogen flushing, unique cuvettes, etc.

3. Learn how to operate the instrument to record sample spectra (sample and reference) at room temperature, in the wavelength range of 250 to 190 nm. Also, learn how to process the data to obtain protein spectra.

4. Learn to record the protein spectra under native buffer conditions, and after denaturing the protein with high temperature. Look out for changes in the CD spectrum of the protein upon denaturation.

5. Record the denaturation curve at 222 nm. This will be followed by recording the renaturation curve on lowering the temperature to observe the reversibility of the protein denaturation.

6. Obtain the recorded spectra, denaturation curves, and temperature versus. CD signal data in XY format. Learn how to calculate thermodynamic parameters.

7. Obtain the data in two buffer conditions to compare their stability: these conditions may be at different pH, different salt conditions, presence and absence of 2 M urea, with and without 20% glycerol.

Data analysis and report

You will need to combine results from this demonstration in your report (2–3 pages) and provide your comments on the following:

(a) CD spectra of native and denatured protein.

(b) Determine the T_m of the protein.

(c) Calculate equilibrium denaturation constant at different temperature to estimate ΔG.

(d) Plot the van't Hoff graph to obtain ΔH and ΔS.

(e) Compare thermodynamic parameters in two buffer conditions.

4.6   FTIR Spectroscopy

The complete three-dimensional structure of a protein at high resolution can be determined by X-ray crystallography. This technique requires the molecule to be in the form of a well ordered crystal which is not possible for all proteins. An alternative to X-ray crystallography is multidimensional nuclear magnetic resonance (NMR) spectroscopy. Using NMR spectroscopy the structures of proteins in solution form can be determined. The interpretation of the NMR spectra of large proteins is very complex, so its present application is limited to small proteins (~45 KDa and less). These limitations have led to the development of alternative methods that can provide structural information on proteins (especially on secondary structure). These methods include circular dichroism (CD) and vibrational (Infrared and RAMAN) spectroscopy.

The technique of FTIR (Fourier Transform Infra Red) spectroscopy requires only small amounts of proteins (1 mM) in a variety of environments. Therefore, high quality spectra can be obtained relatively easily without problems of background fluorescence, light scattering, and problems related to the size of the proteins. The omnipresent water absorption can be subtracted by mathematical approaches. Methods are now available that can separate subcomponents that overlap in the spectra of proteins. These developments have made practical biological systems amenable to study by FTIR spectroscopy.

IR spectroscopy works through the measurement of the wavelength and intensity of the absorption of infrared light by a sample. Infrared light is energetic enough to excite molecular vibrations to higher energy levels. The infrared spectra usually have sharp features that are characteristic of specific types of molecular vibrations, making the spectra useful for sample identification. For a molecule of N atoms, 3N-6 fundamental vibrations (or normal modes) exist (3N-5 if the molecule is linear). Therefore, for the linear CO_2 molecule 4 normal modes have to be expected.

It can be shown that if the intensity of light is measured and plotted as a function of the position of the movable mirror, the resultant graph is the Fourier Transform of the intensity of light as a function of wave number. In FTIR spectroscopy, the light is directed onto the sample of interest, and the intensity is measured using an infrared detector. The intensity of light striking the detector is measured as a function of the mirror position, and this is then Fourier-transformed to produce a plot of intensity versus. wave number.

The IR spectral data of polymers are usually interpreted in terms of the vibration of a structural repeat unit. The polypeptide and protein repeat units give rise to nine characteristic IR absorption bands, namely amide A, B, and I-VII. Of these, the amide I and amide II bands are the two most prominent vibrational bands of the protein backbone (Figure 4.46). The most sensitive region is the amide I band (1700–1600 cm-1), which is due to mainly C=O stretching vibration of the peptide linkage. The frequencies of amide I band are found to correlate with secondary structure element of the protein. The amide-II band derives mainly in-plane NH bending and from the CN stretching vibration. Other amide bands are complex which mainly depends on other forces, H-bond and nature of the side chain (Table 4.6).

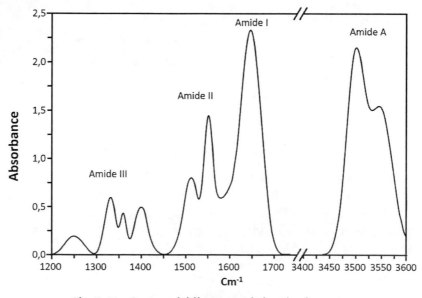

Fig. 4.46 Region of different amide bands of protein.

Table 4.6 Characteristic infrared band of peptide linkages.

Band	Vibration	Approximate Frequency (cm⁻¹)
Amide A	3300	N-H Stretching
Amide B	3100	N-H Stretching
Amide I	1600–1690	C = O stretching
Amide II	1480–1575	CN stretching, N-H bending
Amide III	1229–1301	CN stretching, N-H bending
Amide IV	625–767	OCN bending
Amide V	640–800	Out-of-plane N-H bending
Amide VI	337–606	Out-of-plane C=O bending

4.6.1 Analysis of Protein FTIR Data

Several methods have been developed to assign different secondary structure elements of protein from amide I band including FSD (Fourier self-deconvolution) curve fitting, second derivative analysis, partial-least square methods, and principle component analysis. FSD and second derivative analysis are the two most popular methods for analyzing FTIR spectra.

The important requirement of analysis in FSD method is to select a condition that achieves the maximum band narrowing while keeping the increase in noise and the appearance of side lobes at a minimum. Second derivative spectra allow the qualitative and quantitative determination of the various secondary structures present in the protein. A curve fitting procedure can be applied to calculate the secondary structure element (Figure 4.47).

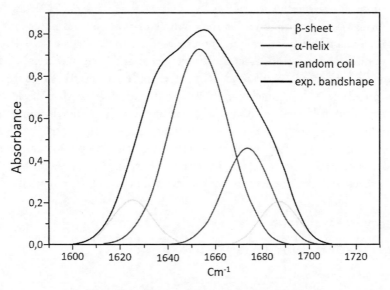

Fig. 4.47 Deconvolution of amide–I band.

4.7   Electrophoretic Techniques

The word *electrophoresis* is derived from the word *electric* and the Greek word *phoresis,* which means "being carried." In electrophoresis, charged particles are carried across a medium under an electric field. Because the movement of charged particles depends on their size and charge, particles with varying charges and sizes can be separated by electrophoresis. In biological systems, such variations are commonly encountered in amino acids, proteins, nucleotides, nucleic acids, and such. Biochemists are constantly required to separate biological molecules either for analytical or for preparative purpose. Biomolecules, in general, possess ionizable groups and, therefore, they can exist as cations (+) or anions (-), depending on the pH of solution, and this forms the basis of separation by an applied electric field. Electrophoresis has, therefore, become a very common biochemical tool over the last half century. Electrophoretic separation can be achieved either in solution (e.g., as in capillary and free flow systems) or in a support matrices (e.g., agarose or polyacrylamide gels) (Figure 4.48).

There are several electrophoresis techniques commonly applied in the analysis of biological molecules. For example, paper (or filter paper or cellulose acetate) electrophoresis is used to separate amino acids. Agarose gel electrophoresis is usually employed to separate nucleic acids. Polyacrylamide gel electrophoresis is commonly used for the analysis of proteins and polypeptides. Capillary electrophoresis, a relatively new technique, is being used for the analysis of a variety of molecules including proteins, peptides, amino acids, nucleic acids, and pharmaceuticals. Many of these techniques are used under specialized conditions for separation of specific molecules. For example, in immunoelectrophoresis (IE), proteins are first separated on a polyacrylamide electrophoresis gel followed by the detection of separated proteins by specific antibodies. This electrophoretic method is also known as the Western blot technique. In another example, pulse field gel electrophoresis (PFGE), large DNA molecules are separated on agarose gels by a pulsed (in duration and strength) electric field as opposed to constant electric field. In iso-electric focusing (IEF), proteins are electrophoresed in a medium possessing a pH gradient that allows determination of the protein iso-electric point.

4.7.1   Theory of Electrophoresis

The movement of a charged particle in an electric field is given by

$$v = Eq/f$$

where, v is velocity of particle (cm/s), E is the electric field (volts/cm), q is the net charge on the particle, and f is the frictional coefficient (a function of size, shape and mass). Thus, the velocity of a charged particle is directly proportional to the electric field I and charge (q), but inversely proportional to the frictional force (f) created by viscous drag. The electric field is defined either by the current or voltage related by Ohm's law

$$V = IR$$

where, V, I and R are voltage, current and resistance, respectively.

The charge, q, is dependent on the molecular structure and the solvent conditions. For example, in a protein molecule, charge will depend on the amino acid composition and the pH of the buffer.

The frictional coefficient, f, is function of the radius of the particle. For a perfect sphere, the frictional coefficient (f_o) is represented by Stoke's law,

$$f_o = 6\pi\eta_o r_o$$

where, η_o is the viscosity of the solvent and r_o is the radius of the sphere (Stoke's radius).

However, most biological molecules are not perfect spheres. For non-spherical particles, the frictional coefficient (f) is given by

$$f = 6\pi\eta_o rA$$

where, r is radius of a sphere, and A is a complex term involving the axial ratio of ellipsoid of revolution. Basically the above terms define the deviation of a biological molecule from an assumed spherical shape. However, since biological molecules are far from being spheres or ellipsoids, it is generally not possible to accurately define their frictional coefficients.

Electrophoresis is carried out either at constant current or constant voltage. Since the velocity of the particle is given by v = Eq/F, at constant E, the velocity depends on q and f. When molecules of similar conformation such as DNA or globular proteins are analyzed, the variable factors become limited to size and not shape. The size factor encompasses two parameters, the volume and the mass. Considering a consistent proportionality constant between mass and volume of a biological molecule (a reasonable assumption), the f will depend only on the mass of the particle.

Under conditions where the biological molecules being analyzed have similar conformations and densities, the frictional coefficient, f, thus depends on the mass of particles. Therefore, the migration of the particles under the influence of an electric field will be proportional to their charges (q) and to their mass (m) ratios.

The migration of a charged particle in an electric field is defined in terms of mobility, μ, which is the velocity per unit electric field and is given by,

$$\mu = v/E$$

substituting v = Eq/f, one can obtain
$$\mu = Eq/Ef$$
$$= q/f$$

Assuming similar conformation and density of a group of particles, their mobility can be defined as

$$\mu_I = q_I/m_I$$

where, μ_I is the mobility of the ith particle, q_I is the net charge on the ith particle, and m_I is mass of the ith particle.

In theory, if we know the net charge on a molecule, its mass can be calculated from the electrophoretic mobility, which can be determined experimentally. However, this has not been possible due to several factors. These factors include interactions between migrating molecules and support medium, uncertainty over the influence of various molecular sizes and shapes on the frictional coefficient, shielding of the molecules by ions in solutions such as buffers.

Therefore, electrophoresis can generally be used to separate molecules for their identification and to check the purity of a molecule. For other applications such as iso-electric point determination or size estimation, the technique is used in combination with standard molecules of known characteristics.

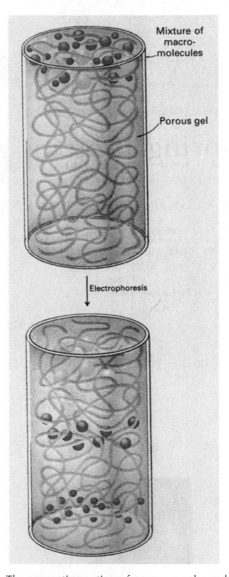

Fig. 4.48   The separating action of a porous polyacrylamide gel.

4.7.2 Polyacrylamide Gel

Polyacrylamide is a support medium for electrophoresis (Figure 4.49). It is prepared by free radical-induced polymerization of acrylamide and a cross-linking agent, N,N′-methylene-bis-acrylamide. An initiator–catalyst system of ammonium persulfate-TEMED (N,N,N′,N′-tetramethylethylenediamine) or Riboflavin (with exposure to UV light)-TEMED produces the free radicals, initiates the polymerization, and catalyzes the polymerization (Figure 4.49).

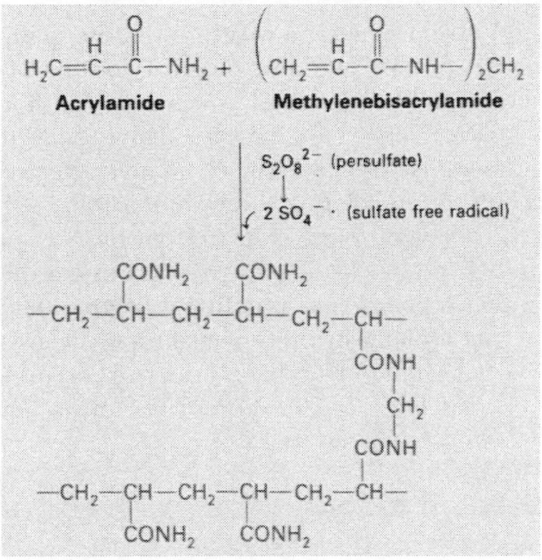

Fig. 4.49 Formation of polyacrylamide gel. The pore size can be controlled by adjusting the concentration of activated monomer (red) and cross-linker (green). [See color plates]

Polyacryl-amide gels are cast either in tubes or on a slab. Polymerization of the acrylamide in the presence of the cross-linker creates a mesh-like structure in the polyacrylamide gels. The pore size in the mesh depends on the concentration of the gel and on the ratio of acrylamide and bisacrylamide. For example, a 7.5% (T; total) polyacrylamide gel could contain 6.75% acrylamide and 0.75% (C; cross-linker) bis-acrylamide. The pore size decreases with increase in the %T polyacrylamide and/or %C bis-acrylamide.

The choice of the polyacrylmide gel concentration and cross-linker concentration is determined by the size of molecules to be analyzed. Lower concentration gels with larger pores allow analysis of relatively high molecular weight proteins, whereas higher concentration gels can resolve relatively low molecular weight proteins better.

4.7.3 Agarose Gels

Agarose is a linear polymer of polysaccharide (~12000 Da) having a basic unit of agarobiose (alternating units of galactose and 3,6-anhydrogalactose). It is naturally isolated from certain seaweeds. Generally, between 1 to 3% agarose concentration is used to prepare agarose gel. Higher concentration of agarose will produce gel of small-pore size, and lower concentration of agarose will produce gel of larger pore sizes. To form agarose gel, agarose is suspended in an aqueous buffer, followed by boiling the mixture to form a clear solution which is then poured into a vessel and allowed to cool to form gel. Both inter- and intra- molecular hydrogen bonding plays a role in the formation of gel and cross-linking. The cross-linking of agarose gel gives it anti-convectional properties.

Although agarose gels can be used for the electrophoresis of both protein and nucleic acids, it is more frequently used in separation of nucleic acids. Its advantages include, ease in handling and sample recovery. Because of its low melting point, agarose gel does not denature the DNA samples.

4.7.4   Sodium Dodecyl Sulfate-Polyacrylamide Gel Electrophoresis (SDS-PAGE)

Electrophoresis is generally one-dimensional (i.e. one plane of separation) or two-dimensional. In biochemical laboratories one-dimensional electrophoresis is used for routine separations of protein and nucleic acid, whereas two-dimensional separation is used for finger printing of protein, and when properly constructed can be extremely accurate in resolving all of the proteins present within a cell (greater than 1,500). Both of these techniques are also used for preparation of sample for mass spectrometry for determination of protein sequence.

In general, gel electrophoresis is used to determine the molecular weight of proteins, to determine the purity of proteins, and to identify proteins by the use of immunoblotting (this technique identifies proteins blotted onto nitrocellulose by the use of antibodies). It has been used as a source of proteins for amino acid sequencing and also as a source of antigen for the immunization of animals to obtain antibodies against the purified protein.

Polyacrylamide is the most commonly used matrix for protein electrophoresis. Casting of the gel is done between two vertical plates. It also reduces influence of oxygen, which can affect the formation of gel.

Polyacrylamide gels are formed from the polymerization of two compounds, acrylamide and N,N-methylene- bis-acrylamide (Bis, for short). Bis is a cross-linking agent for the gels. The polymerization is initiated by the addition of ammonium persulfate along with either -dimethyl amino-propionitrile (DMAP) or N,N,N,N,- tetramethylethylenediamine (TEMED). The gels are neutral, hydrophillic, three-dimensional networks of long hydrocarbons cross-linked by methylene groups.

The separation of molecules within a gel is determined by the relative size of the pores formed within the gel. The pore size of a gel is determined by two factors, the total amount of acrylamide present (designated as %T) and the amount of cross-linker (%C). As the total amount of acrylamide increases, the pore size decreases. With cross-linking, 5%C gives the smallest pore size. Any increase or decrease in %C increases the pore size. Gels are designated as percent solutions and will have two necessary parameters. The total acrylamide is given as a % (w/v) of the acrylamide plus the bis-acrylamide. Thus, a 7½% T would indicate that there is a total of 7.5 gms of acrylamide and bis per 100 ml of gel. A gel designated as 7.5%T:5%C would have a total of 7.5% (w/v) acrylamide + bis, and the bis would be 5% of the total (with pure acrylamide composing the remaining 2.5%).

Protein samples are prepared in SDS (sodium dodecyl sulfate). When the detergent SDS is used with proteins, and separation done on a polyacrylamide gel, the term for the procedure is abbreviated as SDS-PAGE (for Sodium Dodecyl Sulfate PolyAcrylamide Gel electrophoresis). Sodium dodecyl sulfate (SDS), also known as sodium laurel sulfate, is an anionic detergent that binds to proteins. SDS has two important effects on proteins:

(i)   SDS disrupts non-covalent bonds in proteins resulting in their denaturation.

(ii) SDS converts all proteins to negatively charged molecules. As a result all proteins migrate towards the positively charged anode.

These two effects permit one to separate proteins based only on their molecular weights.

Proteins with molecular weights ranging from 10,000 to 1,000,000 may be separated with acrylamide gels, while proteins with higher molecular weights require lower acrylamide gel concentrations. Conversely, gels with higher acrylamide concentration have been used to separate small polypeptides. The higher the gel concentration, the smaller the pore size of the gel and the better it will be able to separate smaller molecules. The percent gel to use depends on the molecular weight of the protein to be separated. Use 5% gels for proteins ranging from 60,000 to 200,000 daltons, 10% gels for a range of 16,000 to 70,000 daltons and 15% gels for a range of 12,000 to 45,000 daltons.

The original use of gels as separating media involved using a single gel with a uniform pH throughout. Molecules were separated on the basis of their mobility through a single gel matrix. This system has only occasional use in today's laboratory. It has been replaced with discontinuous, multiple gel systems (Figure 4.50). In multiple gel systems, a separating gel is augmented with a

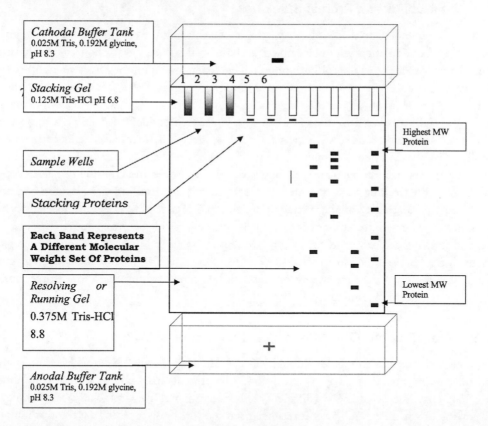

Fig. 4.50 Schematic of basic set-up for polyacrylamide gel electrophoresis. Lanes 1–3 show samples shortly after loading into the wells. Lanes 4–6 show samples after the dye has just entered the stacking gel. Lanes 7–9 show samples that have been resolved into their component parts in the resolving gel. Lane 10 shows molecular weight markers that have been run so that the molecular weights of the resolved components of the samples can be determined. The largest protein is the uppermost band in any lane. The next largest protein would be the second highest band in any lane and so forth. Note the different buffers and the presence of two different gels that compose a discontinuous buffer gel.

stacking gel and an optional sample gel. These gels can have different concentrations of the same support media, or may be completely different agents. The key difference is how the molecules separate when they enter the separating gel. The proteins in the sample gel will concentrate into a small zone in the stacking gel before entering the separating gel. The zone within the stacking gel can range in thickness from a few microns to a full millimeters. As the proteins are stacked in concentrated bands, they continue to migrate into the separating gel in concentrated narrow bands. The bands then are separated from each other on a discontinuous (i.e. disc) pH gel. Once the protein bands enter the separating gel, separation of the bands is enhanced by ions passing through the gel column in pairs. Each ion in the pair has the same charge polarity as the protein (usually negative), but differ in charge magnitude. One ion will have a much greater charge magnitude than the proteins, while the other has a lesser charge magnitude than the proteins. Next section describes the whole process in details.

4.7.4.1 *Ion Mobility and Protein Stacking*

Ion mobility is dependent on the charge density of a molecule and the voltage gradient. At a given pH only part of a population of protein molecules will be dissociated (i.e., charged) at any time. The velocity at which these molecules migrate will be dependent upon the effective mobility and the voltage gradient. Therefore, an ion of lower mobility can migrate as fast as one with higher mobility if the products of voltage and effective mobility are equal. The sample and stacking gel contain Tris-HCl buffer whereas the upper electrode reservoir contains Tris-Glycine buffer. At the pH of the sample buffer and stacking gel (pH 6.7), glycine is weakly ionized and therefore, its mobility is low. Chloride is completely ionized and has a much higher mobility, while the mobility of proteins are intermediate, i.e., between that of glycine and chloride. Once a voltage is applied, chloride (leading) ions migrate away from the glycine (trailing) ions leaving behind a zone of lower conductivity, a higher voltage gradient, and higher pH. The zone accelerates the glycine so it keeps up with the chloride ions. As this glycine/chloride boundary moves through the sample and stacking gel, any proteins in front are rapidly overtaken by chloride ions which have a higher velocity. Behind the moving boundary, the proteins have a higher velocity than glycine. Therefore, the moving boundary sweeps up the proteins, concentrating them into thin zones or stacks in order of decreasing mobility.

4.7.4.2 *What Happens Once the Proteins Have Been Stacked?*

First, the stacked proteins may migrate through a low percentage gel, remaining stacked or unresolved behind the moving boundary or dye front. Second, the proteins may unstack or resolve from the moving boundary. There could be two different methods for unstacking. Unstacking can be achieved by (a) slowing down the protein after it has been stacked, or (b) by speeding up the trailing ions once the protein has been stacked. In the first case, a low percent stacking gel is cast over a higher percentage resolving gel. As the stacked protein enters the higher percentage resolving gel, its mobility is reduced so that it is slower than the glycine ion. Once this occurs, the protein escapes the stack and migrates as if it were in a continuous gel at similar, lower, local field strength. The second case of unstacking uses a shift in pH to accelerate the trailing ions. For the glycine/chloride system, a stacking gel is cast so that the glycine zone will regulate to a lower pH than the resolving gel. When the glycine enters the higher pH resolving gel, its net negative charge will increase its effective mobility. Consequently, the glycine overtakes some of the proteins and now migrates directly behind the chloride ions, causing these proteins to resolve. After this, resolution of different proteins in the sample is achieved because of difference in the molecular weight.

4.7.4.3 *Buffer Systems Used in Gel Electrophoresis*

There are two buffer systems in gel electrophoresis: continuous buffers and discontinuous buffers systems.

4.7.4.3.1 *Continuous Buffer Systems*

Continuous buffer systems consist of a single separating buffer, in which the composition of the gel buffer and running buffer are essentially identical throughout the gel. The buffer has the same pH throughout the gel and reservoirs. Separation is achieved by molecular charge density and gel pore size.

The proteins in a sample applied to a continuous system will move faster in the sample well than in the gel. A concentrated band of sample will form where the molecules are slowed down at the interface of the buffer and the restrictive gel. This type of stacking has limitations, particularly when separating molecules vary widely in size. The smaller molecules have less of a difference between their free solution mobility and their mobility in a gel, so the sharpening factor is not as favorable as in the case of the larger molecules.

4.7.4.3.2 *Discontinuous Buffer Systems*

Discontinuous buffer systems have different buffer ions and pH in the gel and in the electrode reservoirs. Samples are loaded onto a non-restrictive large-pore gel, called a stacking gel, which overlays a smaller pore resolving gel. The major advantages of discontinuous buffer systems are that relatively large volumes of dilute protein samples can be applied to the gel and resolution is much greater than that obtained with continuous systems. This increased resolution is a direct result of the way proteins concentrate, or stack, into narrow zones during migration through the large-pore stacking gel, and destack or resolve, under the given conditions in the small-pore resolving gel.

In the discontinuous buffer system a second or stacking gel is placed on top of the resolving gel; the proteins are loaded into the stacking gel (see Figure 4.51). In the Laemmli system, different buffers are used in the stacking and resolving gels. Both the pH and the concentration of the components are different. These buffers in turn are different from the tank buffer in both concentration and in pH.

There are two particularly attractive features of the discontinuous buffer system. One is that a dilute protein sample in the well is concentrated at the interface of the stacking and resolving gels before entering the resolving gel. The second attractive feature is the ability of this system to resolve proteins into readily distinguishable and relatively narrow protein bands that are readily cut out. Once removed, the protein in the band may be injected as an antigen or micro sequenced.

In conclusion, many studies employing zone electrophoresis of proteins in a polyacrylamide gel use a buffer system designed to dissociate all proteins into their individual polypeptide subunits.

The most common dissociating agent is sodium dodecyl sulfate (SDS), an ionic detergent which denatures proteins by wrapping around the polypeptide backbone. By heating the protein sample at 100°C in the presence of excess SDS and thiol reagent, disulfide bonds are cleaved and the protein is fully dissociated into its subunits. Under these conditions most polypeptides bind SDS in a constant weight ratio (1.4 g of SDS: 1 g of polypeptide). The intrinsic charges of the polypeptide are insignificant compared to the negative charges provided by the bound detergent so that the SDS-polypeptide complexes have essentially the same negative charge and shape, and migrate through the gel strictly according to polypeptide size. The simplicity and speed of this method, plus the fact that only microgram quantities of protein are required, have made SDS-PAGE the most widely used method for determination of molecular mass in a polypeptide sample. Proteins from almost any source are readily solubilized by SDS, so the method is generally applicable. In contrast, non-dissociating native buffer systems, where proteins are electrophoresed in their native form, are designed to fractionate a protein mixture such that subunit interaction, native protein conformation, and biological activity are preserved. Proteins in non-dissociating native systems are separated based on their charge-to-mass ratio.

4.7.4.4 *Safety*

Unpolymerized acrylamide – even in the liquid form – are skin irritants and neurotoxins. Acrylamide may be absorbed through the skin. To prevent absorption through the skin it is important that you wear gloves whenever you are handling acrylamide. Since some unpolymerized acrylamide may be present in the gels it is *important that gloves be worn whenever handling acrylamide gels.*

4.7.5 Isoelectric Focusing (IEF) Gel Electrophoresis

Iso-electric focusing is a special form of electrophoresis technique, which is generally used to estimate iso-electric point of a protein. Proteins are polyelectrolytes due to the presence of different side chains of amino acids in their polypeptide chains with wide ranging pKa values. Thus, under different solution conditions, a given protein could have a net negative, positive or neutral charge. The pH at which a protein has a net charge of zero is referred to the iso-electric point (pI) of that protein. Because of the varying nature and composition of amino acids in their polypeptide chains, different proteins have unique iso-electric points.

Knowledge of a protein's pI of could be used in a variety of ways to understand its structure-function behavior under physiological or in vitro conditions. On a practical side, the pI of a protein is used to design its purification protocol using *ion-exchange chromatography* (see Chapter 2). Briefly, in ion-exchange chromatography, a resin is derivatized with certain acidic or basic groups so that in given solvent conditions, they will be either positively or negatively charged. If under the same solvent conditions, a protein has a net charge opposite to that of the resin, it will bind to the resin and will not elute along with other proteins in a mixture. The bound protein can be eluted by changing the solvent conditions. The protein is ultimately obtained in a purified form. As you can see, if the pI of the target protein is known, an appropriate resin can be selected for its purification.

Other applications of pI include separation and identification of proteins in crude extract mixtures. This process is simply carried out by electrophoresing a soluble mixture of proteins on a polyacrylamide or agarose gel, followed by either staining or by reacting with enzyme substrates or antibodies against proteins. Sometimes, the presence of a protein in a mixture can be derived by simply estimating its pI by comparison with standard proteins of known pIs.

Finally, a mixture of proteins can be separated and identified based on their pIs in one dimension and based on their molecular sizes in the second dimension. This is the basis of two-dimensional electrophoresis commonly used to identify the presence of proteins in complex crude mixture of cellular extract. Two-dimensional electrophoresis is commonly used to identify the expression of unique proteins or changes in the gene expression of cells under conditions that may cause diseases.

Questions to ponder over

1. What will happen if the running buffer is (i) more concentrated? (ii) less concentrated?
2. What is the importance in measurement of the dye front?
3. Explain the reason behind a sharper band in the gradient gel?
4. When trying to distinguish between the bands of a small protein (20–40 kDa), what percentage of cross-linked gel is better and why?

4.7.5.1 *Principles of Isoelectric Focusing*

Proteins under an electric field move towards the cathode or anode, based on their net positive or negative charges, respectively. Under a solution pH condition where a given protein has a net neutral charge, i.e., at its pI, it will not move either to the anode or cathode (Figure 4.51).

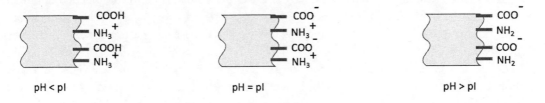

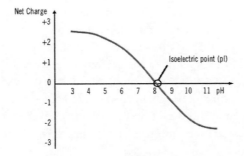

Fig. 4.51 Concept of pI and plot of net charge with respect to pH.

In isoelectric focusing (IEF), proteins are electrophoresed in a medium (polyacrylamide or agarose) that maintains a pH gradient between the cathode and anode. A protein applied at any point on the gel will migrate to the cathode or anode depending on its net charge, until it reaches the place on the gel where the pH of the medium matches with the pI of the protein. Because the protein loses its net charge at that point, it does not migrate any further, and becomes focused; hence the term *focusing* for the process. Since the focusing of the protein is due to its iso-electric point, it is called iso-electric focusing.

4.7.5.2 *The Process of Isoelectric Focusing and the Estimation of pI*

Isoelectric focusing is an electrophoretic method in which proteins are separated by their pI. Protein net charge is determined by pH of local environment. Protein can have a positive, negative, or zero charge depending on its pH environment.

4.7.5.3 *Establishing a pH Gradient*

One of the important steps in IEF is to create a pH gradient. To carry out iso-electric focusing, a gel (e.g., polyacrylamide) is prepared much the same way as for SDS-PAGE, except it is generally of lower concentration to allow relatively hindrance-free movement of proteins in the electric field. Another difference from regular SDS-PAGE is its immobilized pH gradients. This pH gradient is created through addition of ampholytes to the SDS-PAGE gel making buffer. Ampholytes are low molecular weight synthetic polyelectrolytes with varying number of amino and carboxylic groups. Thus a mixture of ampholytes can have a wide range of iso-electric points depending on their nature and number. A mixture of at least 180 individual ampholytes, are required to establish a pH gradient of 4 to 10 between the anode and cathode. Narrower pH gradients can be created with about 30 species of ampholytes per pH unit. Narrower pH gradients are recommended to obtain better resolution in estimating the pI of a protein. In practice, a wider range (pH 3–10) gradient is used first to approximate the pI of a protein, followed by the use of a narrower range (generally within two pH units).

The anode and cathode are placed on filter paper dipped in anolyte (usually a weak acid) and catholyte (NaOH or organic base such as histidine), respectively. The gel is pre-run for 15–20 minutes at low power (20 watts) to create the pH gradient, as the ampholytes with high pI having higher net positive charge will move towards the cathode while low pI ampholytes will move towards the anode. The sample under study is applied on the gel in one lane along with standard pI markers in a separate lane. The samples and markers can be applied at any place on the gel, as migration (to cathode or anode) and focusing will only depend on their net charges and pI, respectively. However, samples are generally applied in the middle of the gel for convenience.

The sample and markers (Table 4.7) are electrophoresed at 250 watts for 3–5 hours. It should be mentioned here that pre-running of the gel to create a pH gradient is not necessary. Sample and markers can be electrophoresed at the same time as the gradient is being formed. This is possible because, ampholytes being smaller in size migrate faster than proteins, and establish the pH gradient ahead of the protein migration.

The focused proteins are then fixed by treating with 20% trichloroacetate for 10 minutes, followed by washing the gel twice in double distilled water for 15 minutes each to remove ampholytes.

Ampholytes must be removed before staining IEF gel, because the Coomassie blue R-250 will otherwise react with them. Staining and destaining of the gel is performed in the same manner as that for SDS-PAGE.

The pI of the sample protein is estimated by plotting a calibration curve of the distance of the marker proteins migration from the cathode end versus their pI, and comparing the distance of the sample protein band from the cathode end.

Table 4.7   IEF Standard Proteins.

Standard Protein	pI	MW (Da)
Phycocyanin (3 bands)	4.45 4.65 4.75	232000
β-Lactoglobulin B	5.10	18400
Bovine carbonic anhydrase	6.00	31000
Human carbonic anhydrase	6.50	28000
Equine myoglobin (2 bands)	6.80 7.00	17500
Human hemoglobin A	7.10	64500
Human hemoglobin C	7.50	64500
Lentil lectin (3 bands)	7.80 8.00 8.20	49000
Cytochrome c	9.60	12200

4.7.6   Two-dimensional Gel Electrophoresis

One of the useful and widely accepted tools in protein research is two-dimensional gel electrophoresis (2-D electrophoresis). It is used for the analysis of complex protein mixtures extracted from cells, tissues, or other biological samples. This technique involves two steps: first, IEF, and second, SDS-PAGE. In the first step iso-electric focusing (IEF), separates proteins according to their iso-electric points (pI); in the second-step of SDS-polyacrylamide gel electrophoresis (SDS-PAGE), proteins are separated according to their molecular weights (MW). In this way, complex mixtures consisting of thousands of different proteins can be resolved and the relative amount of each protein can be determined.

Since this technique involves IEF, it requires placing the sample in gel with a pH gradient, and applying a potential difference across it. In the electrical field, the protein migrates along the pH gradient, until it carries no overall charge. In this step, separation occurs based on their respective pIs.

The separation in the second step by molecular size is performed in slab SDS-PAGE. Before separating the proteins by mass, they are treated with SDS along with other reagents. This denatures the proteins (that is, it unfolds them into long, straight molecules) and binds a number of SDS molecules roughly proportional to the protein's length. Then, an electric potential is again applied, but at a 90 degree angle from the first field. The proteins will be attracted to the more positive side of the gel (because SDS is negatively charged) proportionally to their mass-to-charge ratio. The gel acts like a molecular sieve when the current is applied, separating the proteins on the basis of their molecular weight with larger proteins being retained higher in the gel and smaller proteins being able to pass through the sieve and reach lower regions of the gel.

The result of this is a gel with proteins spread out on its surface. These proteins can then be detected by a variety of means, but the most commonly used stains are silver and Coomassie Brilliant Blue staining.

4.7.6.1 *Sample Preparation*

The IEF is the most critical step of the 2-D electrophoresis process. The proteins must be solubilized without charged detergents, usually in highly concentrated urea solution, reducing agents and chaotrophs. To obtain high quality data it is essential to achieve low ionic strength conditions before the IEF itself. Since different types of samples differ in their ion content, it is necessary to adjust the IEF buffer and the electrical profile to each type of sample.

4.7.6.2 *Protocol for SDS-PAGE*

A. **Sample Preparation:** Samples are prepared by dissolving appropriate amounts in a suitable buffer and adding SDS-sample loading buffer. Samples are then boiled in water for 5 minutes.
B. **Sample Loading:** Place the gel in the electrophoresis unit and fill the chamber holding the gel with running buffer. Remove the well comb by pulling it straight up. Rinse the sample wells with running buffer. Slowly place 5 µl of standard and 10–20 µl of sample in the wells.
C. **Running the gel:** Begin the separation with a constant voltage (150–250 V).
D. **Staining the gel:** After the separation, place the gel in a container with just enough water to cover the gel completely. Remove the water and add staining solution and rock the container gently for 20–30 min. Remove the staining solution and wash the gel with water to remove staining solution until the background has desired appearance.
E. **Analysis:** After proper destaining, measure the distance of standard bands and sample bands from the dye front. Determine relative migration distance, R_f of standard bands and unknown proteins bands. R_f is defined as the migration distance of band through the gel divided by the migration distance of the dye front. Plot a graph of the log of the standard protein molecular mass on the ordinate and the standard protein R_f on the abscissa. From the standard graph, determine the molecular weight of unknown protein band.

4.7.7 Capillary Electrophoresis

Capillary electrophoresis is one of the preferred methods for analyzing complex samples. This technique can be used to separate amino acids, peptides, proteins, DNA fragments, and nucleic acids. It can be also used for the separation of small molecules and metal ions. This technique involves a capillary of very narrow internal diameter tube (~ 50 µm; external tube diameter ~ 300 µm). Using a thin-diameter tube is advantageous, because it has large surface to volume ratio, which allows heat dissipation. This helps in eliminating zone broadening and convection currents. In capillary electrophoresis, such a capillary is filled with a conductive fluid (a buffer) at an appropriate pH.

A sample is introduced in the capillary either by pressure injection or electrokinetic (high voltage) injection. Sample components then move under the influence of an applied electric field (generally > 300 V/cm). The sample components may have positive, negative, and neutral charges. All the components now move through the capillary at different rates. Electrophoretic migration causes the movement of charge molecules towards the electrode of opposite charge. However, separation is due to electrophoretic migration; all the species (components) are drawn towards the cathode due to electro-endosmosis. Since, the flow in the capillary is very strong, therefore, the electro-endosmosis is always strong compared to the electrophoretic mobility, regardless of the charge of the species (components) and neutral charge species always move towards the cathode. Combination of strong fluid flow, electrophoretic mobility and electro-endosmosis results in the separation of bands. In general, ultraviolet detectors are used to detect the components as they approach the cathode (Figure 4.52).

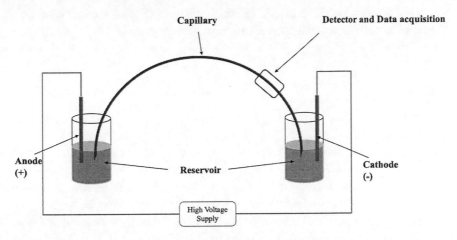

Fig. 4.52   Representation of capillary electrophoresis instrumentation.

As mentioned there are mainly two types of injection techniques for sample introduction in the capillary:

(a) *High voltage injection*: In this method, the anodic side reservoir is replaced by sample reservoir and sample (usually 5–30 µl of a 1 mg/ml solution) is introduced into capillary by applying a high voltage briefly. After application of sample, sample reservoir is replaced with buffer reservoir and voltage is applied again for separation.

(b) *Pressure injection*: In this method capillary is removed from the reservoir and inserted through an air-tight seal of sample solution. A second tube provides pressure to the sample solution, which forces sample into the capillary.

A range of variations are available in capillary electrophoresis, such as:

Capillary zone electrophoresis (CZE): It is also known as a free solution CE. In this only the difference in mobility causes the separation of components.

Capillary gel electrophoresis: In this mode, capillary is filled with gel matrix. Components of different size but same mobility can be separated by this technique.

Non-aqueous capillary electrophoresis: This technique is useful in the separation of samples insoluble in water. Instead of buffer as a migrating fluid, organic solvents are used.

Other related modes: are the chromatographic separation mode, capillary IsoTachophoresis, and the micellar electrokinetic mode.

Questions to ponder over

1. Explain how the presence of a salt in a protein solution could affect the running of an IEF gel of that protein.
2. Explain what is taking place in the gel during the pre-run phase of the analysis.
3. In an IEF gel, a protein migrates to a pH that matches which protein characteristic?
4. What are the different methods of identification of a protein band in SDS-PAGE or IEF?
5. What is the reason behind using narrow capillaries in capillary electrophoresis?
6. Give three advantages of capillary electrophoresis over gel electrophoresis and two advantages of gel electrophoresis over capillary electrophoresis.

References

Bloomfield, V. A. (2000). Survey of biomolecular hydrodynamics. *On-Line Biophysics Textbook: Separations and Hydrodynamics*.

Dingle, A. (2014). *Determining the Energy Pathways in Light Harvesting Complex II using Femtosecond Laser Techniques at Two Excitation Wavelengths*. Department of Physics and Electronics, Rhodes University.

Galyuk, E. N., Wartell, R. M., Dosin, Y. M. and Lando, D. Y. (2009). DNA denaturation under freezing in alkaline medium. *Journal of Biomolecular Structure and Dynamics*, 26(4), 517–523.

Garriga, P., Sági, J., Garcia-Quintana, D., Sabés, M. and Manyosa, J. (1990). Conformational Isomerizations of the Poly (dA-dT) and Poly (amino2dA-dT) Duplexes Involving the Unusual X-DNA Double Helix: A Fourth Derivative Spectrophotometric Study. *Journal of Biomolecular Structure and Dynamics*, 7(5), 1061–1071.

Greenfield, N. J. (2006). Using circular dichroism spectra to estimate protein secondary structure. *Nature Protocols*, 1(6), 2876.

Kelly, S. M., Jess, T. J. and Price, N. C. (2005). How to study proteins by circular dichroism. *Biochimica et Biophysica Acta (BBA)-Proteins and Proteomics*, 1751(2), 119–139.

Ragone, R., Colonna, G., Balestrieri, C., Servillo, L. and Irace, G. (1984). Determination of tyrosine exposure in proteins by second-derivative spectroscopy. *Biochemistry*, 23(8), 1871–1875.

Sancho, M. I., Almandoz, M. C., Blanco, S. E. and Castro, E. A. (2011). Spectroscopic study of solvent effects on the electronic absorption spectra of flavone and 7-hydroxyflavone in neat and binary solvent mixtures. *International Journal of Molecular Sciences*, 12(12), 8895–8912.

Shukla, M. K. and Leszczynski, J. (2007). Electronic spectra, excited state structures and interactions of nucleic acid bases and base assemblies: a review. *Journal of Biomolecular Structure and Dynamics*, 25(1), 93–118.

Singh, B. R. and Das Gupta, B. R. (1989). Molecular topography and secondary structure comparisons of botulinum neurotoxin types A, B and E. *Molecular and Cellular Biochemistry*, 86(1), 87–95.

Wilson, K. and Walker, J., eds. (2010). *Principles and Techniques of Biochemistry and Molecular Biology*. Cambridge: Cambridge University Press.

Yan, D., Domes, C., Domes, R., Frosch, T., Popp, J., Pletz, M. W. and Frosch, T. (2016). Fiber enhanced Raman spectroscopic analysis as a novel method for diagnosis and monitoring of diseases related to hyperbilirubinemia and hyperbiliverdinemia. *Analyst*, 141(21), 6104–6115.

Molecular Biology*

5.1 Introduction

Molecular biology is the study of the molecular basis of biological processes in living organisms. These include understanding the interactions between biomolecules that form the basis of life as well as the regulation of these interactions. Of particular significance to molecular biology are the nucleic acids (DNA/RNA), proteins and their synthesis. Nucleic acids are the fundamental constituents of a living cell where they function to encode and transmit genetic information needed for the continuity of life in every tissue and organism.

In just over 60 years since the discovery of the structure of DNA by James Watson and Francis Crick, and 40 years since venturing into the revolutionary area of genetic engineering, the concepts of molecular biology have gained a strong foothold in routine household conversations. DNA, RNA, 23andMe, and enzymes have become the subject of interesting discussions on television, newspapers, and business weeklies. The field of microbiology is important not just for scientists and practitioners in the field, but even common people seem curious for insights into the genomics, diagnostics and serology of pathogens, for example, after the outbreak of Covid-19 in 2019. The astonishing scientific discoveries in the field of molecular biology have led to an understanding of the complex biological processes of life and its evolution.

Heredity is the transmission of characteristics from one generation to the other in all forms of life on earth. Much of the understanding of heredity originated in the 1800s, from the pioneering research of Gregor Mendel, an Augustinian monk. He studied the characteristics of parents and offspring in pea plants and defined the "law of combination of different characters" which described the gene as a carrier of hereditary traits. The relation between genetic material and DNA, however, was not demonstrated until the middle of the twentieth century during which time scientists continued to explore the nature of genes, study the behavior of chromosomes during cell division, and the chemical composition of the nucleic acids. Several lines of evidence from a combination of studies carried out within a living organism (in vivo) and those performed in cell or tissues grown in culture or in cell extracts (in vitro), converged to define DNA as the unvarying bearer of heredity. This realization led to the elucidation of the structure of DNA, the molecule of life, and marked the beginning of the development of molecular biology.

---

* Roshan Vijay Kukreja, co-authored this chapter, contributing significantly to the writing of this book.

Molecular Biology has since emerged as the combination of two complementary approaches to the study of life: *biochemistry*, which deals with the chemistry of molecules and the vital processes of life, and *genetics* which is the study of genes, genetic variation, and heredity in organisms; to become one of the most exciting and vibrant fields in science. The intriguing question of how the information encoded in DNA is expressed and used for the construction of a polypeptide has led to the invention of numerous technologies for studying these complex processes at the molecular level. Molecular biology remained a pure science with few practical applications until the discovery of certain enzymes in the 1970s that could cut and recombine desired segments of DNA in the chromosomes of certain bacteria. The resulting recombinant DNA technology and genetic engineering revolutionized this field and led to the development of powerful tools to isolate, analyze, and manipulate nucleic acids. This had astonishing scientific and practical implications in the fields of biotechnology, genome mapping, phylogenetics, molecular medicine, and gene therapy.

Since the completion of the human genome project, which is regarded as a major landmark event in science, thousands of individual human genomes, and those of numerous other species have been sequenced. Studying these sequences has enabled us to understand the cellular and molecular nature of diseases and the relationship of humans to the tree of life. Advances in the development of molecular genetics techniques have revolutionized plant and animal breeding for agricultural needs. As the frontiers expand with the ever-growing databases of nucleic acid and protein sequences and with the advent of powerful technologies to investigate the structure and function of these biomolecules, molecular biology is certain to continue its exciting growth for centuries to come. This chapter is our humble effort to provide an overview of the structure and biological functions of nucleic acid(s), the various techniques used in its isolation and analysis and it's forever increasing applications in the field of science.

5.2   Structure of Nucleic Acids

5.2.1   The Nature and Components of Nucleic Acids

Nucleic acids are the fundamental constituents of a cell and the building blocks of all living organisms. They act as repositories and transmitters of genetic information for every cell, tissue and organism, and hence are key to the continuity of life. The blueprint of an organism is encoded in its nucleic acid as much of the organism's physical development throughout life is programmed in these molecules. There are two types of nucleic acids: deoxyribonucleic acid (DNA) and ribonucleic acid (RNA). While the acronyms DNA and RNA are considered standard nomenclature these days, their names have undergone a long evolution, from nuclein to thymus nucleic acid to nucleic acid to deoxyribonucleic and ribonucleic acid.

Nucleic acids are composed of a long chain of repeating subunits, called nucleotides. Nucleotides are the building blocks of nucleic acids. Each nucleotide subunit is composed of a nitrogenous base, a pentose (5-carbon) sugar and a phosphate group.

Nitrogenous bases, as their name suggests, are heterocyclic nitrogen containing molecules with the chemical properties of a base. Nucleic acids are made up of two kinds of these bases, Purines which have a fused five and six member rings as shown in Figure 5.1a and Pyrimidines that are composed of a six member ring as shown in Figure 5.1b. DNA consists of two purines, adenine (A) and guanine (G), and two pyrimidines, cytosine (C) and Thymine (T). RNA consists of the same bases except that uracil (U) is found instead of thymine in RNA. The only difference between uracil and thymine is the presence of a methyl substituent at position C5 as seen in Figure 5.1b.

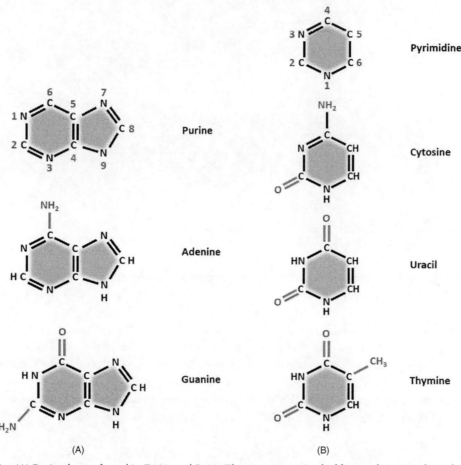

(A)   (B)

Fig. 5.1   (A) Purine bases found in DNA and RNA. They are comprised of five and six membered carbon rings joined together. (B) Pyrimidine bases found in DNA and RNA. They have a six-carbon ring. DNA is made up of bases A, G, C and T; whereas RNA contains A, G, C and U.

Two types of pentose sugars exist in nucleic acids. Nucleotide subunits of RNA contain a pentose sugar called ribose whereas DNA is comprised of the sugar 2-deoxyribose (Figure 5.2). The difference between the sugars lies in the presence or absence (deoxy) of an oxygen atom at position 2 of the ring, and this difference dramatically influences the function of these two nucleic acids. DNA stores the genetic information while the RNA plays a vital role in the transmission of this information for the synthesis of polypeptides. These functions are described in detail in the subsequent sections of this chapter. In order to avoid ambiguity between the carbon atoms in the pentose sugar and the heterocyclic rings of the bases, the positions on the pentose sugars are designated by prime (').

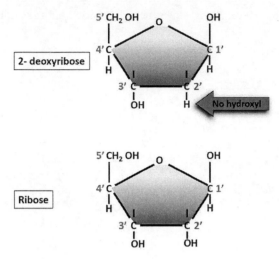

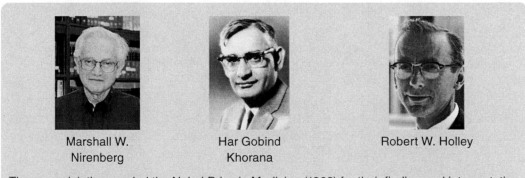

Fig. 5.2   Chemical structures of ribonucleic acid (RNA) and deoxyribonucleic acid (DNA). 2-Deoxyribose is the sugar molecule in DNA whereas ribose is the sugar in RNA.

The connection between the successive subunits in nucleic acids occurs through a phosphate moiety attached to the hydroxyl group on the 5' carbon of one sugar and 3' hydroxyl of the next, forming a 5' to 3' phosphodiester link between adjacent sugar residues. This process can be repeated indefinitely resulting in long polynucleotide chains (Figure 5.3). Every phosphate group in the DNA or RNA is a strong acid (carries a negative charge) at physiological pH and hence the name nucleic *acids*. A base linked to a sugar is called nucleoside and the bond between the 1' carbon of the sugar and the base is referred to as the glycosidic bond. When a phosphate group is added to the nucleoside, it is called a nucleotide. Hence a nucleotide is a 5' mono-phosphorylated derivative of the nucleoside. The nomenclature of the individual subunits in DNA is detailed in Table 5.1.

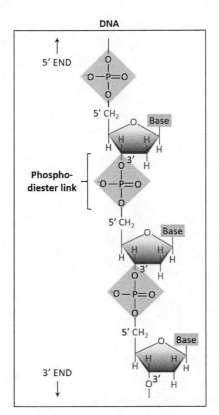
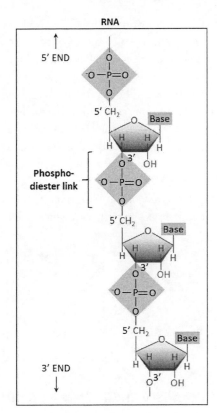

Fig. 5.3 A polynucleotide chain made up of a series of 5'-3' ribose-phosphate or deoxy-ribose phosphate backbone.

Table 5.1 Nomenclature of nucleic acid base derivatives.

Base	Nucleoside		Nucleotide	
	DNA	RNA	DNA	RNA
Adenine	2-deoxyadenosine	adenosine	2-deoxyadenosine-5-monophosphate (dAMP)	adenosine-5-monophosphate (AMP)
Cytosine	2-deoxycytidine	cytidine	2-deoxycytidine-5-monophosphate (dCMP)	cytidine-5-monophosphate (CMP)
Guanine	2-deoxyguanosine	guanosine	2-deoxyguanosine-5-monophosphate (dGMP)	guanosine-5-monophosphate (GMP)
Thymine	2-deoxythymidine		2-deoxythymidine-5-monophosphate (dTMP)	
Uracil		uridine		uridine-5-monophosphate (UMP)

5.2.2 Primary Structure of Nucleic Acids

The phosphodiester linked sugar residues form the backbone of the nucleic acid molecule. As mentioned above, the phosphodiester bond between the nucleotide subunits is between the 3' hydroxyl of one nucleotide and the 5' phosphate of the other (Figure 5.3). Thus, the two ends are distinguishable, and the polynucleotide possesses a sense of directionality 5' to 3' which plays a significant role in its function. The terminal nucleotide at one end of the chain has an unreacted or free phosphate which is negatively charged, while the terminal nucleotide at the other end carries a free 3' hydroxyl group. The negatively charged phosphates being extremely insoluble in lipids ensure the retention of nucleic acids within the nucleus or cell.

In addition, every polynucleotide also carries a sense of individuality which is determined by the sequence of its bases. This defined sequence of a polynucleotide forms its primary structure (Figure 5.4). The sequence or the notation for such a molecule would be ATGCGT and is conventionally written from the 5' end at the left to the 3' end at the right. The genetic information is stored in the primary structure of DNA. A gene represents a defined sequence of DNA that encodes and conveys the information via this sequence of bases.

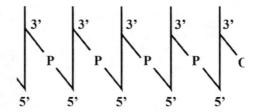

Fig. 5.4   Primary structure of a polynucleotide.

5.2.3   Secondary and Tertiary Structures of Nucleic Acids

The discovery of DNA as the substance that genes are made up of has a long history. The first isolation of DNA was accomplished by a German biochemist Friedrich Miescher in the 1800s. Subsequent studies showed DNA to contain only four kinds of monomers and it was deemed too simple a molecule to direct the development in an organism. It was therefore assumed that genes were made of proteins which were then beginning to be recognized as complex molecules. It was not until the mid 1900's, when a series of crucial experiments by Avery and his colleagues led to the conclusion of DNA indeed being the genetic material. They found that DNA from the pathogenic strains of bacterium *Pneumococcus* could be transferred to non-pathogenic strains, making them pathogenic. They demonstrated that purified DNA was sufficient to cause this transformation, and that the transforming factor could be destroyed by enzymes that degrade DNA (deoxyribonucleases), but not by proteases or ribonucleases. This was followed by an elegant set of experiments by Hershey and Chase who showed that it was the DNA of bacteriophage T2 that entered the bacterial cell. Through these and other similar experiments, by 1952, the evidences were strongly supportive of DNA being the genetic material.

5.2.3.1   *A Model for DNA Structure: The Double Helix*

Several lines of evidence converged in the ingenious conception of the double helical model for the secondary structure of DNA by Watson and Crick in 1953.

1. X-ray diffraction studies demonstrated that DNA was helical and because the layer line spacing was one-tenth of the pattern repeat, there must be 10 nucleotides per turn.

2. Data on the density of DNA fibers by Linus Pauling suggested that the helix must contain two strands.

3. Discovery by biochemist Erwin Chargaff which showed that irrespective of the actual amounts of each base, certain pairs of bases are always found in a 1:1 ratio. The proportion of A is always same as that of T, and the proportion of G is always same as that of C, i.e., [A] = [T] and [G] = [C]. Furthermore, the amount of the purine bases is always equal to the pyrimidine bases; [Pyrimidines] = [Purines]. Chargaff also noted that the base composition of DNA of any species can be described by the proportion of its bases G+C, which ranges from 22 to 74% in different species.

Watson and Crick proposed that the two polynucleotide strands in the double helix are aligned in opposite directions (antiparallel) and are stabilized by hydrogen bonding between the nitrogenous bases on the opposite strands, if they were paired in a certain way; A can form a hydrogen bond with T, and G can form a hydrogen bond specifically with C. This bonding is known as base pairing and the two strands are said to be complementary. As seen in Figure 5.5, one strand runs in the 5'-3' direction while the other runs in 3'-5' direction. The sugar phosphate backbone sits on the outside while the bases lie on the inside, stacked in pairs perpendicular to the axis of the helix. If this structure was to be considered in terms of a spiral staircase, the bases form the treads of the staircase stacked one above the other. The hydrophobic interactions resulting from such stacking of the base pairs and the Van der Waals forces further stabilize the double helix. Each base pair is rotated ~ 36° with respect to the next. The helix has ten base pairs per turn and rises 0.34 nm in each turn. The twisting of the two DNA strands around one another forms the double helical structure, leaving gaps between each set of phosphate backbones resulting in a minor (narrow) groove (~12 Å across) and a major (wide) groove (~22 Å across) as can be seen in the model of DNA in Figure 5.6. This

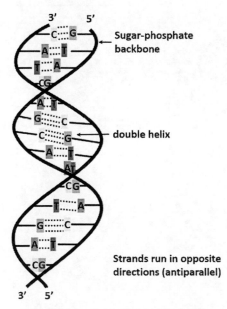

Fig. 5.5 The DNA double helix.

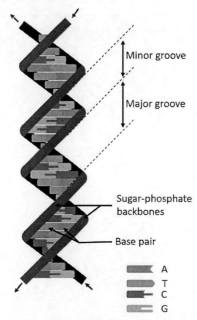

Fig. 5.6 The double helical DNA molecule modeled by Watson and Crick.

wide major groove is easily accessible to DNA-binding proteins. The double helix is right-handed and is the most favored conformation of DNA in the cellular environment commonly referred to as the **B-form** of DNA.

DNA is also known to exist in other forms of helical structures such as the **A and Z forms**. Although the B helix is the structure of DNA in cells with the genome being majorly organized in this conformation, the A helical structure is the conformation that the double-stranded RNA molecules adapt as do the DNA–RNA hybrid molecules. This may be due to the presence of the 2'-hydroxyl group in RNA that poses a steric hindrance to organization in the B form. As seen in Figure 5.7, even though the helices in both A and B forms are right-handed, these structures are very different. In the relatively compact A helix, the bases lie farther to the outside and instead of lying flat, are strongly tilted with respect to the axis, with more bases per turn (Table 5.2). The major groove in the A form is much deeper and less accessible in comparison to the B form. The Z form of DNA represents a different structure which was discovered under in vitro conditions by Alexander Rich and colleagues in 1979. The Z form is strikingly different from the other classical forms as in it is left-handed, has the most base pairs per turn, is slender and least twisted and has a single groove with higher density of negative charges in comparison to the other forms. It gets its name from the zigzag path that the sugar phosphate backbone follows along the helix. The Z form is most often found in polynucleotides with alternating purines and pyrimidines in each strand.

The flexibility or the ability to change its organization under physiological conditions is a crucial aspect of the functionality of DNA. For DNA expression or replication, the strands of parental DNA need to unwind, with each strand serving as the template for the synthesis of a new complementary strand. The specificity of this is determined by base pairing and the resulting two double stranded DNA molecules are an exact copy of the original. This concept of self-replication via base pairing is

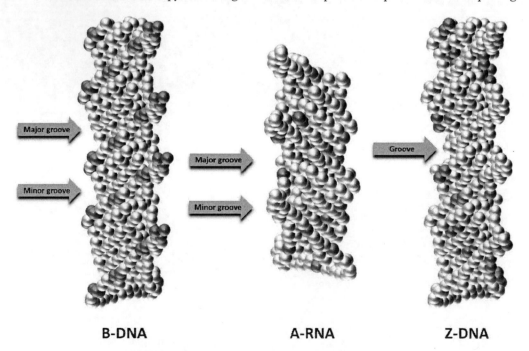

B-DNA   **A-RNA**   **Z-DNA**

Fig. 5.7   Different forms of DNA helical structures.

crucial for the transmission of genetic information during cell division. The ability of the strands to separate without disrupting the covalent bonds, and reform into a double helix at rapid rates needed to sustain genetic functions, is the central property of the helical structure of the DNA.

Table 5.2 Comparison of parameters in the different forms of helical structures of nucleic acids.

	B DNA	A DNA	Z DNA
Orientation of helix	Right-handed	Right-handed	Left-handed
Bases per turn	10	11	12 (6 dimers)
Rotation per residue	36°	33°	~30° per residue
Rise in helix per residue	0.34 nm	0.26 nm	0.37 nm
Helical pitch	3.4 nm	2.8 nm	4.5 nm
Major groove	Wide	Deep and narrow	Very shallow
Minor groove	Narrow	Wide and shallow	Very deep and narrow

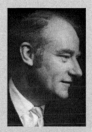 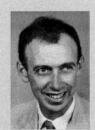 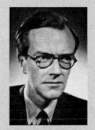 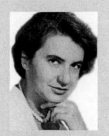

Francis Crick   James Watson   Maurice Wilkins   Rosalind Franklin

1962 the Nobel Prize for medicine was awarded to James Watson, Francis Crick, and Maurice Wilkins. Rosalind Franklin made a crucial contribution in the discovery of the double helix structure of DNA.

The single-stranded molecules of DNA can base pair with a complementary sequence within the single-strand by forming a hairpin intramolecular complex resulting in double helical regions. This special sequence of double-stranded DNA that corresponds to such structures is called a **palindrome** or an **inverted repeat**. This structure also referred to as a double hairpin or **cruciform** consists of two copies of an identical sequence present in the reverse orientation. It is defined as a sequence of the double-stranded DNA that is same when read in opposite direction as seen below:

5' ATTGCG 3'
3' GCGTTA 5'

Formation of such structures results in presence of a few unpaired bases at the ends which renders it less stable than the extended structure under physiological conditions. Alternatively, single-stranded DNA molecules can base pair with another complementary single-stranded molecule (DNA/RNA) to form an intermolecular duplex resulting in hybrids.

5.2.3.2 *Structures of Single-Stranded Nucleic Acids (RNA)*

Although DNA is usually found in the double helical form, genomes of certain viruses and other nucleic acids like RNA exist in single-stranded forms within the cells. RNA is abundant throughout the cell and distributed most commonly in small organelles called ribosomes. Ribosomal RNA (rRNA) forms the major component of ribosomes. Messenger RNA (mRNA) and Transfer RNA (tRNA) are the other forms with a smaller size compared to rRNA. The primary structure of RNA is similar to that of the DNA with a polynucleotide chain consisting of a sugar phosphate backbone that extends in the 5'-3' direction. These molecules can base pair with a complementary sequence in the immediate vicinity within the molecule and can loop back upon itself to form an antiparallel, double-stranded helical structure called a **hairpin loop**. This structure consists of a base paired, double-stranded helical region (stem) with a loop of unpaired bases at one end (Figure 5.8a). If the complementary sequences are distant within the single-stranded molecule, they juxtapose to create a double-stranded region with a stem and a long single-stranded loop. Single-stranded RNA such as transfer RNA (tRNA) which is involved in protein synthesis as described in the next section, organizes itself in conformations wherein in addition to the secondary structure resulting from the folding of the chain with self-complementary regions, a more complex folding of the helices is found. Such higher order folding imparts a defined shape and internal organization that is essential for its function, thereby generating a complex **tertiary** structure.

At high temperatures or under denaturing conditions, the single-stranded nucleotides largely exist in the form of a **random coil** which is constantly changing and is characterized by plasticity and freedom of rotation of bonds in the molecule (Figure 5.8b).

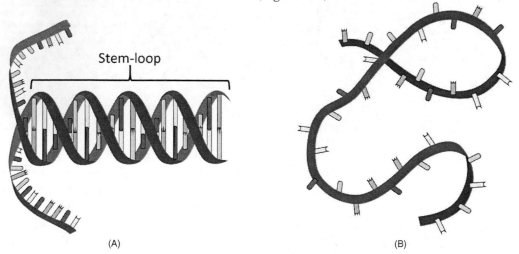

(A)   (B)

Fig. 5.8 (A) Hairpin loop structure of RNA. (B) Random coil conformation of RNA.

5.2.3.3 *Super Coiled Tertiary Structures of Closed DNA*

Although the double helical structure represents DNA as a monotonous linear molecule, many naturally occurring DNA molecules within the nucleus are circular with no free 5' or 3' ends. Genomes of certain small viruses consist of circular DNA wherein two circles of the single strands of DNA are twisted around each other, whereas within the genomes of bacteria and eukaryotes,

DNA is organized in large circular loops. The circular DNA molecules are supercoiled where the duplex is twisted in space around its own axis. This involves a higher order of folding of the elements of the secondary structure and places the molecule under torsion, which can only occur in closed molecules, because an open structure will tend to release the tension by unwinding.

Hence these twisted three-dimensional conformations are energetically more favored and are known to play a very important role in genetic processes such as replication and transcription. Most naturally occurring circular DNA molecules within both prokaryotic and eukaryotic cells have left-hand super-helical twists known as negative supercoiling. Negative supercoils twist the DNA about its axis in the direction opposite to the turns of the right-handed double helix, enabling the DNA to release the pressure by adjusting the structure of the helix by slight unwinding of the two strands (Figure 5.9). This helps in separation of the two strands making it easier to open replication origins and gene promoters. Positive supercoils in which the DNA is supercoiled in the same direction as the double helix, tend to tighten the structure by winding the double helix further and occur ahead of the formation replication fork and transcription complexes.

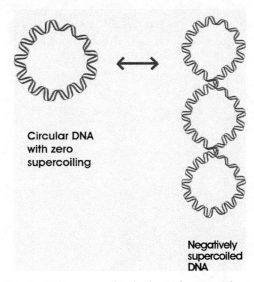

Fig. 5.9   Supercoiling in DNA causes the duplex to be twisted around itself in space.

5.2.4   Stability of Secondary and Tertiary Structures of Nucleic Acids

Under physiological conditions, the A and B forms of the helices confer stability to the nucleic acid molecules. However, for these molecules to perform important biochemical functions such as replication and transcription for example, the double helix needs to unwind. The non-covalent forces that stabilize the helix can be disrupted by heat or by exposure to lower salt concentrations, leading to the separation of the two strands. This loss of secondary structure of the nucleic acid molecule is known as denaturation or melting. Such transition from helix to random coil is sharp and occurs over a very narrow temperature range. It can be monitored spectroscopically by observing the absorbance of ultraviolet light at 260 nm. The stacked bases in the double helix conformation are able to absorb light to a lesser degree in comparison to when they are in a less constrained environment. This phenomenon is called *hypochromism* or the hypochromic effect and results from the interactions between the electron systems of light absorbing heterocyclic purine and pyrimidine rings of the nucleotides. Any departure from the helical structure is reflected by a decline in the hypochromic effect, leading to an increase in optical density towards a value characteristic of free bases. The midpoint of the temperature range over which the DNA is denatured is referred to as the melting temperature (T_m) and is influenced by the base composition of the DNA as well as the conditions employed for denaturation (Figure 5.10). The T_m values are highest for the DNA molecules that have higher proportions of cytosine and guanine in them. Since the G-C pair is bonded by three hydrogen bonds, it is more stable than the A-T pair which has only two hydrogen bonds. The higher the predominance of G-C pairs in the DNA, the greater the energy that would be required to separate the two strands, thus resulting in higher T_m. The T_m is known to increase by ~0.4°C for every 1% increase in the G-C content, and under physiological conditions it usually lies in the range of 85–95°C.

If the melted DNA is cooled, the separated strands can re-associate to form the double helix in a process is called renaturation. Renaturation results from the ability of the complementary strands to base pair and generate a short helical region which then extends along the molecule to form a lengthy duplex molecule. This property of the nucleic acids can be extended to allow any two complementary sequences to anneal with each other and form a helical structure. This process is known as hybridization and as described in detail in the subsequent sections of the chapter, is extremely useful for isolating a specific sequence of DNA from a complex mixture.

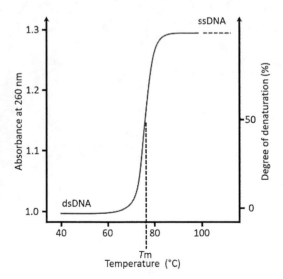

Fig. 5.10   Melting curve of DNA. Denaturation of DNA can be followed by monitoring the absorbance at 260 nm and is indicated by Tm.

5.2.5   Physical Organization of DNA within the Nucleus

As described above, DNA is comprised of a sugar-phosphate backbone and nitrogenous bases. The enormous amount of DNA in eukaryotic cells needs to be compacted in order to be packed within the nucleus. This is achieved by having the DNA complexed with a set of DNA binding proteins resulting in the formation of a protein–DNA complex called chromatin. As seen in Figure 5.11, the twisted double helical shape of DNA is initially wound around a core complex of four small proteins named histones (H2A, H2B, H3, and H4). These basic proteins, rich in lysine and arginine, are the building blocks of the chromatin structure. Approximately 150 bp of DNA is wrapped twice around an octamer of histone molecules to form a nucleosome. Nucleosomes further associate in a second order of compact packaging to form chromatin fibers. These structures are further coiled condensed into chromosomes.

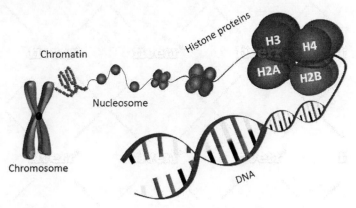

Fig. 5.11   Compact organization of DNA in the nucleus.

Questions to ponder over

1. What are the two types of nucleic acids and how do they differ in structure?
2. What is a nucleotide comprised of and how is it different from a nucleoside?
3. The backbone of a DNA molecule is made up of which two components?
4. Which forces stabilize the DNA double helical structure under physiological conditions?
5. According to Chargaff's rule, in a double-stranded DNA, A+G = C+T. Is this statement correct?
6. What would be the complementary strand for the DNA fragment 5'-ATGCATGGCTA-3'?
7. In what forms do the DNA helices exist in nature and what is the difference between them?
8. What conformations do the different types of RNA molecules adapt in a cellular environment?
9. What is hypochromic effect? What factors affect the melting temperature of a DNA molecule?

5.3   Functions of Nucleic Acids

The fundamental role of nucleic acids is storage and transmission of genetic information. Gene expression is a process by which information stored in the DNA is converted to RNA and then to a protein. This description of the flow of genetic information within a biological system is referred to as the central dogma of molecular biology and is depicted in Figure 5.12. It was first stated by Francis Crick, in 1957, as "once information has passed into protein it cannot get out again."

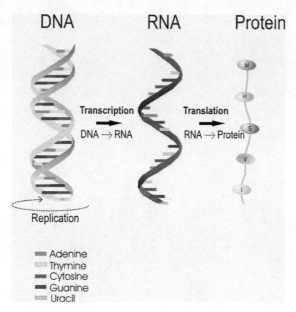

Fig. 5.12   The central dogma of molecular biology: DNA to RNA to protein.

Each of the biological processes that govern the flow of genetic information is detailed below:

5.3.1   Replication: DNA to DNA

The process that is crucial for the continuation of life on earth and the one that passes the genetic information from cell to cell or from generation to generation is DNA replication. Before a cell duplicates and is divided into new daughter cells, DNA within the nucleus must be replicated in order to ensure that each new cell receives the correct number of chromosomes. This process of DNA duplication or replication is vital for the growth, repair, and reproduction of cells in organisms.

The replication of DNA is accomplished by a complex of enzymes as represented in Figure 5.13 and in the steps outlined below:

Formation of Replication Fork: The double-stranded nature of DNA provides a means of replication during cell division since both strands act as templates for the formation of new DNA molecules. Before DNA can be replicated, it has to be unwound or "unzipped" into two single strands and this is usually achieved by the enzyme DNA helicase. DNA helicase disrupts the hydrogen bonding between the complementary base pairs resulting in the separation of the strands and creating a Y shaped structure called a replication fork. The replication fork is bi-directional with one strand oriented in the 3' to 5' direction (towards the replication fork) and is termed as the leading strand, while the other which is oriented in the 5' to 3' direction is the lagging strand. Due to the different orientations, the two strands are replicated differently. In order to prevent the single strands from re-annealing small proteins called single-stranded binding proteins (SSBs) bind to the single DNA strands.

Binding of Primers: Once the DNA strands have been separated, a short sequence of RNA, around 10 nucleotides in length (called the primer), binds to the 3' end of the leading strand. This primer acts as the starting point of DNA synthesis and is synthesized by the enzyme DNA Primase.

Elongation: Enzymes such as DNA polymerase are responsible for the creation of new DNA strands during this process of elongation. There are five different types of DNA polymerases found in bacteria and human cells. DNA polymerase III is mainly responsible for replication whereas polymerase I, II, IV, and V are involved in checking of errors and repair. DNA polymerase binds to the leading strand at the site of the primer and begins adding new nucleotide bases that are complementary to the DNA strand. Since replication proceeds in the 5' to 3' direction on the leading strand, this process is continuous. The lagging strand begins replication by binding with numerous RNA primers at various points along the strand. DNA polymerase then adds pieces of DNA called Okazaki fragments to the lagging strand. This process of replication is discontinuous as the Okazaki fragments are disjointed.

Termination: Once the base pairs have matched up on the strands, an enzyme called exonuclease strips away the primers from the original strands. This gap is filled with complementary nucleotides. The new DNA strand is proofread by another exonuclease to check and remove any errors. Finally, an enzyme called DNA ligase joins the Okazaki fragments together to form two continuous strands. The ends of the DNA strands consist of tandemly repeated DNA sequences called Telomeres. They act as protective caps at the end of the chromosome by maintaining its length during replication and preventing it from fusing with nearby chromosomes. DNA telomerase catalyzes the synthesis of telomere sequences at the ends of the DNA segments. Once this process is completed, the two DNA strands, one new and the other newly formed complementary strand wind up into the double helix.

5.3.2 Transcription: DNA to RNA

In every organism the expression of genetic information involves the DNA being "transcribed" or "read" to direct the synthesis of RNA and protein molecules. Transcription is the process by which information in a strand of DNA is copied into a new molecule of messenger RNA (mRNA). These molecules are named messenger RNAs as they carry information from the DNA to the protein-synthesizing machinery of the cell. The process of transcription takes place in the nucleus of the cells and is carried out by an enzyme RNA polymerase and a number of accessory proteins called transcription factors. It is described in the steps outlined below and depicted in Figure 5.13.

Initiation: Transcription begins with the binding of RNA polymerase to a specific region of DNA called promoter, thereby resulting in the formation of a closed-promoter complex. The promoter region serves as a recognition site for DNA binding proteins called transcription factors which are responsible for controlling gene expression. All eukaryotic enzymes require these transcription factors to initiate transcription. RNA polymerase then unwinds several bases of DNA to form a partially unwound open-promoter complex. The partially exposed single-stranded DNA is referred to as a "transcription bubble." Having located a promoter and formation of a transcription initiation complex, RNA polymerase is ready to begin synthesizing an RNA chain at a start site within the transcription bubble. The process of transcription in eukaryotes is much more complicated due to the fact that eukaryotic cells have several different RNA polymerases which are designated as I, II, and III, each with a specialized function. RNA polymerase I catalyzes the synthesis of rRNA molecules. All of the structural genes that code for proteins in eukaryotes are transcribed by RNA polymerase II. This enzyme also transcribes some of the small nuclear RNAs that are involved in splicing. RNA polymerase III, the largest and the most complex of all eukaryotic polymerases, catalyzes the synthesis of tRNA molecules as well as small RNA genes.

Elongation: During this step the RNA polymerase begins mRNA synthesis by traversing the original or template DNA strand and adding nucleotides that are complementary to this strand. The monomers required in transcription are different from those required in replication. Instead of deoxyribonucleoside triphosphates, the ribonucleoside triphosphates ATP, GTP, CTP, and UTP are needed to make RNA. During this process, an adenine (A) molecule in the DNA binds to a uracil (U) in the RNA and guanine is paired with cytosine. The mRNA molecule is elongated during the process which also involves a proofreading mechanism to check for mistakes/mutations and replace any incorrectly incorporates bases.

Termination: During this step, RNA polymerase comes across a stop or termination sequence in the gene. The mRNA strand is complete, and it detaches from DNA.

RNA Processing

When a eukaryotic gene is transcribed in the nucleus, the primary transcript or the newly synthesized RNA is considered to be an "immature" molecule called a pre-mRNA. The pre-mRNAs undergo extensive processing before they can be translated into proteins. The additional steps involved in eukaryotic mRNA maturation results in a molecule with a much longer half-life than that of a prokaryotic mRNA. These include:

5' Capping: During the synthesis of pre-mRNA, a cap moiety is added to the 5' end of the growing transcript by a phosphate linkage. This cap is a modified guanine nucleotide and it protects the nascent mRNA from degradation. In addition, the cap plays a role in initiation of the translation process by ribosomes.

3' Poly-A tail: Once elongation is complete, the 3' end pre-mRNA is cleaved off by an endonuclease. An enzyme called poly-A polymerase then adds a chain of approximately 200 adenosine residues, called the *poly-A tail* to the RNA. This modification makes the RNA more stable and protects it from degradation. In addition, the poly-A tail aids in the export of mature mRNA from the nucleus to the cytosol to be translated into a protein by the ribosomes.

Pre-mRNA Splicing: Eukaryotic transcripts are composed of protein coding sequences or *exons* (*ex*pressed), and non-coding sequences called ***introns*** (*int*ervening). Intron sequences in mRNA do not encode functional proteins. Before protein synthesis, all of the pre-mRNA's introns must be completely removed or spliced. If the process errs by even a single nucleotide, the reading-frame of the rejoined exons shifts resulting in a dysfunctional or mutated protein molecule. The process of removing introns and reconnecting exons is called *splicing*. Splicing occurs in a sequential manner from the 5' to 3' end and is carried out by specific protein-RNA complexes called spliceosomes. In some cases, the pre-mRNA transcript may be processed differently to produce mRNAs that code for different proteins. This process in known as alternative splicing, wherein different portions of mRNA can be selected for use as exons. This process is regulated by certain proteins that may be expressed differently in various cell types leading to different exon combinations and thus production of different proteins.

The newly formed mRNA copies of the gene then serve as blueprints for protein synthesis during the process of translation.

5.3.3   Translation: RNA to Protein

Translation is the process by which the nucleotide sequence of messenger RNA in translated into the amino acid sequence of proteins within the cytosol. This is accomplished by transfer RNA (tRNA) molecules, certain special enzymes and RNA-protein complexes called ribosomes. The ribosomes in eukaryotes are larger than in prokaryotes, wherein the 40S and 60S subunits combine to form a functional 80S ribosome whilst prokaryotic cells have 70S ribosomes. tRNAs are small noncoding RNA sequences that transport amino acids to the ribosome. Each tRNA is covalently linked to a specific amino acid, forming an aminoacyl tRNA and has a triplet nucleotide sequence that is complementary to the code for that amino acid. A *codon* is a sequence of three RNA or DNA nucleotides that specifies a particular amino acid in a protein.

The translation process proceeds in three stages as described below, represented in Figure 5.13.

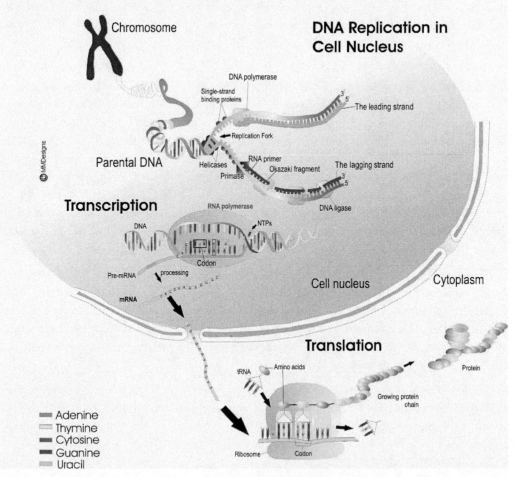

Fig. 5.13   Schematic view of the role of nucleic acids in transmission of genetic information. [See color plates]

Initiation: This process involves the assembly of the two subunits of ribosome around the mRNA. In prokaryotic cells, the ribosome binds to the 5' end of mRNA at a sequence known as Shine–Dalgarno sequence, which corresponds to the Kozak sequence in eukaryotes and is located around the initiation codon. The transfer RNA molecules bring amino acids to the ribosome one at a time. The first tRNA carrying the amino acid methionine is attached at the start codon.

Elongation: In this step, the mRNA is read one codon at a time, and each tRNA identifies the appropriate codon on the mRNA, adding the matching amino acid to the growing protein chain. The ribosome travels along the mRNA and the mRNA is shifted one codon over, each time exposing a new codon so that the genetic message can be read and translated into a protein. The sequence of nucleotides in the template mRNA chain determines the sequence of amino acids in the generated polypeptide chain.

Termination: When the tRNA encounters a stop codon in the ribosome and the final amino acid has been attached to the polypeptide chain, the ribosome subunits separate, and the mRNA is released along with the polypeptide chain. The mRNA may go through translation again and the ribosome can be reused. The polypeptide may be subjected to post-translational modifications and directed to specific cellular compartments or exported outside the cell. These proteins form the major structural and functional molecules of a cell's working machinery.

The basic principle of DNA Replication: At the origin of replication, a replication fork is formed by separation of the double-stranded DNA into two single-strands by the enzyme DNA helicase. The strands are coated with single-stranded binding proteins in order to keep them unwound. DNA replication occurs in both directions. An RNA primer that is synthesized by the enzyme DNA primase binds to the 3' end of the leading strand and the enzyme DNA polymerase III begins elongation of the leading strand by adding nucleotides that are complementary to the strand. The leading strand is synthesized continuously, whereas on the lagging strand, DNA is synthesized in short stretches called Okazaki fragments. Once the complementary nucleotides are incorporated, the RNA primers are removed by the enzyme exonuclease and the Okazaki fragments are joined by DNA ligase resulting in formation of two continuous DNA strands that wind to form a double helix.

The basic principle of Transcription: Following replication of DNA within the nucleus, the enzyme RNA polymerase travels along the DNA molecule, unwinding the double-strand and making an RNA transcript by adding one ribonucleotide at a time that is complementary to the original template. After the enzyme passes, and the pre-mRNA strand is synthesized, the DNA rewinds. In eukaryotic cells, the pre-mRNA undergoes extensive processing resulting in formation of a mature mRNA which is further translated to proteins.

The basic principle of Translation: In the cytosol, the mRNA molecule binds to the ribosome and transfer RNA molecules bring the amino acids to the ribosome one at a time. Each tRNA molecule identifies the appropriate codon on the mRNA and adds a corresponding amino acid to the growing polypeptide chain. The ribosome traverses through the mRNA, so that the genetic message can be read and translated into a protein.

Questions to ponder over

1. Which enzyme unzips the DNA for replication and which enzyme is responsible for synthesizing RNA?
2. Which RNA bases would pair with the DNA segment TAGCTACGAT during transcription?
3. What would be the nucleotide sequence (5'-3') of the coding DNA strand from which the following mRNA segment was transcribed 5'-UAGUCAGAGUUCCGAU-3'
4. What is added to the 3'-end and to the 5' end of eukaryotic mRNAs after transcription?
5. What is pre-mRNA splicing? Which enzymes catalyze this reaction and why is it important?
6. What are the different types of RNA and what roles do they play in transmission of genetic information?
7. In a eukaryotic cell, where are the following proteins located and what is their function: (a) DNA polymerase, (b) RNA polymerase, (c) DNA ligase, and (d) ribosome?
8. How many nucleotides in DNA or mRNA code for a specific amino acid and what are they called?

5.4 Genes and Genome

5.4.1 Introduction

A gene is the basic physical and functional unit of heredity. The essential attributes of genes were defined by Mendel more than a century ago wherein he recognized the gene as a "particulate factor that passes unchanged from parent to progeny." Each gene is a small segment/sequence of DNA that contains the code or information required to build specific proteins or RNA in an organism. The sequence of a gene specifies the sequence of the polypeptide and hence its molecular structure and subsequent localization. The relationship between the sequence of DNA and the sequence of the corresponding protein is called the **genetic code**.

A genotype consists of the complete set of genetic information inherited by the organism and its expression is responsible for generating the phenotype, which is the physical form of the organism. The genotype includes many genes packaged in chromosomes and each chromosome consists of hundreds to thousands of genes. Each gene is located at a particular position termed as locus, on the chromosome. The nucleus of every human cell has 23 pairs of chromosomes, with one chromosome of each pair inherited from each parent, for a total of 46 chromosomes. A gene may exist in alternative forms that govern the expression of some particular characteristic in an organism, for example, the color of the eye. These forms of the same gene with minor differences in their DNA sequence are called alleles. When an organism has two identical alleles it is said to be homozygous, and if the alleles are different, the organism is heterozygous. Alleles could be either dominant or recessive. The occurrence of different alleles at the same site in the genome is termed polymorphism. A gene is a stable entity but can suffer alterations in sequence commonly referred to as a mutation. Changes in the nucleotide sequence lead to changes in the amino acid sequence of the resulting protein, thereby altering or abolishing its activity.

The entire set of genes in a cell or an organelle forms its genome. Genome represents the entire set of DNA or the genetic instructions for the building and functioning of an organism. All living beings have a unique genome and there is a tremendous diversity in the size and organization of genomes in different organisms. In humans, the entire genome consists of around 200,000 genes which is approximately 3.2 billion base pairs of DNA that exists in all cells which have a nucleus.

5.4.2 Genome Complexity

Prokaryotes like bacteria and viruses do not need large amounts of genetic information in order to function. *E. coli*, being a unicellular organism only carries the genetic information that is required by it in order to maintain itself in a limited environment. For replication, a virus extensively borrows from the genetic information carried by the host.

In higher eukaryotes, the vast amount of information needed to direct the development of this multi-cellular organism from the original cell (embryo) to all the varied tissues and cells is carried in its genome. Since the DNA must code for all the specialized proteins found in different tissues, such organisms are expected to have a considerably larger and more complex genome than that of prokaryotes. Most eukaryotic cells organisms consist of 10 to 100,000 times more DNA than *E coli*. However, in many eukaryotes, no direct correlation is found between the size of the genome and its genetic complexity. As seen in Figure 5.14, a plant or an amphibian is certainly not more complex than a human, yet their genomes contain 10 to 50 times the amount of DNA than that of a human genome. Within eukaryotic organisms, much of the basis for variation in genomic size was deduced from the discovery that apart from functional genes, a substantial portion of eukaryotic genomes consists of DNA sequences that do not code for proteins. The thousand-fold greater size of the human genome compared to that of *E. coli* thus may be not solely due to a larger number of human genes. The large size of genome of salamander in comparison to a human genome may reflect the presence of a large amounts of non-coding DNA, rather than more genes. In the human genome, only 2% of DNA is made up of protein-coding functional genes, while the remaining 98% is non-coding and often referred to as "junk DNA."

Thus, complexity of eukaryotic genomes results from the abundance of large amounts of such different classes of repetitive non-coding DNA sequences that are either dispersed or arranged in tandem. Some of these non-coding elements are detailed below:

Transposable Elements: Among repetitive sequences, Transposable Elements (TEs) are found in large numbers in almost all organisms and are mostly responsible for the pronounced differences between their genomes. Transposable elements, also known as transposons, are DNA sequences that move (or jump) from one location in the genome to another. These were discovered over 60 years ago by a geneticist, Barbara McClintock, at the Cold Spring Harbor Laboratory in New York. They make up approximately 12% of the *C. elegans* genome, 50% of human genome, and more than 80% of maize plant genome. TEs have been known to play a major role in the evolution of eukaryotic genomes. They are powerful forces of genetic alterations since TE mobilization can promote or repress gene activation, modulate gene expression, create or reverse mutations, produce duplications of the same genetic material, shuffle regulatory sequences to new locations, thus altering the genome.

Satellite DNA: In addition to TEs, tandems of highly repetitive short sequences of non-coding DNA, called Satellite DNA, also contribute largely to genomes. When separated on a density gradient, these repeat-sequence of DNAs band as "satellites", different from the main band of bulk DNA, and hence are frequently referred to as satellite DNAs. These sequences are repeated millions of

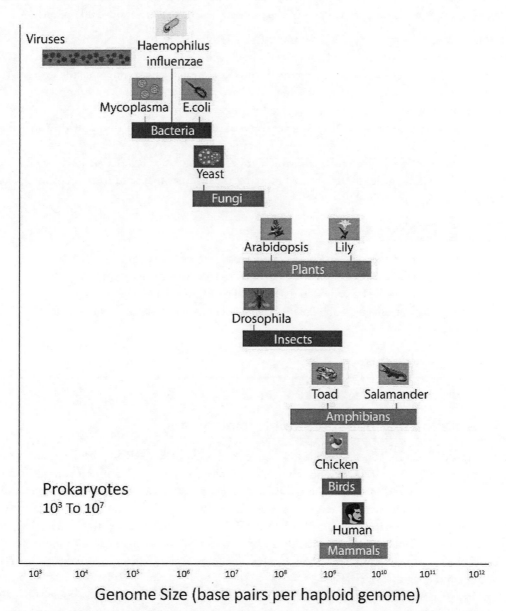

Fig. 5.14   Size of haploid genomes of different organisms represented in logarithmic scale.

times per genome, accounting for 10 to 20% of the DNA of the higher eukaryotes. Satellite DNAs are not transcribed but are the main components of functional centromeres and considered to be important for the packaging of DNA in the heterochromatin region, which plays an important role in controlling gene activity and maintaining the structure of chromosomes.

Alu Elements: Alu elements form another kind of repeated DNA sequences that do not code for proteins but are scattered throughout the genome rather than being clustered like satellite DNA. Their function remains uncertain although they may be origins for DNA replication. These sequences exist as hundreds of thousands of copies in the human genome and are about 300 bp long.

Introns: Introns also account for a substantial fraction of total genomic DNA in the genomes of higher eukaryotes. Introns are non-coding sections of a gene, transcribed into the precursor mRNA sequence, but ultimately removed by splicing during RNA processing to only include exons. Most introns have no known cellular function but may have helped accelerate evolution by facilitating genetic recombination between the protein-coding regions (exons) of different genes.

Other classes of non-coding DNA sequences serve as functional genes as they provide instructions for production of much needed transcripts. Examples include genes for formation of ribosomal RNAs and transfer RNAs, microRNAs which are short lengths of RNA that block the process of protein production, genes for much used proteins like histones that bind to eukaryotic DNA in order to form the chromatin structure.

Questions to ponder over

1. What role does a gene play in heredity and what is the genetic code?
2. How many pairs of chromosomes exist in each cell and why are they paired?
3. What is the difference between the genomes of prokaryotic and eukaryotic organisms?
4. Why do certain plants and amphibians have a larger genomic size as compared to humans?
5. What are the different non-coding elements present in eukaryotic genomes and what is their purpose of existence?

5.5   Isolation and Separation of Nucleic Acids

The process of isolation of nucleic acids involves extraction of DNA or RNA from various sources and is the most basic procedure routinely used in molecular biology. Common sources include bacteria, living or conserved tissues, plants, blood, hair, bones, saliva, urine, semen, etc. The methods employed to isolate nucleic acids target the separation of DNA present in the nucleus of the cell from other cellular components, and the choice of which would depend on the source, size, and age of the sample. Isolation of nucleic acids is a crucial step for downstream application in various types of biological research including molecular diagnostics, gene expression analysis, forensics, pathology, and drug discovery.

The very first isolation of DNA dates back to 1869 and was performed by a Swiss physician Friedrich Miescher. Since then with our ever-increasing knowledge of genetic material and cellular environment and the discovery of different forms of RNA, there has been a tremendous advancement in the introduction of specialized methods for extraction and purification of nucleic acids. Generally, they are divided into solution-based or column-based protocols. These protocols have been further developed into convenient commercial kits that contain most of the components for isolation of pure nucleic acids, in order to ease the extraction process of these biomolecules. Automated systems for carrying out high-throughput screening have been designed as an alternative to labor-intensive manual methods. They have increased productivity and reliability while minimizing contamination related issues and human errors.

Nucleic acid isolation involves three basic steps: cell lysis, separation of DNA/RNA from contaminating proteins, salts, DNases, RNases, and finally the recovery of purified nucleic acid. The first step in isolation of nucleic acids is effective disruption of cell walls or membranes enabling release of the genetic material from the nucleus. This can be accomplished by chemical and/or mechanical methods such as use of a lysis buffer, mechanical homogenization, sonication, grinding, shearing, etc., depending on the properties of the sample. Lysis buffers consist of detergents that breakdown cell membranes, and enzymes (such as proteinase K) that help digest the protein components. EDTA may be used to deactivate DNases by chelating Mg^{2+} ions that are essential for their enzymatic activity. RNases can be removed by the use of ribonucleases. DNA is isolated from cells in the gentlest and cleanest possible manner, and at lower temperatures in order to prevent its fragmentation by mechanical shearing, and to minimize sample contamination and crossover.

Given below are some of the most commonly used procedures used for purification of nucleic acids:

5.5.1 Conventional Chemical Nucleic Acid Extraction Methods

Phenol-Chloroform-Isoamyl alcohol extraction method: Separation of DNA from other cellular components by using organic solvents is one of the oldest and widely employed methods. Lysed cells are mixed with a phenol-chloroform-isoamyl alcohol (PCIA) reagent causing the solution to separate in organic/hydrophobic phase and an aqueous phase. Centrifugation of the emulsion formed by this mixture results in a lower organic phase containing phenol, an upper DNA containing the aqueous phase, and denatured proteins which form a cloudy interface. Purified DNA is recovered by precipitation with ethanol or isopropanol in the presence of high salt concentrations. This method is very efficient, yielding a clean double-stranded DNA sample. However, it is labor intensive, and the use of organic solvents pose health and safety concerns. The quality of the DNA from this procedure is usually not suitable for more sensitive downstream analytical techniques like PCR or sequencing. Easy-DNA® Kit (Invitrogen) is one example that utilizes this technique.

Alkaline extraction method: Alkaline lysis can be employed to isolate plasmid DNA from bacterial cultures such as that of *E. coli*. It uses Sodium Dodecyl Sulfate (SDS) and NaOH to selectively denature high molecular weight chromosomal DNA and bacterial proteins by coating it with the sulfate. Plasmid DNA is then recovered after removal of denatured material by centrifugation. This technique is considered to be one of the quick and reliable methods to obtain plasmid DNA from cells.

Cetyltrimethylammonium Bromide (CTAB) method: For extraction of DNA from plants, samples are frozen in liquid nitrogen and ground to disrupt the cell wall giving excess to nucleic acids without enzymes and chemical activation. Cetyltrimethylammonium bromide (CTAB), a non-ionic detergent, is used for the precipitation of nucleic acids and acidic polysaccharides in low ionic strength solutions. The CTAB-nucleic acid precipitated complex is further solubilized at high-salt concentrations, leaving behind the acid polysaccharides in the precipitate. Organic solvents and alcohol precipitation are then used for the extraction of purified DNA.

Chelex® method: A related method routinely used in forensic laboratories for DNA extraction from various sources, such as hair, blood stain, buccal swabs utilize a Chelex® ion-exchange resin. Chelex® (Bio-Rad Laboratories, CA, USA) is a styrene divinylbenzene copolymer containing paired iminodiacetate ions, that act as chelators for polyvalent metal ions which cause DNA degradation at high temperatures and lower ionic conditions. In this technique, the impurities from the solution bind to the resin while the single-stranded DNA remains in the solution after centrifugation

RNA extraction: The methods used for extraction of RNAs are similar to those mentioned above. However, extra care and precautions are taken during the process since RNA molecules are easily susceptible to degradation and have a very short half-life once extracted from cell or tissues. RNA is vulnerable to digestion by RNases that are ubiquitously present in bacteria, tissues, and blood. Strong detergents that denature endogenous RNases and proteins are incorporated in the isolation medium. Guanidinium thiocyanate, a chaotropic agent and potent inhibitor of RNase is most commonly used in RNA extraction.

5.5.2   Solid Phase Nucleic Acid Extraction using Silica-based Technology

This method is widely employed in commercially available kits for nucleic acid purifications. Under optimal chaotropic salt concentrations and pH, DNA is captured by adsorption to silica on membranes/particles/beads while other cellular components such as protein fragments, etc., flow through the membrane and are removed by subsequent washings. DNA/RNA is eluted in a low salt or elution buffer. The principle of this technology is based on the high affinity of the negatively charged phosphate backbone of DNA towards the positively charged silica particles under high salt concentrations. This method has been incorporated in micro kits and spin columns wherein the reagents are tested and standardized thereby providing a high degree of reliability, with one such example being the Qiagen QIAmp DNA micro kit. The use of this technology results in an increased yield of purified DNA, is easy, quick, cost- effective, and can be automated. However, the process involves use of many buffers, solvents, and multiple tube changes with the probability of introducing contamination during the process. The kit-based methods for isolation of RNA have become increasingly popular as they overcome some of the problems of RNA extractions such as RNase contamination.

5.5.3   Magnetic Beads-based Nucleic Acid Isolation

In recent years, technologies incorporating superparamagnetic particles and magnetic beads have been increasingly used to purify nucleic acids. This method eliminates the need for columns and centrifugation, thus enabling high-throughput automated extraction from a large quantity of samples. This method is based on the reversible binding of nucleic acids to magnetic particles/beads that have been coated with a DNA binding antibody or a functional group which interacts specifically with DNA, under optimal salt concentrations. The superparamagnetic nature of the particles allows them to be manipulated by an external magnet to retain the particles and draw them to the outer edges of the tube or to the bottom of the tube, while the contaminating proteins and salts are washed away. After subsequent wash steps, the purified DNA/RNA is released from the magnetic particles using an elution buffer and is ready for quantification and analysis. Attachment of target oligonucleotides to the magnetic beads allows for the isolation of specific sequences of ssDNA or RNA. These methods are rapid and can be automated, but could be costlier than other methodologies.

5.5.4 Anion Exchange Technology

This method is based on the specific interaction between negatively charged phosphate groups of the nucleic acids and positively charged diethylamino ethyl cellulose (DEAE) groups on the resin. Salt concentrations and pH are determining factors for binding or elution of nucleic acids with the anion exchange resin. DNA from cellular lysates can bind to the DEAE groups on the resin over a wide range of salt concentrations. Contaminants such as RNA and proteins can be removed by washing with a low to medium salt buffers. Purified DNA can then be eluted using a high-salt buffer. This method yields high quality of DNA in comparison to silica-based methods but since it involves use of high salt concentration for DNA elution, desalting may be required for downstream applications. This technology is more commonly employed in plasmid isolation kits such as PureLink® HiPure Plasmid DNA Purification Kits from Invitrogen, Qiagen plasmid mini/midi kits, and Genomic tip.

5.5.5 Automated Extraction Systems

The advent of newer technologies and increasing demand for high-quality nucleic acid molecules for use in downstream applications in molecular diagnostics and genetic analysis, have driven the market, towards incorporation of automated instrumentation for high throughput sample processing. Automated nucleic acid extraction systems tend to simplify the process while increasing quality, yield, reproducibility and safety, reducing work time, and decreasing labor costs. They tend to reduce inconsistencies in sample yield and minimize cross-contamination providing uniform quantities of material for downstream PCR applications and sequencing analyses. Automated instruments may utilize the same principle used in solid-phase or magnetic bead based nucleic acid extraction. However in contrast to manual kits, these can process large amounts of samples in minimal time, thereby drastically reducing the cost and effort required to complete the process. The automated extraction machines are extensively being used in life science and clinical diagnostics labs where raw samples such as blood and other specimens are robotically analyzed in 96- or 384-well microtiter plates. High quality samples can be rapidly processed and extracted in minimal time without any manual intervention.

5.5.6 Electrophoresis for Separation of Nucleic Acids

Gel electrophoresis is a standard technique used in molecular biology for the detection and separation of nucleic acids, based on their size. Since nucleic acids have a uniform charge distribution due to the negatively charged phosphate backbone, these macromolecules can be separated by application of electric fields wherein the negatively charged molecules move through a matrix of agarose towards the positively charged anode. Shorter strands of DNA move through the pores in the gel more quickly and therefore travel farther than larger fragments, and this difference in the rate of migration separates the fragments on the basis of their size. The different sized molecules form distinct bands on the gel. To visualize the DNA, the gel is stained with a fluorescent dye such as ethidium bromide that intercalates into the double-stranded DNA and exhibits strong fluorescence upon illumination with ultraviolet light. The separated DNA fragments appear as bright bands on the gel matrix. A DNA marker/DNA ladder with fragments of known lengths is usually run through the gel alongside with the samples. The approximate length of the DNA fragments in the sample can be calculated by comparing it with those of the DNA marker (Figure 5.15).

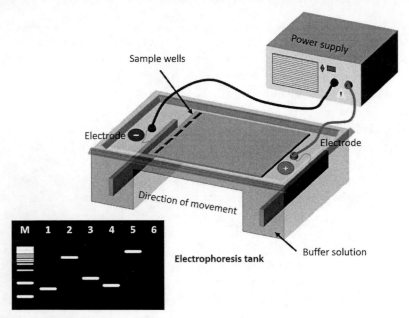

Fig. 5.15   Schematic representation of DNA gel electrophoresis technique.

The gel used in electrophoresis is usually made of agarose, which is a gelatinous substance extracted from seaweed. Agarose gel electrophoresis is used for the resolution of DNA fragments ranging from 100 bp to 25,000 bp in length. The distance between DNA bands of different lengths is influenced by the concentration of agarose in the gel, the higher the agarose concentration the smaller is the average pore size of the gel, making the matrix denser and thus requiring longer run times. The concentration of agarose used to make the gel depends on the size of the DNA fragments that need to be separated. Smaller fragments separate efficiently in higher concentrations of agarose whereas larger molecules require a lower concentration of agarose. Agarose gels are commonly used in the concentration ranges of 0.7–2%.

Larger fragments of DNA such as chromosomes can be separated by using a modified form of electrophoresis called pulsed field gel electrophoresis. This technique developed by Schwartz and Cantor in 1984 efficiently separates DNA fragments in the mass range of 200–3000 kb. In contrast to applying a constant and unidirectional electric field as used in regular electrophoresis, the direction of the electric field is varied continuously during separation of DNA in this method. This is usually achieved by pulsing the applied field in short time intervals and changing its directions in between pulses causing the DNA molecules to reorient themselves in the direction of the field. It is assumed, that during reorientation, the helical structure of DNA is alternately stretched and compressed, and the time required for this is dependent on its molecular weight. Smaller molecules reorient themselves to the changed electric field more quickly than the larger molecules, causing the latter to migrate slowly through the gel.

DNA gel electrophoresis is widely used as an analytical tool in PCR, gene analysis, DNA sequencing, cloning, in blotting techniques for analysis of macromolecules, DNA profiling, DNA fingerprinting in forensic sciences, and many other techniques.

Questions to ponder over

1. What are the three basic steps in nucleic acid isolation and how are they accomplished?
2. What chemicals are conventionally used for extracting nucleic acids and what is their mechanism?
3. How does a salt solution help in extraction of DNA?
4. Which characteristic feature of the DNA is primarily responsible for movement of the DNA molecules in an electric field?
5. What factors determine the rate at which DNA fragments migrate through the gel in electrophoresis?
6. How does pulse field electrophoresis differ from the standard gel electrophoresis?

5.6 Manipulation and Detection of Nucleic Acids

5.6.1 Enzymes Used to Manipulate Nucleic Acids in Molecular Biology

Extensive developments in recombinant DNA technology in the last few decades have led to efficient manipulation of nucleic acids in the fields of molecular biology and genetic engineering. Many of these have resulted from the isolation and characterization of numerous key enzymes that have the ability to manipulate biological DNA. Nucleic acids are manipulated in order to acquire specific characteristics and properties. Such manipulations include digestion, ligation, and amplification of DNA or addition or removal of specific chemical groups such as phosphate or methyl groups. These modifications are catalyzed in vitro by purified DNA modifying enzymes that hold the key to the essence of genetic engineering. Such manipulations have not only increased our knowledge about gene structure and control of gene expression but have also provided a means for detection and identification of various disease markers. This development has resulted in the formation of a huge industry involved in the production and supply of high-quality purified DNA modifying enzymes, some of which are listed below.

5.6.1.1 *Nucleases*

Nucleases cut or digest the DNA molecules by cleaving the phosphodiester bond in the backbone of the DNA molecule. Deoxyribonucleases are specific for DNA whereas ribonucleases digest RNA.

Based on their mode of action, there are two main classes of nucleases:

Exonucleases: They digest the phosphodiester bonds present at the ends of the nucleic acid molecules. Different exonucleases can be distinguished based on the number of strands in the DNA molecule that they are capable of degrading. For example, Bal31 removes nucleotides from both the strands of the DNA molecule, whereas exonuclease III catalyzes the removal of nucleotides only from the 3' end of the double-stranded DNA. The enzyme is not active on single-stranded DNA, and thus 3'-protruding termini are resistant to cleavage.

Endonucleases digest the phosphodiester bonds present in the middle of the DNA molecule. They can be further categorized into three major classes:

i. Enzymes that exclusively digest single-stranded DNA (S1 nuclease).
ii. Those that cleave both single- and double-stranded DNA (e.g. DNase I).
iii. This special group of enzymes, called *Restriction Endonucleases*, cleave double-stranded DNA but only at specific recognition sites called restriction sites. In bacteria, these enzymes provide a defense mechanism against invading viruses, while its own DNA is protected from cleavage by a modification enzyme (a methylase) that modifies the nucleotides at the recognition site. Together, these two processes form the restriction-modification system. There are three types of restriction endonucleases that can be distinguished from each other based on their structure, features of their restriction and cleavage site and the co-factors required for their activity. Type I and III are large enzymes with complex structure and recognition sites. They cleave the DNA in a non-specific manner. Type II restriction enzymes are most commonly used in molecular biotechnology and genetic engineering since they have clearly defined cleavage sites close to or within the recognition sequence. They are smaller in size and require Mg^{2+} ions as co-factors in order to function. They usually bind to DNA as homodimers. Restriction enzymes recognize four to eight nucleotides long palindromic sequences in DNA, and either make staggered cuts to generate sticky ends or straight cuts to generate blunt ends. Over 3000 restriction enzymes, isolated from number of species, have been studied and more than 600 of these are available commercially. These enzymes are routinely used for DNA modification in laboratories and are a vital tool in molecular cloning.

Table 5.3   Some examples of frequently used type II restriction endonucleases.

Enzyme	Organism	Recognition Sequence	Products	Ends
HaeIII	*Haemophilusaegyptius*	5'-GGCC 3'-CCGG	5'-GG CC-3' 3'-CC GG-5'	Blunt
PyuII	*Proteus vulgaris*	5'-CAGCTG 3'-GTCGAC	5'- -CAGCTG- -3' 3'- -GTCGAC- -5'	Blunt
AluI	*Arthrobacter luteus*	5'-AGCT 3'-TCGA	5'-AG CT-3' 3'-TC A-5'	Blunt
EcoRI	*Escherichia coli*	5'-GAATTC 3'-CTTAAG	5'-G AATTC-3' 3'-CTTAA G-5'	Sticky
HindIII	*Haemophilus influenzae*	5'-AAGCTT 3'-TTCGAA	5- -AAGCTT- -3' 3'- -TTCGAA - -5'	Sticky
BamHI	*Bacillus amyloliquefaciens*	5'-GGATCC 3'-CCTAGG	5'-G GATCC-3' 3'-CCTAG G-5'	Sticky
HpaI		5'-GTTAAC-3' 3'-CAATTG-3'	5'-GTT AAC-3' 3'-CAA TTG'5'	Blunt
PstI	*Providensiastuartii*	5'-CTGCAG 3'-GACGTC	5'-CTGCA G-3' 3'-G ACGTC-5'	Sticky

5.6.1.2 *Ligases*

Ligases are enzymes that act as biological glue and join the nucleic acid molecules by forming phosphodiester bonds between the 5' phosphate of one nucleotide and the 3' hydroxyl group of the other. In nature, the function of DNA ligase is to repair single-strand breaks in DNA that arise as a result of replication and/or recombination. DNA ligase uses the complementary strand of the double helix as a template to fix the single-strand breaks by creating a final phosphodiester bond that is essential for the complete repair of the DNA strand. Some forms of ligases such as DNA ligase IV isolated from bacteriophage T4, may specifically repair breaks in both the strands of the DNA molecule. They can achieve both blunt end and sticky end ligations. In recombinant DNA technology, ligases catalyze the joining of DNA of interest called as "insert", with the vector molecule in the reaction known as ligation. DNA ligases are extensively used in molecular biology laboratories for recombinant DNA experiments and find applications in both DNA repair and replication.

5.6.1.3 *Polymerases*

DNA polymerases are enzymes that synthesize a new strand of DNA complementary to an existing DNA or RNA strand which acts as a template. For its activity, DNA polymerase requires the template DNA strand, a primer with a free 3'-OH group that hybridizes with the template in order to form a double-stranded region thereby initiating the polymerization, and a pool of all the four dNTPs needed to synthesize the new DNA strand. Different types of DNA polymerases are used in recombinant DNA technology.

E. coli DNA polymerase I enzyme has both polymerase as well as bidirectional exonuclease activity. It can be cleaved to produce a fragment called the Klenow fragment that only has polymerase and 3'-5' exonuclease activity. This Klenow fragment can synthesize the new DNA strand complementary to the template but cannot degrade the existing strand. Klenow fragments are predominantly used in DNA sequencing.

Thermostable DNA polymerases are a class of polymerases that are resistant to denaturation by heat and remain functional at high temperatures. *Taq* polymerase, an enzyme isolated from bacterium *Thermus aquaticus,* finds extensive applications in amplification of DNA using a technique called polymerase chain reaction (PCR) which is discussed in detail in the subsequent sections of this chapter.

Reverse transcriptase (RT) is RNA dependent DNA polymerase found in RNA viruses also known as retroviruses. Instead of DNA, RT uses mRNA as a template for synthesizing a complementary DNA strand (cDNA). Formation of a double-stranded cDNA using RT finds applications in genetic engineering. The cDNA formed from any mRNA molecule can be cloned in an expression vector and used for protein expression in large quantities.

5.6.1.4 *DNA Modifying Enzymes*

There are numerous enzymes that modify DNA molecules by adding or removing specific chemical groups. Four such enzymes that are routinely used in research laboratories for performing such modifications are:

Alkaline phosphatases: This group of enzymes removes the phosphate group from the 5' terminus of the DNA molecule. As the name suggests, alkaline phosphatases are most effective within an alkaline environment. Alkaline phosphatases are important in molecular biology as the removal of phosphate groups from the 5' end of the DNA molecule prevents them from ligating (the 5' end attaching to the 3' end), thereby keeping DNA molecules linear until the next step of the process for which they are being prepared. Removal of the phosphate groups and subsequent labeling also facilitates radiolabeling (replacement by radioactive phosphate groups) in order to measure the presence of the labeled DNA during the experiment. Commercially, it is obtained from three major sources, viz., *E. coli* (bacteria), calf intestine, and arctic shrimp. Another important use of alkaline phosphatase is as a label for enzyme immunoassays.

Polynucleotide kinase (PNK): These enzymes, extracted from *E. coli* infected with bacteriophage, catalyze the transfer of a phosphate group from ATP to the 5' end of the DNA molecule.

Terminal transferase: This group of enzymes, obtained from calf tissue, catalyze the addition of one or more deoxyribonucleotides to the 3' terminus of the single-stranded or double-stranded DNA molecules. The enzyme is commonly used for labelling the 3'ends of DNA as well as for addition of complementary homo-polymeric tails to the DNA molecules.

Topoisomerases: These enzymes change the confirmation of covalently closed circular DNA molecules such as plasmids by removing the supercoils present within them.

Questions to ponder over

1. What was one of the most significant discoveries that allowed development of recombinant DNA technology?
2. Which endonuclease cleaves both single- and double-stranded DNA molecules in a non-specific manner?
3. Enzyme Bal31 is an example of what class of DNA manipulating enzymes and what is its mode of action?
4. How do restriction enzymes know where to cut DNA?
5. Which enzyme is used to achieve blunt end ligations in a double-stranded DNA molecule?
6. The Klenow fragment is the truncated version of which enzyme and how does it manipulate the DNA?
7. What are the different types of DNA modifying enzymes and how do they function?

5.6.2 Nucleic Acid Mutagenesis

Site-directed mutagenesis is a fundamental technique in molecular biology and protein engineering now being used for introducing defined mutations in the DNA sequence and investigating the resulting protein following *in vitro* expression. It is a powerful tool used to probe gene regulation and to study the structural and functional role of amino acid residues in a protein by comparing the mutant protein that carries the altered amino acids to the wild-type protein.

Two methods are commonly used in vitro site directed mutagenesis:

5.6.2.1   *Oligonucleotide-directed Mutagenesis*

This traditional method of incorporation of mutation in a gene requires that the DNA that needs to be mutated, be cloned into a single-stranded vector such as M13. This technique involves synthesis of an oligonucleotide complementary to the sequence of interest, but with one base mismatch. This oligonucleotide acts as the primer and is annealed to the single-stranded DNA in presence of a DNA polymerase and dNTPs. The DNA polymerase produces a complementary DNA strand that now incorporates the oligonucleotide consisting of the base mutation capable of transforming cells. This produces multiple copies of the recombinant DNA molecule, half of which contain the wild-type sequence and the other half contain the sequence with the desired mutation, as illustrated in Figure 5.16.

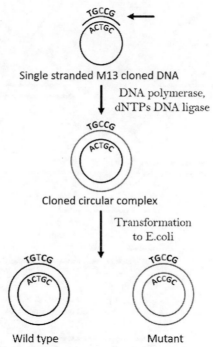

Fig. 5.16   Oligonucleotide extension mutagenesis. In the first step, the template DNA fragment inserted in an M13 phage vector is annealed to a synthetic oligonucleotide primer that contains the mutation. This is followed by extension of the primer by DNA polymerase and synthesis of the second strand. DNA ligase seals the nicked site resulting in a closed circular double-stranded DNA molecule. One strand contains the original sequence while the other is comprised of the mutated sequence. The double-stranded DNA is further transformed into *E. Coli* cells wherein subsequent replication results in some double-stranded circular DNA molecules with the wild type sequence and the rest containing the mutated sequence.

5.6.2.2   *PCR-based Site-directed Mutagenesis*

PCR-based techniques have become largely popular to generate arrays of predefined mutations within the sequence of interest. This method relies on the base mismatch between the primers and template DNA to be incorporated into the amplicon following thermal cycling, thus replacing the original sequence.

The basic PCR technique also known as the overlap extension method makes use of two primary PCR reactions to produce two overlapping DNA fragments that contain the mutation in the overlap region. Each reaction uses one flanking primer and one internal primer with the desired mutation. The two overlapping DNA fragments are annealed to generate a new duplex fragment that is extended by DNA polymerase and amplified by subsequent rounds of PCR to generate a full-length mutated segment (Figure 5.17). This technique can be used to incorporate site-specific insertion and deletion mutations and also for introducing multiple mutations within the same template.

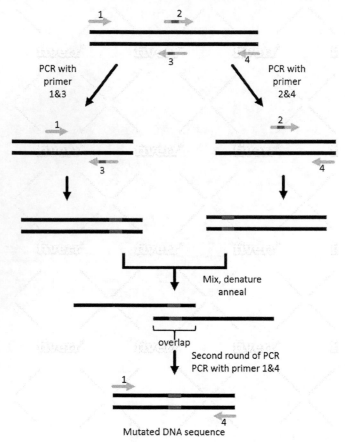

Fig. 5.17 PCR-based mutagenesis. Two external primers (1 and 4) that are complementary to the forward and reverse DNA strands, respectively, and two internal primers (2 and 3) that contain the desired mutations are used in the two PCR reactions that are carried out in separate tubes under the same reaction conditions. The products of the two reactions are allowed to mix, denature, and reanneal where some strands from the first PCR product anneal with those obtained from the second PCR reaction leading to regions of overlap corresponding to the sequences of primers 2 and 3. Subsequent PCR reactions lead to amplification of the full length fragment of the mutated DNA. [See color plates]

A modification of this technique, known as the megaprimer PCR method utilizes long, double-stranded DNA fragments as primers to introduce any combination of point mutations, deletions, or insertions. This method uses three oligonucleotide primers to perform two rounds of PCR on a DNA template. One oligonucleotide contains the mutation and the other two serve as the forward and reverse primers. The first PCR uses the external primer and the mutagenic primer to generate an amplified double-stranded DNA fragment containing the desired mutation. This amplified fragment, the megaprimer, is used in the second round of PCR in conjunction with the other external primer to amplify a longer region of the template DNA (Figure 5.17).

In addition, random mutations and deletions can be introduced in a gene by use of "error-prone" or low fidelity PCR amplification, or by treating DNA with chemical mutagens to generate enzymes, proteins, entire genomes, or entire metabolic pathways with desired or improved properties. This in vitro directed enzyme evolutionary approach to protein engineering using random mutagenesis has been employed for the development of novel enzymes, proteins, and catalytic antibodies.

5.6.2.3   *CRISPR/Cas-9 Technology*

More recently, the development of the CRISPR/Cas-9 technology has enabled scientists to make changes to the DNA of an organism by permitting in vivo mutagenesis. Genetic material can be added, altered, or removed at desired locations within the genome using these gene/genome editing techniques.

CRISPR/Cas-9 (short for clustered regularly interspaced short palindromic repeats CRISPR-associated protein 9) technology was adapted from the naturally occurring genome editing systems of prokaryotic organisms like bacteria. The bacteria capture DNA fragments from invading viruses and use these to create DNA sequences called CRISPR arrays. These arrays are used to detect and destroy the DNA from similar viruses during subsequent infections thereby providing a form of acquired immunity. The bacteria then use Cas-9 to cut apart the DNA thus disabling the virus.

In the lab, scientists replicate this system by creating a short "guide" RNA sequence that binds to a specific complementary sequence of the DNA in the genome. This RNA then guides the Cas-9 enzyme to the same location where it cuts across both strands of the DNA. At this stage the cell tries to repair the damaged DNA and scientists are able to use the cell's DNA repair machinery to add, delete, or introduce changes to the existing DNA by replacing it with a customized sequence within the genome of interest (Figure 5.18). Although Cas9 is the enzyme that is commonly used, other enzymes such as Cpf1 and Cas-12a have also been explored.

Genome editing is of great interest in biological research and for the prevention and treatment of diseases. CRISPR/Cas-9 technology has been explored to functionally inactivate genes in human cell lines for the treatment of a wide variety of diseases such as sickle cell disease, hemophilia, and cystic fibrosis; to genetically modify crop strains and to modify yeasts used to make biofuels. Ethical concerns limit the use of these technologies for alteration of human genomes.

Questions to ponder over

1. What is site-directed nucleic acid mutagenesis and where does this technique find its application in science?
2. What is the difference between the commonly used methods of introducing mutations within DNA sequences?
3. CRISPR can change DNA in humans and animals? What did scientists observe that helped them create this technology?
4. What is the role of guide RNA in CRISPR gene editing, and which enzymes aid this process?

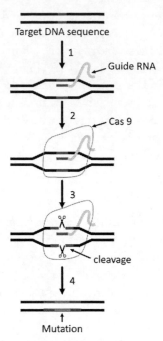

Fig. 5.18 Mechanism of CRISPR/Cas9 genome editing. This technology uses a short guide RNA molecule that directs the Cas-9 enzyme to a specific region of the genomic DNA resulting in a double-strand cut/break. The double-strand break is then repaired by the host cell leading to introduction of desired changes to the fragment of interest. [See color plates]

5.6.3 Nucleic Acid Hybridization

Nucleic acid hybridization is a basic technique in molecular biology which exploits the ability of individual single-stranded nucleic acid molecules (DNA/RNA) to form double-stranded complex hybrids by base pairing with similar molecules that have a high degree of complementarity in their sequence. These hybrids can be formed between two strands of DNA, two strands of RNA or between a DNA and RNA. Nucleic acid hybridization is used to determine the degree of sequence identity between the nucleic acids and for the detection of specific sequences within them.

The hybridization assays can be carried out in solution or by immobilization of one component on a nitrocellulose/nylon membrane and involves the use of a labeled nucleic acid probe that detects complementary DNA or RNA sequences in the target molecule. Nucleic acid probes may be DNA/RNA probes or synthetic oligonucleotides. These probes can be modified or labeled, which enables the identification of the complementary sequence that they bind to. The two methods commonly used to label the nucleic acid probes are isotopic labeling, which is carried out using radioactive labels, and non-isotopic labeling, which makes us of non-radioactive labels.

Isotopic labeling: In molecular biology the most common radioactive label used is 32-phosphorus (^{32}P) although ^{35}S is also used in certain techniques. The incorporation of the radioisotopes can be detected by autoradiography, where the labeled probe bound to the target sequence is exposed to an X-ray sensitive film which reveals the location of the label and thus the nucleic acid to which it is bound.

Non-radioactive labeling: These are becoming increasingly popular for labeling nucleic acid probes due to their safety and improved sensitivities. The labeling technique can be either direct or indirect.

Direct labeling involves incorporation of modified nucleotides containing a fluorophore such as rhodamine, fluorescein, ATTO dyes, etc., that can be detected directly by fluorescence spectroscopy (Figure 5.19).

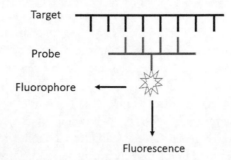

Fig. 5.19   Direct labeling of nucleic acid probes by fluorescent nucleotides.

Indirect labeling involves chemical coupling of a modified reporter group to the nucleotide. After incorporation into the DNA fragment, the reporter groups can be bound to specific binding proteins or ligands that have high affinity for it. These ligands are conjugated to a marker or reporter enzyme which can be detected in an assay. For example, the detection of biotin (which acts as a reporter) incorporated in a DNA molecule relies on its high affinity to streptavidin. The latter may be coupled or conjugated to reporter enzyme such as alkaline phosphatase which allows signal amplification by converting a colorless p-nitrophenol phosphate (PNPP) to a yellow colored p-nitrophenol (PNP) as seen in Figure 5.20A. Alternatively, digoxygenin, a steroid found in digitalis plants can be incorporated into the DNA and detected by monoclonal antibodies that are conjugated to secondary reporter molecules such as alkaline phosphatase or fluorescent dyes (Figure 5.20B).

The labeling strategy is generally determined by the sensitivity required for the downstream application. While the speed of detection and ease of quantification are major advantages of fluorescent labels, indirect methods with secondary reporter molecules allow signal amplification with resultant increased sensitivity.

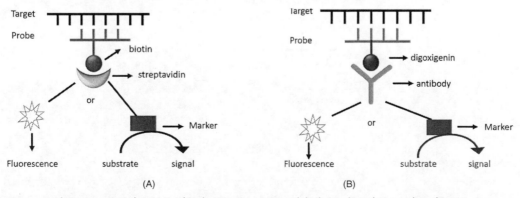

Fig. 5.20   Mechanism of indirect non-isotopic labeling of nucleic acid probes.

Some techniques commonly used in nucleic acid hybridization are listed below:

5.6.3.1 *Blotting*

Blotting is a molecular biology technique used for the identification of nucleic acids and genes, and is widely employed for diagnostic purposes. Electrophoresis allows separation of nucleic acids based on size. However, it provides no indication of the presence of a specific desired sequence in the sample. Blotting enables the transfer of nucleic acid fragments from the electrophoresis gel onto a membrane, resulting in immobilization of the fragments in a banding pattern similar to that on the gel. After immobilization, the DNA can be subjected to hybridization, enabling detection of the desired fragments.

Southern blot, a technique named after its inventor Edwin Southern, is used to detect specific sequences of DNA from a mixture of DNA samples for example a particular gene within a genome or repeat expansions within specific genes. As seen in Figure 5.21, following electrophoresis, the DNA fragments on the gel are denatured by alkaline treatment and transferred via capillary action onto a nylon or nitrocellulose membrane placed in contact with the gel. Subsequent immobilization occurs by UV irradiation (for nylon membranes) or by baking for 2 hours at 80°C in case of nitrocellulose membranes. Following fixation, the membrane, now containing a replica of the original DNA gel is treated with a labeled DNA probe which hybridizes to its complementary single-stranded DNA sequence on the gel. Conditions for hybridization, including temperature and salt concentrations, are chosen to achieve optimal hybridization. The membrane is then washed extensively to remove any unbound probe and is developed auto-radiographically if the probe was radioactively labeled; or treated with chemiluminescent substrate if non-isotopically labeled with biotin or digoxigenin, resulting in detection of the desired DNA sequence.

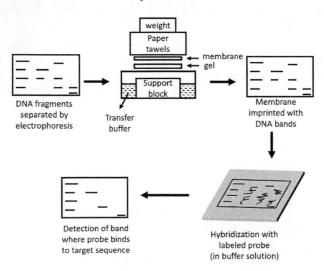

Fig. 5.21   Southern blot apparatus and method.

Northern blot, a variant of the southern blot enables detection of specific RNA (or isolated mRNA) molecules in a sample. It is widely used to study expression of RNA in particular genes in a tissue or organ under different stages of differentiation and morphogenesis as well as abnormal, infected, or diseased conditions. In this method total cell RNA is resolved electrophoretically, with subsequent transfer and probing with radiolabeled DNA. This is followed by radio-autographic detection of DNA-RNA hybrid complexes.

5.6.3.2 *Colony Hybridization*

It is a rapid method for selecting a colony of bacteria which contain a specific sequence of DNA from a mixed population. Bacterial colonies are cultured on a nutrient rich agar plate. These colonies are then replicated on a nitrocellulose filter disc from the surface of the agar plate. The bacterial cells on the filter membrane are lysed by alkaline hydrolysis to release and denature the DNA which in turn binds to the nitrocellulose membrane. The DNA clusters on the nitrocellulose are hybridized with a labeled nucleic acid probe. The probe chosen is complementary to the desired DNA sequence. After washing off the excess unbound probe, the filter is screened by autoradiography and the colonies containing the DNA molecules of interest are identified (Figure 5.22).

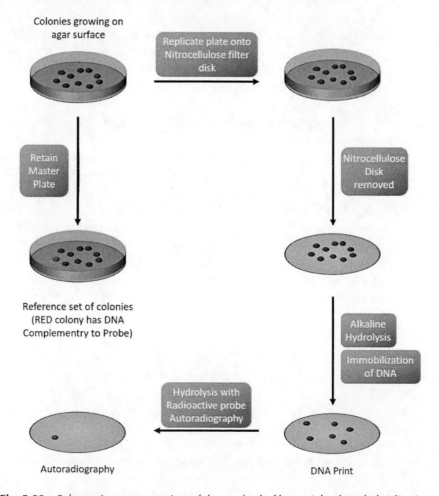

Fig. 5.22 Schematic representation of the method of bacterial colony hybridization.

5.6.3.3 *Fluorescence in situ Hybridization*

FISH is a cytogenetic technique used for the detection and localization of specific nucleic acid sequences within tissues or cells. It involves hybridization of fluorescent probes that are complementary to the sequence of interest and visualized in situ by fluorescence or confocal microscopy.

The fluorescent probes are constructed and labeled either directly by using fluorescent nucleotides, or indirectly, by incorporation of reporter molecules that can subsequently be detected by fluorescent antibodies or other affinity molecules (Figure 5.23). Probes must be large enough to hybridize specifically with the target. The probe and the DNA sample are denatured to single-strands and incubated for several hours to permit hybridization. After washing off unbound or non-specific probes, the results are visualized and quantified by detecting the fluorescence signal emitted by the labeled DNA either by microscopy or flow cytometry. If the probes were labeled indirectly, the results can be monitored by using an enzymatic or immunological detection method. It is a valuable tool for understanding a variety of chromosomal abnormalities and other genetic mutations.

Three types of probes are commonly used in fluorescence in situ hybridization, each of which have different applications. Locus specific probes bind to a particular region of the chromosome and are used to determine the location of a specific gene on the chromosome. Repeat probes are generated from repetitive sequences located in the middle of each chromosome and are used to verify if an individual has correct number of chromosomes. Whole chromosome probes are a collection of smaller probes each binding to a different sequence along the length of the chromosome. Spectral karyotyping can be carried out by using multiple probes that are labeled with different dyes to visualize the entire colored map of the chromosome. This is useful for monitoring chromosome arrangements and detecting any abnormalities therein.

FISH is a valuable tool in gene mapping studies for understanding chromosomal abnormalities, genetic mutations, identifying regions of deletion or amplification and translocation, identification of non-random chromosomal rearrangements, identification of novel oncogenes, etc. It has been successfully used in the detection of the BCR/ALB1 translocation in chronic myeloid leukemia, augmentation of human epidermal growth factor receptor 2 (HER2) in breast cancer, down syndrome, 22q13 deletion syndrome, and many other diseases. As a result, FISH has found diverse applications in the various fields of research including reproductive medicine, clinical genetics, oncology, neuroscience comparative genomics, etc. FISH is also popularly used in the genome comparison of different biological species to deduce evolutionary relationships.

> ### Questions to ponder over
>
> 1. What is DNA hybridization and how is it useful?
> 2. What are the various methods used for labeling nucleic acid probes and how do they differ?
> 3. If the nucleic acid fragments generated by enzyme restriction endonuclease are separated by gel electrophoresis and transferred onto a membrane filter and probed with a radioactive DNA fragment, what is this procedure called?
> 4. How is fluorescence in situ hybridization (FISH) technique used for detection of breast cancer?

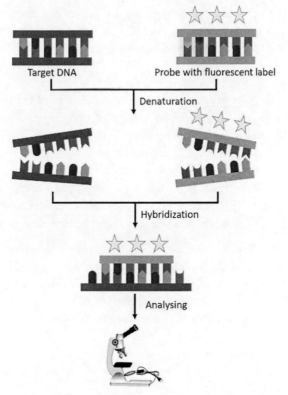

Fig. 5.23 Illustration of fluorescence in-situ hybridization technique.

5.7 Polymerase Chain Reaction

5.7.1 Introduction

Polymerase chain reaction (PCR) is a rapid and extensively used technique in molecular biology for selective amplification of defined target regions of DNA present within the DNA source, thereby generating thousands to millions of copies of that particular DNA sequence. The polymerase chain reaction was developed in 1985 by an American biochemist Kary Mullis for which he was awarded the Nobel Prize in 1993. PCR is routinely used in clinical and biological research laboratories for a wide range of applications including gene expression, genotyping, cloning, mutagenesis, target detection, sequencing, forensic sciences, and clinical diagnostics amongst several others.

A basic PCR reaction requires several components and reagents such as the DNA template which contains the target region to be amplified, a heat resistant DNA polymerase such as *Taq* polymerase that polymerizes the new DNA strands, two oligonucleotide primers that are complimentary to the 3' ends of each of the sense and anti-sense strands of the target DNA, a mixture of deoxynucleoside triphosphates or dNTPs which are the building blocks from which the DNA polymerase synthesizes a new DNA strand, buffer solutions providing a suitable environment for optimum activity and stability of the DNA polymerases, and divalent cations such as magnesium or manganese ions that act as a co-factor for *Taq* polymerase thereby increasing its polymerase activity. The method in general involves repeated cycles of heating and cooling of the reaction mixture to enable template DNA denaturation, primer hybridization and annealing in order to achieve enzymatic replication of the DNA strand.

Designing appropriate oligonucleotide primers is crucial to the successful outcome and specificity of the PCR experiment. In order to execute selective amplification of the target DNA, some prior DNA sequence information is required for the design of two primers which are specific to the target DNA sequence. The oligonucleotide primers should flank the DNA fragment intended to be amplified from the DNA template. The forward primer will anneal with the antisense DNA strand which is oriented in the 3' → 5' direction and the reverse primer will anneal with and should complement the 5′ → 3' DNA strand. It is imperative to minimize the possibility of the primers binding to locations within the DNA other than the desired one. Hence several factors are taken into consideration while designing effective primers to be used for the reaction:

a. Primers should not be very long or short in length. Short primers produce non-specific DNA amplification products resulting from hybridization at non-target sites, and long primers result in a slower hybridizing rate. The optimal length of the primers should be 18–25 nucleotides. This ensures adequate specificity for optimal binding to the template.

b. The G-C content should ideally be between 40 to 60%, with an even distribution of all four nucleotides.

c. The melting temperature of the primers, i.e., the temperature at which half of the DNA strands are double-stranded, should ideally be between 50–60°C. The T_m values for the two primers should be similar and not differ by more than 5°C.

d. The structure of the primers chosen should be relatively simple with no significant secondary structure in order to avoid internal folding. Inverted repeats or self-complementary sequences > 3 bp in length (e.g., GCGCGC or TATATATA) and single base runs (e.g., AAAAA or CCCCC) should be avoided as this could result in a hairpin or loop formation which may lead to primer-primer annealing and improper hybridization to the target thus disrupting the amplification process.

Increasing use of a plethora of publically available bioinformatics resources such as PrimerQuest, Oligo, Gprime, Gene Fisher, amongst several others, for designing primers has made the process much more straightforward and efficient.

5.7.2   Steps in PCR

PCR is a chain reaction wherein the newly synthesized DNA strands act as templates for further DNA synthesis in subsequent cycles. It comprises of a series of thermal cycles with each cycle consisting of three successive stages namely denaturation, annealing, and extension. Each of these steps is repeated 20–40 times doubling the number of DNA copies each time. The temperatures used and the duration of each cycle is determined based on a variety of parameters, including the type of DNA polymerase used, the melting temperature (T_m) of the primers, and the concentration of bivalent ions and dNTPs in the reaction. The individual steps common to most PCR methods are indicated in Figure 5.24 and are described below:

Denaturation: In this first cycle, the double-stranded template DNA is denatured or separated into two single-strands by heating the reaction chamber to over 90°C for a few minutes. The high temperatures result in melting of the DNA template by disruption of hydrogen bonds between the complementary bases within the two strands of the template DNA yielding single-stranded DNA molecules. These separated strands then act as templates for production of new DNA strands in subsequent cycles.

Annealing: At this stage the reaction temperature is lowered to 50–65°C for 20–40 seconds to allow annealing of the primers to each of the single-stranded DNA templates. Two different primers are typically included in the reaction mixture, one for each of the two single-stranded complements containing the target region. Stable hydrogen bonds between complementary bases are formed only when there is high sequence complementarity between primer and the template sequence. Selection of a proper temperature for the annealing reaction is crucial for the efficiency and specificity of the reaction. The temperature must be low enough to enable hybridization between the primers and the template DNA but high enough for the hybridization to be specific and prevent formation of mismatched hybrids. The primer should only bind to a complementary part of the strand, and nowhere else. A typical annealing temperature is about 3–5°C below the calculated T_m of the primers used.

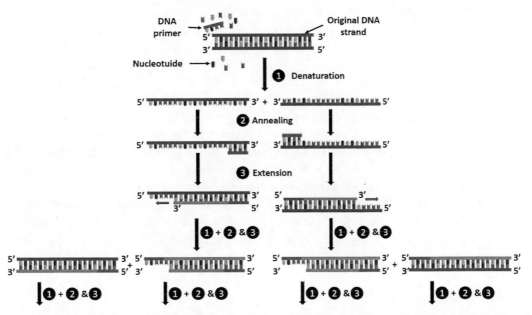

Fig. 5.24   The polymerase chain reaction. In each cycle the double-stranded DNA is denatured and separated to two single strands. The reaction mixture is cooled to allow annealing of synthetic DNA primers to the complementary segment on each strand. The primers are extended by the enzyme DNA polymerase and the process is repeated for numerous cycles.

Extension: During this step the DNA polymerase synthesizes a new strand of DNA complementary to the template DNA strand in the 5' to 3' by addition of dNTPs from the reaction mixture. The temperature at this step depends on the DNA polymerase used. The commonly used enzyme is *Taq* polymerase which is obtained from the thermostable bacteria *Thermus aquaticus*. This bacterium normally lives in hot springs and can withstand high temperatures up to 80–90°C. The temperature of 72°C is commonly used in the reaction with this enzyme. The precise time required for this step depends both on the DNA polymerase used and on the length of the DNA sequence being amplified. Conventionally at their optimal temperature, most DNA polymerases polymerize a thousand bases per minute. Under optimal conditions with each successive cycle of denaturation, annealing and extension, the original template strands and all newly generated strands act as templates resulting in an exponential amplification of the specific DNA target region. The number of copies of a DNA fragment formed after a given number of PCR cycles can be calculated by using the formula 2^n where n is the number of cycles. Thus, a reaction set for 20 cycle's results in 2^{20} or 1073741824, copies of the original double-stranded DNA target region.

Final elongation and hold: The final elongation step is occasionally performed at a temperature of 70–74°C for 5–15 minutes after the last PCR cycle to ensure amplification of any remaining single DNA strands. The final hold step is carried out at 4°C to cool the reaction chamber and may be used for short term storage of PCR products.

5.7.3   Variations of PCR

Over the years various modifications to the conventional PCR technique have been introduced to improve its efficiency and specificity. Some of these are described below:

5.7.3.1   *Nested PCR*

Nested PCR is a modified form of PCR designed to improve the specificity of DNA amplification by reducing the contamination in products that occurs due to non-specific amplification or non-specific primer binding sites. Nested PCR makes use of two sets of amplification primers used in two successive PCR reactions. In the first reaction, one pair of primers is used to generate DNA fragments which, in addition to the intended target, may contain products amplified from non-specific regions. The DNA molecules generated from the first reaction serve as an amplification target for the next PCR which uses a second set of primers whose binding sites are located or "nested" within the original set of primers thereby increasing the specificity of the reaction as can be seen in Figure 5.25.

5.7.3.2   *Quantitative PCR (qPCR)*

Quantitative PCR is the most widely used application of PCR which is used to amplify and simultaneously quantify absolute or relative amounts of target DNA sequence in a sample. It is also known as Real Time PCR as it allows real time monitoring of the exponential increase in the amounts of DNA as it is being amplified. The DNA or RNA molecules are tagged using fluorescent probes whose signal increases in direct proportion to the amount of PCR products generated in the reaction. The concentrations of the amplified products are monitored and quantified in real time as the reaction progresses by tracking the fluorescence signal.

Two methods that are commonly employed for the detection of amounts of amplified PCR products in real-time are:

1. Use of fluorescent dyes such as SYBR green that intercalates with double-stranded DNA molecules. In solution, this dye exhibits very little fluorescence. But upon binding to the double-stranded DNA molecules in the reaction, the enhancement of the fluorescence emission can be detected and measured during the reaction. With the amplification of DNA during the early exponential phase of the reaction, the amount of fluorescence increases above the background level. The point at which the signal exceeds/crosses this detection threshold and becomes measurable is known as the Threshold Cycle (CT) or crossing point. By using multiple dilutions of a known amount of standard DNA, a standard curve of log concentration against CT can be generated and the amount of DNA or cDNA present in an unknown sample can then be calculated from its CT value. SYBR green probes monitor the total amount of double-stranded DNA molecules but cannot distinguish between different sequences

2. Use of sequence-specific DNA probes such as TaqMan probe, Molecular beacons, or Scorpion primers which consist of oligonucleotides labeled with a fluorescent reporter and permit detection only upon binding with specific target DNA sequences.

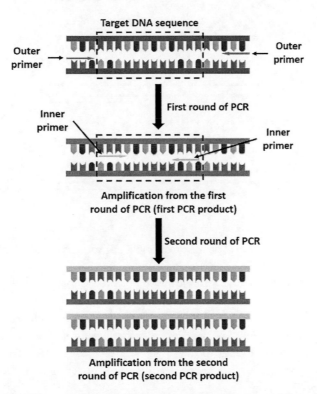

Fig. 5.25 Nested PCR. This method utilizes two sets of amplification primers. The first set/external primers are used to generate a PCR product. The second set of primers whose binding sites are situated inside or "nestled" within the first set are used for the next PCR cycle. These internal primers generate a shorter PCR product thereby increasing the specificity and fidelity of the PCR.

The *TaqMan probe* consists of an oligonucleotide specific to the target DNA that is labeled with a fluorescent probe at one end and a quencher at the other. This probe is designed to bind to the center of target DNA during the annealing step. As the *TaqMan* polymerase extends the second complementary strand during PCR, its 5' to 3' exonuclease activity degrades the probe into single nucleotides thus removing the close proximity between the fluorophore and the quencher. A fluorescence emission signal is detected which increases in direct proportion to the number of newly synthesized DNA strands detected and can be measured in real time (Figure 5.26).

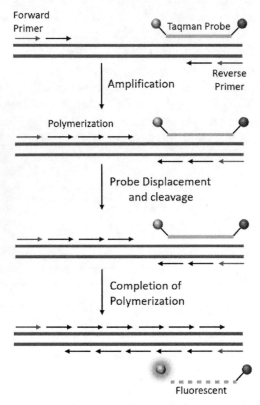

Fig. 5.26   Schematic representation of detection of amplified products in real time using TaqMan probe.

Molecular beacons are oligonucleotides that contain both the fluorophore and quencher groups at opposite ends. They form stem-loop structures wherein the central region is complementary to the target DNA sequence and the stem arms are complementary to each other. In the closed-loop conformation, the quencher, being in close proximity to the fluorophore, prevents the fluorescence emission of the latter. Upon binding to the target sequence, the molecular beacon is linearized separating the quencher from the fluorophore leading to the restoration of fluorescence that can be quantified (Figure 5.27).

Scorpion probes are similar to molecular beacons but contain a PCR primer covalently linked to the probe. The Scorpion probe maintains a self-complementary stem-loop configuration in the un-hybridized state with a fluorophore and quencher attached at either ends. It is attached to the 5' end of the PCR primer via a non-amplifiable "blocker" moiety. In the initial PCR cycles, the polymerase extends the PCR primer synthesizing a complementary strand of the specific target sequence. During the next cycle, the hairpin loop unfolds, and the loop-region of the probe hybridizes intra-molecularly to the newly synthesized DNA strand. This leads to separation of the fluorophore from the quencher resulting in detection of a fluorescence signal which is in direct proportion to the amount of target DNA (Figure 5.28).

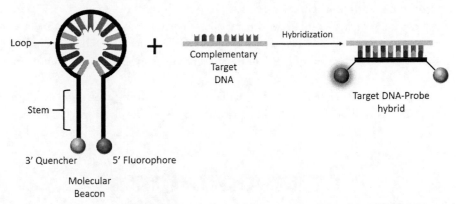

Fig. 5.27 Illustrating how a molecular beacon is used for quantification of amplified PCR products in real time.

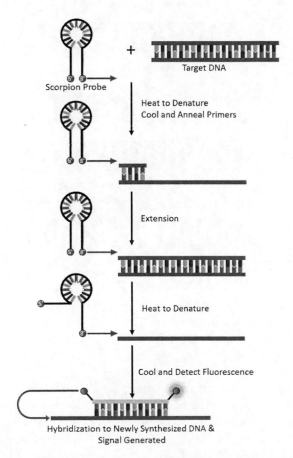

Fig. 5.28 Mechanism of detection of amplified products in real time using Scorpion probes.

5.7.3.3 *Reverse Transcription PCR (RT-PCR)*

Reverse Transcriptase PCR (RT-PCR) is a variation of the polymerase chain reaction that is used to amplify or identify a sequence from cellular or tissue RNA. As seen in Figure 5.29, the RNA strand is first reverse transcribed to its complementary cDNA by using the enzyme reverse transcriptase, and the latter is subsequently amplified using PCR. Thermo-stable DNA polymerases such as Tth polymerase isolated from *Thermus thermophilus*, which have has the ability of catalyzing high-temperature reverse transcription of RNA in the presence of manganese ions, and so, are used for the reaction.

RT-PCR is widely used in gene expression studies such as obtaining exon sequences from mature mRNAs and can be combined with qPCR to quantify expression levels of specific RNA molecules in a tissue or cell. It is employed clinically for the diagnoses of genetic disorders and to monitor drug therapy.

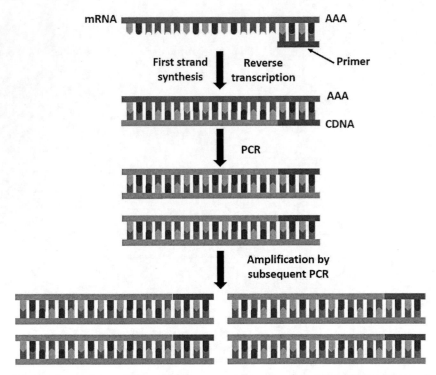

Fig. 5.29 Reverse transcriptase PCR. mRNA is converted to complementary DNA (cDNA) using enzyme reverse transcriptase. The cDNA is then used for PCR.

5.7.3.4 *Inverse PCR*

The standard PCR is used to amplify a DNA fragment that lies between two inward-pointing primers. Inverse PCR (also known as inside-out PCR), on the other hand, is used to amplify DNA sequences that flank only one end of a known DNA sequence and for which no primers are available. It follows standard PCR protocol, but the primers are oriented in the reverse direction with respect to the normal orientation. Inverse PCR involves restriction endonuclease mediated digestion of target

DNA that contains the known sequence and its flanking region. This generates a DNA fragment containing the known sequence flanked by two regions of unknown sequence. These restriction fragments that self-ligate to form a circle, serve as the template in PCR. The unknown sequence is amplified by two primers that bind specifically to the known sequence but are oriented in opposite directions. The product of the amplification reaction is a linear DNA fragment wherein the central unknown region remains flanked by two short known sequences (Figure 5.30).

Inverse PCR is commonly used in molecular biology for the identification of genomic inserts and for the identification and amplification of sequences flanking transposable elements.

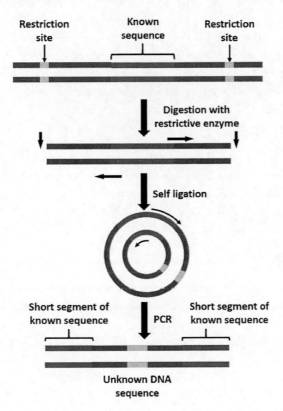

Fig. 5.30 Mechanism of inverse PCR for amplification and characterization of unknown sequences in a DNA molecule.

5.7.3.5 *Multiplex PCR*

Multiplex PCR is a widespread technique used for the amplification of multiple DNA sequences simultaneously in a single reaction. In a multiplexing assay, multiple primer sets within a single PCR reaction mixture are used to produce amplicons that are specific to different DNA sequences. By targeting multiple sequences at once, more information is obtained from a single experiment than would otherwise accrue, saving significant time and resources within laboratory settings. However, for accuracy and specificity, the primer design of all the primers needs to be optimized for them to work simultaneously within a narrow range of annealing temperatures and buffer concentrations in the reaction mixture. Multiplex PCR is a rapid and convenient technique commonly used in clinical and research settings for identification of pathogens, detection of RNA, for studying gene mutations and deletions, and in forensic sciences.

5.7.3.6 *Touchdown PCR*

Touchdown PCR is a variation of conventional PCR that enables simple and rapid optimization of specificity and sensitivity without compromising the yield. Touchdown PCR involves the use of high initial annealing temperatures which permit the formation of only perfectly matched primer-template hybrids, and is then progressively reduced to lower, more tolerant temperatures in successive PCR cycles. As the copies of the target sequence begin to accumulate over the first few cycles, high annealing temperatures are not critical for specificity as these products are unlikely to have any mispriming sites. Touchdown PCR has widespread applications in the construction of cDNA libraries and in the detection single nucleotide polymorphisms.

5.7.3.7 *Asymmetric PCR*

This technique involves preferential amplification of one of the strands of the target DNA molecule. One of the primers is left out or is introduced with a limiting concentration. When the limiting primer is exhausted, exponential increase in replication occurs through elongation of the excess primer. This variant of PCR is used to generate one DNA strand as a product for use in downstream application such as sequencing and for probing hybridization.

Questions to ponder over

1. What is the purpose of PCR and what is the function of a primer in this process?
2. From which source is the enzyme *Taq* polymerase obtained and why does PCR require this polymerase?
3. What happens during the denaturation step in PCR and at what temperature does it occur?
4. If two double-stranded DNA molecules are used at the beginning of a polymerase chain reaction, and you perform eight cycles of PCR, how many double-stranded copies of the DNA will you end up with?
5. What is the difference between a basic PCR and Inverse PCR?
6. How does Nested PCR work and what advantages does it offer over the traditional PCR?
7. What is real time PCR and what are the different types of probes that are used for the detection of the amplified products in this technique?

5.8 Nucleic Acid Sequencing

Nucleic acid sequencing is used to determine the sequence of nucleotides or bases along the length of DNA/RNA fragments and is one of the major techniques in molecular biology. The nucleotide sequence is the blueprint that encodes information that is essential for the development of an organism and hence, is the most fundamental requirement for the study of the genes or genome. Knowledge of nucleic acid sequences has become indispensable in numerous applied fields including basic research, biotechnology, identification of pathogens, forensic sciences, detection and diagnosis of different diseases, and for the development of potential therapies for the treatment of those diseases, study of gene expression, mutations, polymorphisms, etc.

In the mid-1970s, two methods were developed for sequencing DNA: the chain termination or Sanger sequencing method, which was developed by an English biochemist Frederick Sanger and the Maxim-Gilbert sequencing method developed by American molecular biologists Allan Maxim and Walter Gilbert. In the year 1980, both Walter Gilbert and Frederick Sanger were awarded the Nobel Prize in Chemistry for their contributions. Both the Sanger sequencing and Maxim–Gilbert methods represent the first generation of DNA sequencing methods.

5.8.1 First Generation Sequencing

5.8.1.1 *Chain Termination/Sanger Sequencing Method*

The classical chain termination method makes use of a single-stranded DNA template that needs to be sequenced, a short nucleotide primer complementary to the target sequence, enzyme DNA polymerase, four deoxyribonucleoside triphosphates (dNTP) and four di-deoxyribonucleoside triphosphates (ddNTP) that lack a 3' hydroxyl group required for the formation of a phosphodiester between the nucleotides. The DNA sequencing reaction mixture is divided into four separate parts each including the standard dNTPs (dATP, dGTP, dCTP and dTTP) and the DNA polymerase, a low level of only one of the ddNTPs (ddATP, ddGTP, ddCTP and ddTTP), and the synthesis is allowed to proceed. When a ddNTP is incorporated into the chain of nucleotides, the reaction terminates as the 5' to 3' phosphodiester link fails to form between the nucleotides. Since the incorporation of ddNTP is a random event, the synthesis terminates at different points for each of the reactions. This produces four sets of DNA fragments, each terminating at a different type of base. The products of these four reactions are denatured by heating and separated by polyacrylamide gel electrophoresis. Electrophoresis is performed in the presence of urea to prevent renaturation of DNA which may alter the electrophoretic mobility of the DNA molecule. The gels used, tend to be very long in order to achieve maximum resolution in separation of fragments of different lengths. The DNA bands may then be visualized by autoradiography or UV light and the DNA sequence can be directly read off the X-ray film or gel image. In each lane the bands represent the DNA fragments that have terminated after incorporation of a particular ddNTP. The DNA sequence of the newly synthesized strand can be determined by reading the relative positions of the band across all lanes starting at the bottom of the gel to the top.

5.8.1.2 *Maxim and Gilbert Sequencing*

This technique of DNA sequencing also referred to as chemical degradation method is based on the base-specific chemical modification of DNA and subsequent cleavage of the DNA backbone at sites adjacent to the modified nucleotides.

This method involves radioactive labelling of the 5' end of a double-stranded DNA segment that needs to be sequenced. The labeled DNA is subjected to chemical reagents that cleave in a base specific manner either by methylation or removal of the base. Formic acid typically cleaves at sites occupied by either A or G, while guanines are methylated using dimethyl sulfate. Hydrazine cleaves at T and C sites and the addition of sodium chloride to the hydrazine reaction allows for a C-specific reaction. The concentration of the modifying chemicals is chosen such that each molecule is modified at only one position along its length and every base in the DNA fragment has had an equal chance of being modified. The modified DNAs are then cleaved by piperidine which breaks the phosphodiester bond at the 5' end of the nucleotide whose base has been modified. Thus, a series of cleaved fragments of different lengths are generated, all with a labeled end in common and the other "cut" end; the latter indicating the position of the base that was cleaved. The strands are separated by electrophoresis under denaturing conditions and the sequence of the DNA can be inferred in a way similar to the one described in the Sanger sequencing method.

Although based on simple principles this method is time consuming and requires working with large amount of radioactive material and toxic chemicals. With the advancements in the Sanger sequencing methods and advent of next generation sequencing technologies, this method has lost its popularity in present times.

5.8.1.3   *Automated Fluorescent DNA Sequencing*

As originally developed, both the Maxim-Gilbert and the chain termination methods of DNA sequencing employ radioactive labels and the fragments generated are visualized by autoradiography. In addition to posing health risks and disposal issues, this approach is not well suited to automation. Advances in fluorescent dye labeling technologies have led to the development of high throughput automated DNA sequencing techniques.

Using this technique each of the four dideoxynucleotides is labeled with different fluorophores. Since each dideoxynucleotide is associated with a different label, it is possible to carry out all the four sequencing reactions in a single reaction tube. The four chain terminated products are run on just one track of the denaturing electrophoresis gel. Each fragment with base specific fluorescent label is excited by a laser and from the detection of light emitted by the dyes at their characteristic wavelength, the sequence can be interpreted.

In addition to the reduction in cost and time for sequencing, this technique offers real time detection of the sequence, making this approach the preferred method used by most laboratories. Capillary electrophoresis is increasingly used for the sequencing of DNA molecules instead of the gels, thus allowing high throughput to be achieved. Commercially available kits that contain all the components necessary to perform the sequencing reaction in a "master mix" format wherein the addition of template and primer is all that is required to complete the reaction, are being widely used in laboratories. Many large-scale sequence facilities employ fully automated systems that use the 96-well microtiter plates, to derive the DNA sequences.

5.8.2   Next Generation (Second Generation) Sequencing

Next generation sequencing (NGS) comprises of a number of different modern sequencing techniques that allow for massively parallel DNA sequencing reactions. These new technologies have largely supplanted first generation techniques by virtue of their speed, reduced cost, and high throughput capabilities. Major advantages of these NGS technologies are that they do not require bacterial cloning of DNA fragments and electrophoretic separation of sequencing products. Since the completion of sequencing of the human genome in year 2003, that took over decade to complete and cost around 3 billion dollars, automation and advances in the field of genomics and technological improvements have enabled scientists to rapidly sequence entire genomes or specific regions of interest such as exomes, in a matter of hours and for less than $1000. This powerful platform has revolutionized the fields of molecular biology, genomics, personalized medicine, and clinical diagnostics. The second-generation sequencing systems are based on the principles of either "sequencing by synthesis" or "sequencing by ligation."

5.8.2.1 *Pyrosequencing*

Pyrosequencing, also popularly known as the "454" method, is a DNA sequencing technique based on the "sequencing by synthesis" principle. This technique derives its name from the detection of light upon release of a pyrophosphate molecule during DNA synthesis.

This method involves a cascade of enzymatic reactions wherein light is generated in an amount proportional to the number of incorporated nucleotides. As seen in Figure 5.31, the chain starts with the DNA polymerization reaction when one of the four types of added deoxynucleotide triphosphates (dNTPs) are incorporated into the single-strand DNA template, thereby releasing inorganic pyrophosphate (PPi). This serves as a substrate for ATP sulfurylase which converts PPi to ATP that further drives the luciferase-mediated oxidation of luciferin to generate light. Unincorporated nucleotides and ATP are degraded by the enzyme apyrase in between dNTP additions, allowing the reaction to start again with another nucleotide. This process is repeated by adding each nucleotide in continuation until the synthesis is complete. A detector picks up the intensity of light emitted by the process, which is then used to infer the number and type of nucleotides added, as illustrated in Figure 5.31.

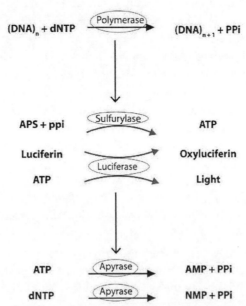

Fig. 5.31   General mechanism of pyrosequencing reaction method.

The method is limited to sequencing 300–500 nucleotide base pairs, in comparison to the over 1000 base pairs achievable by Sanger sequencing. It however offers potential advantages of accuracy, flexibility, low cost, and ease of automation. Pyrosequencing is used for the detection of single nucleotide polymorphisms, insertion-deletions, or other sequence variations, in addition to being able to quantify DNA methylation and allele frequency.

5.8.2.2 *Illumina*

The Illumina NGS sequencing technology is based on the principle of "sequencing by synthesis" and infers the sequence of a DNA template by stepwise incorporation of reversibly fluorescent and terminated nucleotides. The nucleotides used for this technology are modified such that each nucleotide is reversibly attached to a single fluorescent molecule with a unique emission wavelength, and in addition, each nucleotide is reversibly terminated ensuring incorporation of a single nucleotide into the growing DNA strand.

In this technique, smaller DNA fragments of the genome to be sequenced are constructed as a library wherein each fragment is tagged with custom adapters and index sequences. Clonal bridge amplification is carried out on solid surface where primer sequences that are complimentary to the adapter sequence are immobilized across a proprietary flow cell. This results in generation of DNA clusters with 1000 identical copies of each template fragment. Modified nucleotides that are fluorescently labeled and have reversible 3'-OH blockers are added simultaneously to the flow cell along with DNA polymerase. After each round of synthesis and nucleotide incorporation, the unused bases and DNA polymerase molecules are washed away. The fluorescence signal is read and recorded at each cluster strand extension following which both the 3' terminator group and the fluorescent molecule are cleaved and washed away. This process in repeated until the entire sequencing reaction is complete. The end result is a rapid and highly accurate (99.9%) base-by-base sequencing of the entire genome in a massively parallel manner, as illustrated in Figure 5.32.

This sequencing by synthesis technology based on reversible dye terminators, now used by Illumina, was developed by Shankar Balasubramanian and David Klenerman at the University of Cambridge. In order to commercialize this method, they founded the company named Solexa in 1998 which was acquired by Illumina in the year 2007, and has since built upon, rapidly and constantly improving the technology. Currently, the company offers MiSeq, NextSeq 550 and 2000, HiSeq3000/4000, Novaseq 6000 platforms that find a wide variety of applications in DNA sequencing (whole genome, exome, and targeted de novo sequencing), as well as RNA sequencing (total RNA, mRNA, and small RNA).

This innovative and flexible technology is the most commonly used next generation sequencing platform and finds a broad array of applications in the field of genomics, transcriptomics, and epigenomics. In comparison to the Pyrosequencing and Ion Torrent platforms, this technique offers additional advantages in sequencing of homopolymeric regions since it only allows incorporation of a single nucleotide at a time. Certain limitations of this technology include substitution errors due to the background noise levels resulting from incomplete removal of the fluorescent signal, issues with regions of extreme GC% being inefficiently amplified by PCR, and read length limitation which presents obstacles in de novo sequencing.

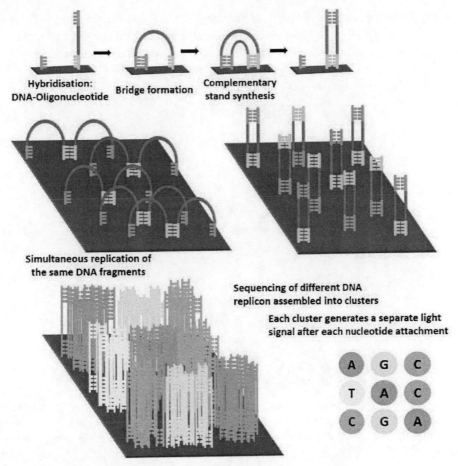

Fig. 5.32 Next generation sequencing on an Illumina platform. DNA fragments to be sequenced are amplified and bound to a flow cell generating clusters with about 1000 copies of each fragment. Upon nucleotide incorporation, the fluorescence signal corresponding to each base is measured and the imaging of tens of millions of clusters is carried out in parallel resulting in a rapid and cost-effective sequencing of the entire genome. [See color plates]

5.8.2.3 *Ion Torrent Sequencing*

Unlike Illumina and Pyrosequencing, Ion Torrent sequencing also known as ion semiconductor sequencing does not make use of optical signals. Instead, it measures the direct release of H⁺ ion upon incorporation of dNTP into a growing DNA strand.

This technique involves construction of a library by DNA fragmentation and adapter ligation. The molecules are clonally amplified on the beads by emulsion PCR. The beads carrying the amplified DNA clusters are immobilized on the surface of an ion chip consisting of a semiconductor transistor designed to detect changes in the pH as the reaction progresses. The DNA clusters are sequentially flooded with a single species of dNTP. The dNTP is incorporated into the new strand by DNA polymerase if complementary to the nucleotide of the leading strand. This results in the release of H⁺ ion leading to a change in the pH of the solution which is detected by the semiconductor

(Figure 5.33). If the introduced nucleotide is not complementary to the target strand, no voltage change is recorded. The series of electrical pulses transmitted from the chip to a computer is translated directly into a DNA sequence thus avoiding any optical measurements. This results in sequencing technology that is simpler, rapid, cost effective, and marketed in the form of a compact economical personal genomic machine (PGM) utilized as a bench top instrument in various research and clinical laboratories.

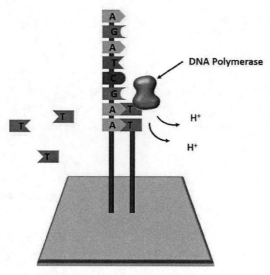

Fig. 5.33 Principle of Ion Torrent Sequencing Reaction. DNA clusters on the ion chip are flooded with single species of dNTP along with polymerase. Changes in pH are recorded as each H+ ion is released upon successful incorporation of a complementary dNTP to the leading strand inferring the sequence of the target DNA.

In the presence of homo-polymer repeats of the same nucleotide (e.g., AAAA) on the template sequence, multiple dNTP molecules are incorporated in a single cycle resulting in a greater pH change and a proportionally higher electronic signal. This is a limitation of the system (shared by other techniques that detect single nucleotide additions, such as pyrosequencing) in that it is difficult to enumerate long repeats. While short stretches can be differentiated, signals generated from high repeat longer stretches become increasingly difficult to differentiate. Another limitation of this system is the short-read length compared to Sanger sequencing or pyrosequencing. Ion Torrent semiconductor sequencers produce an average read length of approximately 400 bp with an average error rate of approximately 1%. Ion Torrent platforms are best suited for small-scale applications and can be used mainly for targeted sequencing, amplicon sequencing, microbial genome and transcriptome sequencing, exome, de novo, and small RNA sequencing.

5.8.2.4 *Solid*

SOLiD (Sequencing by Oligonucleotide Ligation and Detection) is a second-generation nucleic acid sequencing platform that utilizes base-pairing mismatch sensitivity of enzyme DNA ligase to determine the sequence of nucleotides in the target DNA molecule. As against other commonly used sequencing technologies, this method does not make use of DNA polymerase for incorporation of nucleotides. Instead it relies on short oligonucleotide probes that are ligated to one another.

Library construction, for sequencing by ligation, is similar to the one used for pyrosequencing. Emulsion PCR is utilized for clonal amplification of a ssDNA primer-binding region/adapter that has been conjugated to the target sequence on a bead. These beads are then immobilized on a glass surface and exposed to a library of octamer nucleotide sequences that are used as detection probes and for the activity of DNA ligase. These oligonucleotides consist of 8 bases with a different fluorescent dye attached at the 5' end of the probe. They comprise of two probe specific bases that are complementary to the nucleotides to be sequenced, and six degenerate bases. The sequencing reaction commences with the binding of the universal sequencing primers to adapter sequences followed by hybridization of the complementary probe. DNA ligase is introduced in the flow cell which anneals the fluorescently tagged probe to the primer. After ligation of specific octamer to the template, unbound nucleotides are washed away and three nucleotides at the 5' end, that are linked with a specific fluorescent dye for detection of two bases annealed to target molecule, are removed. This cleavage allows for the measurement of the fluorescent signal, which indicates that there is a nucleotide at that position, while simultaneously regenerating a 5' phosphate at the end of the ligated probe thereby preparing the system for another round of ligation.

The process begins again by sequencing another position with a different sequencing primer that is offset by one base from the previous primer (length n-1). This is due to the fact that the first base at the 3' end of the second primer binds to the second base at the 5' end of the adapter sequence. The sequencing process is repeated and completed using 5 universal primers that are one base shifted each time until the entire target sequence has been determined.

Using this approach, since each base is effectively sequenced twice, this technique is the most accurate (99.99% accuracy rate with a sixth primer) of all other NGS platforms and is also relatively inexpensive. It can complete a sequencing run in 7–14 days and can produce up to 320 Gb of data. Unfortunately, the main disadvantage of this technology is the short-read lengths making it unsuitable for many applications especially for the sequencing of palindromic sequences. Substitutions also form the most common errors encountered in this technology Also short distances between the beads can lead to false reads and low-quality bases. Although this technology can be used for sequencing of whole genome, exome, transcriptome, methylation, small RNA sequencing, the SOLiD platform is best suited for sequencing projects that demand low error rates and for transcriptome sequencing.

5.8.3 Third Generation Sequencing

While NGS technologies are extremely powerful and have dominated the DNA sequencing space since their development, they do suffer from certain drawbacks. Since eukaryotic genomes contain numerous repetitive regions, a major limitation to this class of sequencing methods is the relatively short length of reads they produce. In addition, while small variants such as single-nucleotide variations (SNVs) can be accurately detected using short reads, detection and characterization of larger structural variations (SVs) could pose a challenge with NGS. This is important since SVs are implicated in a variety of diseases. In addition to the limitations mentioned above the fact that these techniques rely on PCR could result in difficulties with regions of extreme GC%, as these are inefficiently amplified by PCR.

In order to overcome these limitations, third generation sequencing technologies have emerged that work by reading the nucleotide sequences at a single molecule level, and in real time, in contrast to the existing NGS methods which require breaking long strands of DNA into small segments and inferring nucleotide sequences following amplification and synthesis. By enabling direct sequencing of single DNA molecules, these technologies are able to produce substantially longer reads and are revolutionizing the field of genome science by enabling researchers to explore genomes at an unprecedented resolution. In addition, these technologies can directly detect epigenetic modifications on native DNA and allow sequencing of whole-transcripts and metagenomes without the need for assembly.

Several companies continue to pursue the development of these third-generation sequencing technologies by applying fundamentally different approaches to sequencing single DNA molecules.

5.8.3.1 *SMRT*

A Single Molecule Real Time (SMRT) sequencing platform which utilizes a zero-mode waveguide (ZMW) was developed by Pacific Biosciences in year 2011. The DNA sequencing is carried out on a chip that contains many ZMWs. A closed, circular single-stranded DNA template (created by ligating hairpin adaptors to the ends of the target DNA) is annealed to a single DNA polymerase affixed at the bottom of a ZMW well which creates an illuminated visualization chamber and allows monitoring of the DNA polymerase activity at a single molecule level. The DNA is sequenced as the incorporation of complementary fluorescently labeled nucleotides to the DNA strand produces fluorescence signals on excitation by a laser and is recorded in real time (a "movie"). Since the DNA template is circular, the polymerase can continue the synthesis and the strands can be sequenced with multiple "passes" in a single continuous long read, which can then be split at the adapter sequences, generating multiple "subreads" and thus yielding higher level of accuracy.

SMRT technology has proven to be a cost effective and an efficient technique that can generate long reads of sequences allowing de novo genome sequencing and easier genome assemblies.

5.8.3.2 *Oxford Nanopore*

This technology is based on the passage of an ionic current through a nanoscale pore structure and monitoring changes in the electric current density, upon translocation of the biological polynucleotide (DNA/RNA) through or near the nanopore. This method involves a simple DNA library preparation wherein the DNA strands are ligated with adapters tightly bound to a polymerase or helicase enzyme ensuring passage of the DNA molecule through the pore. The double-stranded DNA unwinds at the pore allowing one strand to pass through. The voltage applied across the nanopore generates an ionic current which is measured and analyzed upon the passage of the different nucleotides, in order to infer the sequence of the DNA fragment. For increased read accuracy, specialized adapter sequences are used to increase the likelihood of the passage of the second strand thus allowing "base calling" using information from both strands (Figure 5.34). Using nanopore sequencing, and the recently commercialized portable MinION sequencer, a single molecule of DNA or native RNA can be sequenced in a massively parallel fashion without the need for fragmentation, reverse transcription (as carried out in traditional RNA sequencing technologies) and amplification. This enables direct identification of base modifications alongside nucleotide sequences thus offering relatively low-cost, rapid processing of samples in real-time. This technology finds widespread applications in human and plant genome sequencing, RNA sequencing, rapid identification of viral pathogens, environmental and food safety monitoring, amongst others.

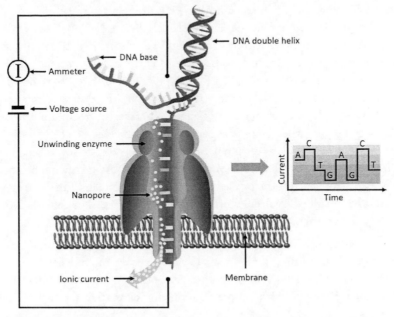

Fig. 5.34 Illustration of mechanism of nanopore DNA sequencing technology. DNA strand is passed through the nanopore. The ionic current generated upon the passage of the DNA bases through the pore is measured and translated into the sequence of the DNA fragment.

Questions to ponder over

1. Which sequencing technology was initially used to sequence human DNA in the Human Genome Project, what were its drawbacks and what methods are being presently employed for the same?

2. During electrophoresis followed by Sanger DNA sequencing, the position of the band on the gel represents the dNTP used as a chain terminator in that mixture. Is this statement correct?

3. Why is the Sanger sequencing method also known as chain termination sequencing?

4. What is involved in the Maxim–Gilbert sequencing method and why is it almost extinct in present times?

5. On what principle are the Illumina and pyrosequencing next generation sequencing technologies based upon? What are the advantages and limitations of each of these methods?

6. How is the SOLiD sequencing technology different from Illumina and why does it have a higher accuracy rate in comparison to the latter?

7. What advantages do the third-generation technologies offer over NGS?

5.9   Analyzing Gene and Gene Expression

In multicellular organisms, approximately 98.5% of genes are junk or of unknown function, only ~ 1.5% of functional genes are expressed in any given cell at any time. Because of gene expression liver cells are different from a muscle cell, and a healthy cell different from the diseased cell. Thus, by collecting and comparing transcriptomes (a sum total of all the mRNA expressed from the genes) of different cells or strains, treated versus untreated, healthy versus diseased, different stages of cellular development, and varied environmental conditions, researcher can gain access to cellular physiology. There are several mechanisms which play their roles in producing different variants of mRNA, such as alternate splicing, RNA editing, or alternative transcription initiation and termination sites. Since transcriptome captures a level of complexity of genes, the researcher can study when and where different types of genes are turned on or off in various types of cells.

As mentioned above, level and expression patterns of mRNA dictate several cellular process and conditions of the cell. Therefore, determination of level of mRNAs is very important to generate a comprehensive picture of gene profile of a cell in a given condition and fulfil the gap between the genetic code and the functional molecules of the cells. Gene expression analysis is generally done by tracking RNA. There are mainly four types of RNA; these are:

i)   mRNA (messenger RNA): encodes amino acid sequence of a protein.
ii)   tRNA (transfer RNA): brings amino acids to ribosomes during translation.
iii)   rRNA (ribosomal RNA): with ribosomal proteins, makes up the ribosomes.
iv)   snRNA (small nuclear RNA): with proteins, forms complexes that are used in RNA processing in eukaryotes.

Other types of RNA and their function are described in Table 5.4.

Table 5.4   Types of RNA and their functions.

Long RNAs	Function
mRNA (0.4–10 kb)	Coding genes
lincRNA (>200 bp)	Regulating basal transcription machinery
rRNA (1898–3898 bp)	Protein synthesis
Small RNAs	**Function**
snRNA	RNA splicing/regulation of transcription
snoRNA (60–300 bp)	RNA modification
miRNA (19–24 bp)	Translational repression, mRNA cleavage
piRNAs (26–31 nt) piwi-interacting RNA	Transposon repression/DNA methylation
tiRNAs (17–18 nt) tini RNAs	Associated with TSS in animals
tRNA (73–95 bp)	Translation
rRNA (5.7 S and 5.0 S)	Protein synthesis
mt-RNA	Mitochondrial Translation
siRNA (small interfering RNA)	RNA silencing
gRNA (guide RNA)	RNA editing
TSSa-RNAs (20–90 bp)	Maintenance of transcription

5.9.1 Methods for the Study of Gene Expression

Several techniques are available for determining gene expression. All these techniques employ DNA–DNA or DNA–RNA hybridization methods. Briefly, in this process, DNA or RNA molecules (single-stranded) are paired with the complementary strands in a complex mixture. Primarily, these techniques can be divided into two types of methods namely, low-throughput methods and high-throughput methods.

5.9.1.1 *Low-Throughput Methods*

(a) Quantitative Northern blot

In a biochemical lab, a most commonly used technique to detect biomolecules, such as DNA, RNA, and proteins, is blotting. As mentioned before, regarding analysis of gene expression, tracking the quantity of RNA is important for the determination of transcription. One of the most commonly used techniques by researchers for the determination of the quantity of mRNA produced by cells due to differences in time or treatment, is the Northern blot. In this technique, cellular membrane is first digested to isolate the biomolecules by lysis of cells. In the next step, expressed mRNAs are then separated from the DNA, proteins, lipids, and other cellular contents. Isolated mRNAs are then separated by gel electrophoresis and transferred by blotting to an immobilizing matrix such as a nylon membrane. A complementary target probe (usually radiolabeled single-strand DNA sequence) is now bound to the mRNA sequence on the membrane, which will then be detected by using an appropriate detection technique (Figure 5.35). The intensity of the resulting band is a direct indicator of expression of the gene of interest.

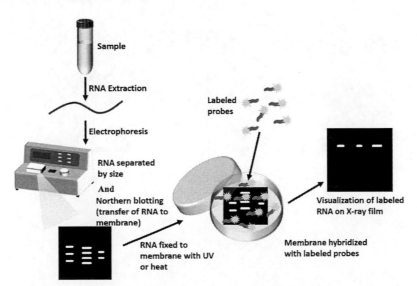

Fig. 5.35 Schematics of Northern blot. The tissue is first homogenized and its RNA is extracted and separated from other biomolecules. RNA sequence is separated using electrophoresis and transferred to a nylon membrane. Fixed RNA will be probed with a reagent which hybridizes with the RNA sequence on the blot corresponding to the sequence of interest. After proper washing of the unbounded probes, labeled RNAs are detected by chemiluminescence or autoradiography.

(b) Nuclease protection assay (NPA)

This technique is not only quantitative but also extremely sensitive, and based upon hybridization of target RNA. This method is used for the detection, quantitation and mapping of specific RNAs in a complex mixture of total cellular RNA. Two types of formats are available in this technique: ribonuclease protection assay (RPA) and S1 nuclease assay. Additionally, this technique is also useful for mapping transcription start sites, studying intron-exon junctions, and detection of small differences in related transcripts.

In this technique, single-stranded antisense RNA probe is allowed to hybridize onto the target RNA. Then RNAses is used to digest other single-stranded RNA that do not hybridize. In general, inactivation of RNAses and the precipitation of hybridized RNA are performed simultaneously. Finally, electrophoresis followed by autoradiography is employed to determine the presence, relative amount, and size of the protected RNA (Figure 5.36).

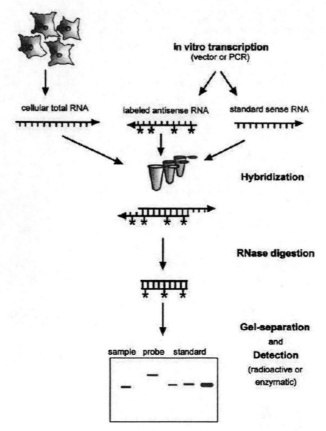

Fig. 5.36 Schematics of RNA protection assay.

(c) PCR-based methods (commonly known as RT-PCR)

As the name suggests, this method uses PCR techniques (described earlier) to estimate the concentration of target RNA. In RT-PCR methods the target RNA is reverse transcribed to complementary cDNA using a reverse transcriptase and a suitable primer. The produce cDNA is now used as a template for the PCR reaction. Other than gene expression analysis, this technique is useful in a variety of applications such as RNAi validation, microarray validation, pathogen detection, genetic testing, and disease research.

There are two different techniques available: (a) one-step assays, in which both reverse transcriptase and PCR reaction are performed simultaneously in one tube, and (b) two-step assays, in which reverse transcriptase and PCR steps are performed in two separate tubes (Figure 5.37). There are advantages and disadvantages in both methods (Table 5.5). If RNA concentration is high, in the initial sample, then it is preferable to perform one-step RT-PCR. However, a careful evaluation should be done to prevent dimer formation because the primers will be present during the lower temperature conditions of reverse transcriptase reaction (RT) and the PCR cycling. Whereas, two-step RT-PCR is advisable when initial RNA concentration is low. Two-step RT-PCR produces sufficient amount of, more, stable cDNA sample that can be archived for future use.

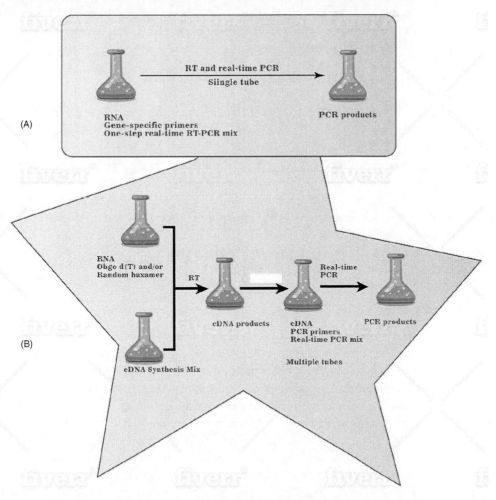

Fig. 5.37 Schematics of (A) one-step PCR and (B) two-step PCR.

Table 5.5 Advantages and disadvantages of one-step and two-step PCRs.

	Advantages	Disadvantages
One-step	• Less experimental variations (simple) • Accurate representation of target copy number • Less risk of error and contamination • Suitable for high throughput methods • Fast and highly reproducible	• Impossible to optimize the two reactions separately (troubleshooting is difficult) • Less sensitive • No stock of cDNA • Detection of fewer targets per sample
Two-step	• A stable cDNA pool is generated which can be stored for long periods of time and used for multiple reactions • Highly sensitive • More efficient • The target and reference genes can be amplified from the same DNA pool • Each reaction can be optimized separately • Flexibility in choosing primers	• More chances of error and DNA contamination • Time consuming • Requires more optimization than one-step • Less favorable for high throughput

(d) Differential display PCR

Sometimes we need to analyze the tissue specific gene expression compared to a control. For this sort of investigation, another RT-PCR based technique, called differential display PCR is employed. A flow chart for this technique is given in Figure 5.38. In brief, a PCR technique is used to amplify cDNAs derived from the mRNAs, using reverse transcriptase, of a given cell or tissue type. Two different oligonucleotides are used: anchored antisense primers (such as the poly(A) tail in eukaryotic cells) and arbitrary sense primers which bind to the 5' end of the transcripts. An anchored primer will anneal to the junction between the poly(A) tail and the 3'-untranslated mRNA template. Then an arbitrary sequence is added to the reaction mixture, producing double-stranded cDNA. The product of this amplification reaction is then separated by gel electrophoresis allowing identification and isolation of the transcripts.

(e) In situ hybridization (ISH)

In situ hybridization is a powerful and versatile technique for localizing specific nucleic acid changes. Gross changes in DNA are quite detectable, although single or restricted number of base substitutions, deletions, rearrangements, or insertions may be difficult to detect. ISH provides temporal spatial information about gene expression and their locus. Here, a labeled RNA or DNA probe hybridizes with a target mRNA or DNA in a sample leading to determination of their distribution or location. ISH can be used on a variety of different samples such as morphologically preserved chromosomes, cells, tissue sections, entire tissue, and circulating tumor cells. Additionally, it is useful in identifying and quantifying specific cellular DNA, mRNA, microRNA (miRNA), noncoding RNA, and other nucleotide entities, thereby providing insight into some of the earliest changes in the cell. When ISH information is combined with histopathological data, it can offer a complete picture of the cellular changes taking place. The main advantage of this technique is that the PCR is carried out directly on the tissue slide with standard PCR reagents.

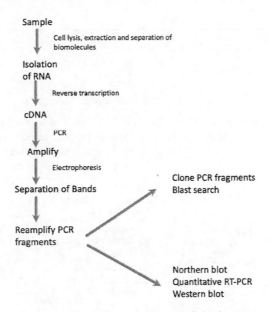

Fig. 5.38 Flow chart of differential display PCR.

In this technique, the target nucleic acid binds to complimentary strands and form hybrids. Hybrids could be DNA–DNA, DNA–RNA, or RNA–RNA, and the probes could either be double-stranded DNA (dsDNA) or single-stranded DNA (ssDNA), RNA (riboprobes), or synthetic oligonucleotides. The labels, either radioisotopes or nonradioactive molecules, such as biotin, digoxigenin, or fluorescent dyes, attach to the probe and are detected by appropriate techniques. In brief, the labeled probe and the target DNA are denatured. Combining the denatured probe and target allows annealing of complementary DNA sequences. These sequences are amplified using PCR and detected by visualization techniques available for gel electrophoresis.

Nonradioactive hybridization methods can be further categorized as direct and indirect methods. In the direct method, a reporter molecule is directly attached to the probe, to be detected after hybridization. In the indirect method, the probe contains the primary reported molecule which will be detected once it binds to the secondary detection molecule containing chromogenic (CISH: Chromogenic in situ hybridization) or fluorescence molecule (FISH: Fluorescence in situ hybridization) (Figure 5.39). In general, FISH is faster and more sensitive with directly labeled probes, whereas indirect labeling offers the advantage of an amplified signal which produces a better signal to noise ratio.

Table 5.6 Comparison of CISH with FISH.

CISH	FISH
Uses peroxidase or alkaline phosphatase-labeled reporter antibodies	Uses directly labeled fluorescent nucleotides or probes with reporter molecules that are detected by fluorescent antibodies or affinity molecules.
Moderately sensitive	Highly sensitive

Contd.

Table 5.6 *contd.*

CISH	FISH
Low cost	Relatively higher cost
Staining is permanent	Staining is temporary. Quenching of fluorescence signal over time.
Gene amplification, gene deletion, chromosomal translocations. Chromosomal number can be detected.	Commonly used for translocations, insertions, inversions, and microdeletions as well as for chromosomal gene mapping and for identifying and characterizing chromosome breakpoints.

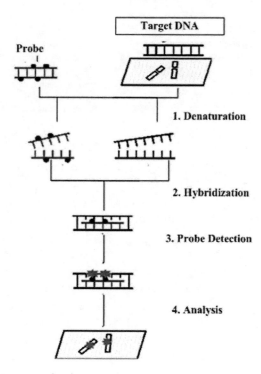

Fig. 5.39   Steps involved in CISH/FISH (many steps are common to both).

1. **Fixation of tissue:** Caution should be taken to ensure target selectivity, stability, and integrity of target DNA or RNA, and proper preservation of sample for examining morphological details.
2. **Probe selection:** Selectivity, specificity, tissue penetration, reproducibility, and stability of hybrids should be considered before selecting probe. Optimum length could be dependent on the application; it could be as small as 20–40 bp to 1000 bp.
3. **Probe labeling:** Two types: radioisotope labeling and non-isotopic labeling. Disadvantages of radioisotope include a long exposure time, poor spatial resolution, risk of exposure to radioactivity, and disposal of radioactive waste. However, non-isotopic labeling is not as sensitive as radioactive labeling.
4. **Target and probe denaturation:** Alkaline or heat denaturation methods are used.

5. **Hybridization:** Depends on the ability of the probe sequence to anneal the complementary sequence just below its melting temperature (Tm).
6. **Controls:** Several controls are being used. Specificity controls that use alternate sequence or sense probe can be used as control. Poly(dT) probes or probes against housekeeping gene sequences are used as controls to detect sample degradation.
7. **Detection:** Autoradiograph (for radioactive probes) and microscopy (for nonradioactive probes).

5.9.1.2 *High-Throughput Methods*

High throughput techniques have to simultaneously analyze the activities of thousands of genes and their products. They may be employed on either stand-alone or combined with other bioanalytical techniques for a more comprehensive analysis of gene expression and related phenomena. The methods include:

(a) Microarray

Traditional low throughput methods are unable to handle a large number of genes simultaneously. The development of DNA microarray techniques in the mid-1990s provided, for the first time, the capability to simultaneously profile and study the transcriptome (a collection of all the mRNA molecules). As such, it enables researchers to better investigate the fundamental aspects of growth, development of life, and genetic cause of anomalies occurring in the cells. In each cell, different genes are turned on and off in response to changes associated with environmental stimuli, physiology, and external/internal factors. So, monitoring and identifying these changes will help in identifying the genetic changes. When a gene is expressed in a cell, it generates messenger RNA (mRNA). Overexpressed genes generate more mRNA than under expressed genes, and DNA microarray techniques are capable of detecting such differentials and are thus useful in determining the expression levels of genes.

Microarray techniques generate a profile of gene expression, which serves as a determinant of protein levels and therefore cellular function between biological samples. A single experiment can provide information on the expression on thousands of genes or potentially the entire genome. Such techniques develop understanding of complex biological systems required for drug discovery, disease diagnosis, and identification of novel genes. It involves hybridizing target molecules to probe molecules that have been fixed as thousands of micro spots on a screen. The fluorescence (or the radioactivity) of target molecules can then be measured (quantified) for each spot to analyze the expression of genes. The log-transformed ratios (generally between Cy3 and Cy5) in each spot reflect the relative mRNA expression levels of the corresponding genes (Figure 5.40).

DNA microarray analysis consists of the following steps:

1. **Isolating and purifying mRNA:** With one sample usually serving as control, another sample would constitute the experimental one (such as healthy versus diseased). Once the tissue samples are obtained, mRNA is isolated and purified. For extraction of RNA, either a column or a solvent such as phenol-chloroform is used. After RNA isolation, mRNA is isolated (from rRNA and tRNA) using a column containing beads with poly-T tails to bind the mRNA (mRNA has a poly-A tail).
2. **Reverse transcription and labeling:** Labeling is necessary for detection and is conducted through a reverse transcription reaction to produce a complementary DNA strand that will

fluoresce. Some protocols do not label the cDNA but use a second step of amplification, where the cDNA from the RT step serves as a template to produce a labeled cRNA strand. For this step, poly-T (oligo dT) primers, reverse transcriptase (to make cDNA), and fluorescently dyed nucleotides are mixed with purified mRNA. In general, a green colored fluorescent dye is used for control sample while a red colored fluorescent dye is used for treated sample. The primer and RT bind to the mRNA first, then the fluorescent dyed nucleotides also bind to create a cDNA.

3. **Hybridization:** The cDNA binds to complementary base pairs in each of the spots on the array, a process known as hybridization. This step involves placing labeled cDNAs onto a DNA microarray where they hybridize to their synthetic complementary DNA probes attached on the microarray. A series of washes are used to remove non-bound sequences.

4. **Scanning the microarray and quantitating the signal:** The fluorescent tags on bound cDNA are excited by a laser and the fluorescently labeled target sequences that bind to a probe generate a signal. The total strength of the signal depends upon the amount of target sample binding to the probes present on that spot. Thus, the amount of target sequence bound to each probe is correlated to the expression level of various genes expressed in the sample. The signals are detected, quantified, and used to create a digital image of the array.

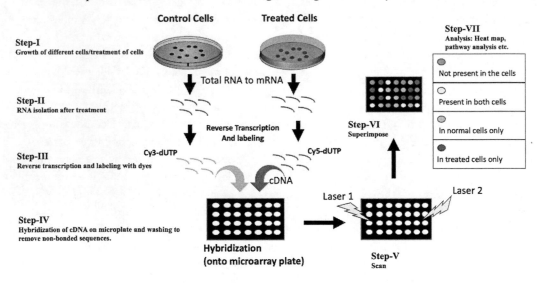

Fig. 5.40 Typical DNA microarray procedure.

(b) Serial analysis of gene expression (SAGE)

Serial analysis of gene expression (SAGE) involves the generation of short fragments of DNA, or tags, from a defined point in the sequence of all cDNAs in the sample analyzed. This short tag, because of its presence in a defined point in the sequence, is typically sufficient to uniquely identify every transcript in the sample. SAGE allows one to generate a comprehensive profile of gene expression in any sample desired from as little as 100,000 cells or 1 μg of total RNA. SAGE generates absolute, rather than relative, measurements of RNA abundance levels, and this fact allows an investigator to readily and reliably compare data to those produced by other laboratories, making the SAGE data set increasingly useful as more data is generated and shared. Software tools have also been specifically adapted for SAGE tags to allow cluster analysis of both public and user-generated data.

Two important aspects form the basis of SAGE analysis: (a) representation of mRNAs by short sequence tags, and (b) concatenation of these tags. Figure 5.41 represents the schematics of the SAGE procedure. Briefly, double-stranded cDNA is synthesized from mRNA with biotinylated oligo(dT) primer. After cleavage with restriction enzyme, called the anchoring enzyme (AE), this is recovered by binding to streptavidin-coated beads. The reaction mixture is then divided into

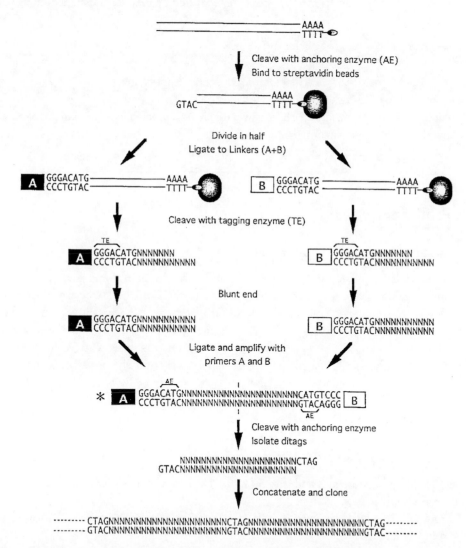

Fig. 5.41 Schematic of the SAGE procedure. The anchoring enzyme (AE) is *Nla*III and tagging enzyme (TE) is *Bsm*FI. Boxed A and B are independent linkers, whose 39 portions are designed to contain TE sequences. Transcript-derived tag sequences are denoted by Ns. Blunt end ligation step is denoted as *, and discussed later in the text.

two portions; two independent linkers that are ligated, digested by a tagging enzyme. Linkers are designed to contain an overlapping cleavage site near to the site of the restriction enzyme used earlier. Release portions are recovered after the digestion, which is then blunt-ended by T4 DNA polymerase. Two portions are mixed now and ligated. Since the 5'-ends of the linkers are blocked by an amino group, only the mRNA derived termini are able to ligate in a tail-to-tail orientation. Ligated products are PCR amplified and cleaved by earlier used restriction enzyme, which is then separated by poly acrylamide gel electrophoresis (PAGE) and isolated. Isolated products are ligated to obtain concatamers (a long continuous DNA molecule that contains the same DNA molecules linked in series). Highly concatenated products are recovered by PAGE, and cloned into a plasmid vector for sequencing.

Questions to ponder over

1. How is RNA transferred to the membrane? Describe its mechanism.
2. Describe NPA. How is unhybridized RNA digested?
3. Compare SAGE with microarray. Explain what may be expected in a comparison of data generated from either platform?
4. Tabulate the differences between SAGE and microarray.

5.10   Protocols

5.10.1   Agarose Gel Electrophoresis

Gel electrophoresis is a standard technique commonly used in laboratories for the separation of charged nucleic acid molecules based on their size. Agarose gels which have a permeable matrix are used for DNA electrophoresis. Upon application of an electric field, the negatively charged nucleic acids migrate through the gel, with shorter DNA fragments moving quicker than the longer strands and these are thus separated based on size. Dyes, fluorescent tags or radioactive labels enable the visualization and analysis of DNA. DNA gel electrophoresis is routinely used as an analytical tool in a wide range of molecular biology techniques such as gene analysis, PCR, nucleic acid sequencing, blotting, DNA fingerprinting, and many more.

The protocol for DNA gel electrophoresis is outlined below:

Preparation of 1% agarose gel for electrophoresis

- Weigh 0.5 g of agarose and add it to 50 ml of 1X Tris-acetate (TAE) or Tris-borate (TBE) buffer and swirl to mix.
- Microwave the solution at short intervals until the agarose has completely dissolved. Allow the solution to cool.
- Pour the gel solution in the electrophoresis tank and remove any air bubbles using a disposable tip.
- Insert the gel comb into the corresponding slots on the gel casting tray.
- Allow the gel to set for 30–60 mins.

Loading and running the gel

- After the gel is set, remove the comb and pour the 1X running buffer into the gel tank to submerge the gel in it.
- Thaw the DNA samples to be analyzed and add the loading dye to each sample so that the migration of the sample through the gel can be monitored.
- DNA marker or DNA ladder (5 μl) is added to the first well of the gel. The DNA fragments in the marker are of known lengths which aid in determining the approximate size of the fragments in the samples.
- Pipet 5 μl the DNA samples into the empty wells of the gel making a careful note of which sample is being loaded in which position of the well.
- Close the gel apparatus by securing the lid in place ensuring that the orientation of the gel and the positive and negative electrodes is right. The negatively charged DNA fragments migrate across the gel to the positive electrode.
- Switch on the power source and run the gel at 50 volts.
- Monitor the progress of the gel by visually monitoring the migration of the marker dye. Stop running the gel by turning off the current when the samples have run approximately ¾ the length of the gel.
- To prevent electrocution, completely switch off the power supply, lift the lid on the gel apparatus and carefully remove the gel from the electrophoresis tank.

Staining the gel and visualizing the results

- Prepare and dilute the staining solution according to the product information. Carefully follow the handling and disposable guidelines.
- If using ethidium bromide or SYBR safe staining solutions, place the gel directly into a container and submerge it entirely in the staining solution.
- Allow the gel to sit in dark for around 30 minutes as the fluorescence dye binds to the DNA fragments.
- Transfer the gel on an ultraviolet trans-illuminator to render the bright DNA bands clearly visible (if the gel ran correctly, the banding pattern of the DNA marker will be clearly visible).
- The size of the sample DNA fragment is estimated by matching it against the closest band of the DNA marker and analyzed using the gel analysis software on the computer.

5.10.2 Extraction of RNA Using the PureLink® RNA Mini Kit

The PureLink® RNA Mini Kit is a reliable and rapid method for isolating high-quality total RNA from a wide variety of sources, including cells and tissue from animal and plant samples, blood, bacteria, yeast, and liquid samples. In general, samples are lysed and homogenized in the presence of guanidinium isothiocyanate, a chaotropic salt that protects the RNA from endogenous RNases. Ethanol is added to the sample which is then processed through a spin cartridge containing a clear silica-based membrane to which the RNA binds. Any impurities are effectively removed by subsequent washing. The purified total RNA is then eluted in RNase medium and may be used for a variety of downstream applications such as RT-PCR, Northern blot, microarray analysis, and such like.

The protocol for isolation of RNA from animal/plant cells is outlined below:

Lysis and Homogenization

- To prepare lysates from $\leq 5 \times 10^6$ suspended cells, transfer the cells to an RNase free tube and centrifuge at 2000 x g for 5 minutes at 4°C.
- Discard the growth medium and using RNase-free pipette tips add 0.6 ml of lysis buffer to the pellet.
- Vortex at high speed until the cell pellet is completely dispersed.
- Transfer the lysate to the homogenizer and insert into a collection tube and centrifuge at 12,000 $\times g$ for 2 minutes.
- Remove the homogenizer and transfer the supernatant to a clean RNase-free tube.

Bind, wash, and elute RNA

- Add one volume 70% ethanol to each volume of cell homogenate and vortex.
- Transfer up to 700 μL of the sample to the spin cartridge (with the collection tube) and centrifuge at 12,000 $\times g$ for 15 seconds at room temperature.
- Discard the flow-through and reinsert the spin cartridge into the same collection tube.
- Repeat until the entire sample is processed.
- Add 700 μL Wash Buffer I to the spin cartridge and centrifuge at 12,000 $\times g$ for 15 seconds at room temperature. Discard the flow-through and the collection tube and place the spin cartridge into a new collection tube.
- Add 500 μL Wash Buffer II with ethanol to the spin cartridge and centrifuge at 12,000 $\times g$ for 15 seconds at room temperature.
- Discard the flow-through and reinsert the spin cartridge into the same collection tube.
- Repeat the two steps given above one more time.
- Centrifuge the spin cartridge at 12,000 $\times g$ for 1–2 minutes to dry the membrane with the attached RNA.
- Discard the collection tube and insert the spin cartridge into a recovery tube.
- Add 30 μL–3 × 100 μL RNase–free water, to the center of the spin cartridge and incubate at room temperature for 1 minute.
- Centrifuge the spin cartridge for 2 minutes at $\geq 12,000 \times g$ at room temperature to elute the purified RNA from the membrane into the recovery tube and store as desired.

5.10.3   Polymerase Chain Reaction (PCR)

PCR is the most commonly used technique in molecular biology for amplification of selective regions of DNA present within the DNA source thereby generating thousands to millions of copies of that particular DNA fragment.

A basic PCR reaction requires several components and reagents including the DNA template that contains the sequence to be amplified, and oligonucleotide primers that are complimentary to the strands of the target DNA. The method in general involves repeated cycles of heating and cooling of the reaction mixture to enable template DNA denaturation, primer hybridization and annealing in order to achieve enzymatic replication of the DNA strand. Parameters for the appropriate design of primers as described in previous sections of the chapter should be followed for the successful outcome of a PCR experiment.

Standard set-up and method for a basic PCR reaction is described below:

- When setting up a PCR experiment wear gloves in order to avoid contamination of the reaction mixture or reagents. All reagents should always be placed on ice and allow them to thaw completely before proceeding with the reaction.
- It is important to create an experimental design that includes a positive and a negative control. Negative control reaction mixture is deprived of the DNA template and a positive control would be a set of oligonucleotide primers and a DNA template that has been shown to successfully work in previous experiments.
- Organize the equipment to be used and the reagents on a workbench.
- Assemble the reaction mixture into 50 μl volume in 0.2 ml PCR tubes placed on ice in the amounts as described in the table below:

Reagent	Concentration of Stock Solution	Volume to be Used	Final Concentration
Buffer	10X	5 μl	1X
dNTPs	10 mM	5 μl	200 μM
MgCl$_2$	25 mM	3 μl	1.5 mM
Forward Primer	20 μM	1 μl	20 pM
Reverse Primer	20 μM	1 μl	20 pM
Template DNA		1 μl	100 ng/μl
Taq DNA Polymerase	5 units/μl	0.5 μl	2.5 units
Sterile H$_2$O		up to 50 μl	

- To prepare the negative control, add all the reagents with the exception of template DNA, to a separate 0.2 ml PCR tube,
- In addition, prepare a positive control reaction mixture containing template DNA and primers previously known to successfully amplify under the same conditions as the experimental PCR tubes.
- Gently pipet the contents in the tube to allow homogenization and very briefly spin the tubes in the centrifuge.
- Program the thermal cycler for the PCR reaction with settings as suggested in the table below:

Step	Temperature	Time	Number of Cycles
Initial Denaturation	94°C	3–5 min	1
Denaturation	94°C	30 sec	25–35
Annealing	3–5°C below Tm	45 sec	25–35
Extension	72°C	1 min/kb	25–35
Final Extension	72°C	5–15 min	1
Hold	4°C	depends on user protocol	1

- Insert the PCR tubes in the thermal cycler. Once the lid on the thermal cycler is firmly shut start the program.
- When the PCR cycle is finished store the PCR tubes at 4°C.
- PCR products can be detected by agarose gel electrophoresis. If the DNA segment is successfully amplified, ethidium bromide will intercalate between the DNA bases illuminating the bands when seen under UV light.

References

Allison, L. A. (2007). *Fundamental Molecular Biology*. New Jersey: Blackwell Pub.

Lewin, B., Krebs, J. E., Goldstein, E. S. and Kilpatrick, S. T. (2014). *Lewin's Genes XI*. Burlington, Massachusetts: Jones & Bartlett Publishers.

Navarro, E., Serrano-Heras, G., Castaño, M. J. and Solera, J. J. C. C. A. (2015). Real-time PCR detection chemistry. *Clinica Chimica Acta*, 439, 231–250.

Shendure, J., Balasubramanian, S., Church, G. M., et al. (2017). DNA sequencing at 40: past, present and future. *Nature*, 550(7676), 345–353.

Tan, S. C. and Yiap, B. C. (2013). Erratum to "DNA, RNA, and protein extraction: the past and the present". *BioMed Research International*.

Templeton, N. S. (1992). The polymerase chain reaction: history, methods, and applications. *Diagnostic Molecular Pathology: The American Journal of Surgical Pathology, part B*, 1(1), 58–72.

van Dijk, E. L., Jaszczyszyn, Y., Naquin, D. and Thermes, C. (2018). The third revolution in sequencing technology. *Trends in Genetics*, 34(9), 666–681.

6

Cell Culture*

6.1 Introduction

Cell cultures are remarkable tools in biological and biochemical research. Cellular models are often used for understanding physiological processes, biochemical production, antibody production, vaccine production, and cancer research, along with a multitude of other uses. Additionally, they are also useful to understand the mechanism of signal transduction, protein synthesis, drug action (pharmacology and toxicology), drug metabolism, cell–cell interactions, and genetics. Furthermore, cell culture also provides future avenues for medical treatment including cell-based therapy and regenerative medicine. These are the reasons why in vitro propagation of cells becomes an essential requirement for every biochemical lab. Such technology provides a user-friendly and relatively cheap tool to examine the biological issues, overriding the legal, moral, and ethical concerns related to in vivo studies. In a cell culture experiment, cells are provided with a conducive environment to grow, different from their native environment. This is widely referred to as cell culturing and consists of several steps of isolating cells from their native environment; they will then be maintained under precise conditions and nurtured with additives, in an appropriate medium.

Cells are the smallest structural and functional units of any organism. After isolation from their respective tissues (plants and animals), they can be grown (cultured and differentiated) in an artificial media (mixture of buffers and nutrients). Ross Harrison (1907) first developed a technique for tissue culture called the "hanging drop technique." He placed a small tissue in a medium (containing serum) from which cells migrated to the surrounding environment. Carrel and Lindbergh (1935), further developed cell culture technique. and then utilized it to build a vaccine. Their research revolutionized the study and improved understanding of cell cultures. In the 1940s and 1950s, several protocols for assays were developed to examine viral growth (Salvador Luria and Renato Dulbecco). Later, more techniques were developed to examine the different characteristics of cells including growth, differentiation, protein production, and cell death. Since its inception in the twentieth century, cell culture based techniques has been invaluable in the development of basic virology, vaccine development, disease modeling, pathogenesis and drug development.

Cells are isolated from animals, microbes or plants. Once isolated, all cells require aseptic techniques, and viable growth and proliferation conditions. Generally, a wide range of compounds

---

* Ghuncha Ambrin, co-authored this chapter, contributing significantly to the writing of this book.

can affect cell characteristics, and so it is very important that cells come in contact with an optimal environment for cell growth requireing a complex mixture of nutrients (sugars, amino acids, minerals, growth factors, metal ion, salts, buffers, and myriad others).

Use of particular cell lines for culturing is determined by:

(a) Age of the cell, species, and gender of the donor tissue.
(b) In case of human cell lines, the medical history of donor.
(c) Culture history, such as passage history, medium used, and the source of tissues.

Each cell line is distinguished by several characteristics, such as growth pattern, morphological appearance, biological markers (protein markers, chromosome marker, specific surface markers, and such), and dividing capacity.

6.2   Cell Structure and Function

All cells share certain characteristics. They are composed of several kinds of living matter enclosed by a barrier separating the cells from the outside environment. The cells are filled with cytoplasm and all contain DNA. Theodor Schwann, Matthias Jakob Schleiden, and Rudolf Virchow conceptualized what is known as the classical cell theory. Schwann and Schleiden (1839) first prposed that **cells** are the basic unit of life and based on their observations they put forward the foundation of classical **cell theory** to which Rudolf Virchow (1855) contributed finishing touches.

The elements of cell theory are:

1. All living things are made of cells.
2. The basic unit of life is the cell and all tissues and organs are made of specific cells with common characteristics.
3. New cells are born of preexisting cells

Cells are complex structures and are highly organized. The genes in the nucleus have all the necessary information to produce new cells. Roles of cells include: enzymatically controlled of chemical reactions, various mechanical activities, response to stimuli, production and regulation chemical and electrical energy, production and modification of several useful molecules, conducting the reproduction-death cycle, and clearing toxins and unnecessary molecules. These activities are carried out by coordinated functions of different organelles whose functions are listed in Table 6.1.

The cells are either prokaryotic or eukaryotic. The two cell types can be differentiated in terms of their mechanism of cell division and locomotion. Complex plants and animals contain membrane bound organelle specializing in specific behavior and function. Prokaryotic and eukaryotic cells are similar in cellular membrane structure and genetic information.

Prokaryotes are thought to have been the first living (primordial) organisms. They are single cell organisms which lack membrane bound nucleus and other organelles. Prokaryotic cells belong to the domain of archaebacteria. They are the simplest cellular organisms lacking complex membranes, chromosomes and cytoskeleton, which are the characteristic of other cells known as eukaryotes. As such prokaryotic cells lack organelles and membrane bound structures inside themselves. But though prokaryotic cells lack defined nucleus, they have a region called nucleoid containing a single chromosome. In general, their cell wall is outside the plasma membrane.

Eukaryotes are complex organisms containing a nucleus surrounded by a membrane. All the genetic material in the form of chromosomes resides within a distinct nucleus. All other organelles like mitochondria are also surrounded by a membrane structure unlike the prokaryotes. Eukaryotes are multicellular organisms where all the cells come together to form tissues or organs. Examples of eukaryotic cells include protists, fungi, plants and animals (Figure 6.1).

Table 6.1   Structure and functions of different parts of a cell.

Cell Component	Types of Cell	Description	Function
Cell Wall	Include plant, fungi, and bacterial cells, except animal cells	• Outermost layer is rigid and strong • built of cellulose	• Supports cellular structure • Hardened cell walls protect the cell • Allows transport of nutrients/wastes such as H_2O, O_2, CO_2
Cell Membrane	All known cells have cell membranes flush with cell wall	• Plant – inside layer of cell wall • Animal – outer layer; containing cholesterol • Also contains various phospholipids and protein molecules • Semi-permeable	• Allows transport of molecules to and fro • Protects cell from unwanted molecules • Supports cell to maintain its organelles • Selectivity • Maintains homeostasis
Nucleus	Except prokaryotes, all cells have a nucleus at their core	• Large membrane bound structure, oval in shape • Contain at least one nucleoli • Holds genetic materials and proteins (such as DNA, Histones, etc.)	• Regulate cellular activities • Responsible for reproduction, cell cycle management and death of a cell.
Nuclear membrane	Except prokaryotes, all cells have a nuclear membrane within	• Bilayer membrane • Semi-permeable	• Transport of molecules from in/out of nucleus
Cytoplasm	Within all cells	• Clear, thick, dense material (cytosol) • Contains several organelles • Contains support molecules such as cytoskeleton fibers	• Protect cell organelles. • Conduct necessary enzymatic functions, protein production, etc.
Endoplasmic reticulum (ER)	Except prokaryotes, all cells have ER within	• Network of several tube shaped membrane bound structures • Attach to nuclear envelope and cell membrane	• Transport materials inside the cell • Synthesize and modify proteins, lipids • Glycosylation
Ribosome	Within all cells	• Made of molecules; rRNA and protein • free or attached to ER	• Synthesize proteins

Contd.

Table 6.1 *contd.*

Cell Component	Types of Cell	Description	Function
Mitochondrion	Except prokaryotes, all cells have mitochondria	• Shaped like peanut • Bilayer membrane • Covered by inner and outer impermeable membrane	• Centre of oxidative metabolism, catabolism, energy storage, electron transport, cellular respiration • Power house of the cell
Vacuole	Although characteristic of plant cells (large vacuoles) but animal cells also have small vacuoles.	• Filled with fluid • Largest organelle in plant cells	• Storage space for food, sugar, water, metabolic and toxic/non-toxic wastes • Creates turgor pressure • Site for Intracellular digestion mediated by acid hydrolases
Lysosome	Uncommon in plant, it is found in animal cell.	• Single membrane bound small organelle.	• Breaking down food molecules • Digesting older cellular matter
Chloroplast	Found in plants and algae	• oval in shape containinga green pigment, chlorophyll • Double membrane with inner membrane modified into sacs called thylakoids • Stacks of thylakoids called grana which are interconnected • Gel like innermost substance called stroma	• Convert energy from Sun to make food (glucose) for the plant, i.e., photosynthesis • Generating oxygen
nucleolus	All cells except prokaryotes	• Found inside the cell's nucleus • May have more than one • Disappear during cell division	• Make ribosomes
Golgi Apparatus	All cells except prokaryotes	• Stacks of flattened sacs • Have both **c**is and trans orientation •	• Modify proteins made by the cells • Package and export proteins • Synthesis of complex • polysaccharide that make up the cell wall
Cilia	Animal cells, Protozoans	• Have a 9–2 arrangement of microtubules • Short, but numerous	• Locomotion
Flagellum	Bacterial cells & Protozoans	• Have a 9–2 arrangement of microtubules • Long, but few in number	• Locomotion

Contd.

Table 6.1 *contd.*

Cell Component	Types of Cell	Description	Function
Centrioles	Animal cells	• Paired structures near the nucleus • Made of a cylinder of microtubule pairs	• Separate chromosome pairs during mitosis
Cytoskeleton	All cells	• Made of microtubules and microfilaments	• Strengthen cell and maintains its shape • Transports organelles, neurotransmitters within the cell • Provides force required for locomotion

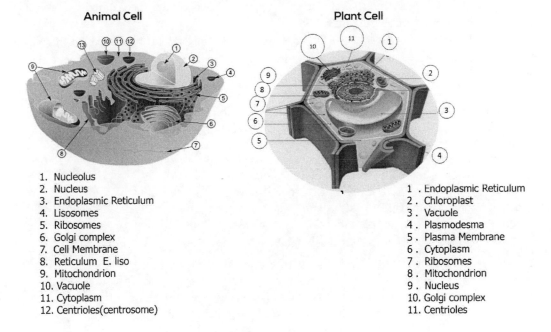

Animal Cell

Plant Cell

1. Nucleolus
2. Nucleus
3. Endoplasmic Reticulum
4. Lisosomes
5. Ribosomes
6. Golgi complex
7. Cell Membrane
8. Reticulum E. liso
9. Mitochondrion
10. Vacuole
11. Cytoplasm
12. Centrioles(centrosome)

1. Endoplasmic Reticulum
2. Chloroplast
3. Vacuole
4. Plasmodesma
5. Plasma Membrane
6. Cytoplasm
7. Ribosomes
8. Mitochondrion
9. Nucleus
10. Golgi complex
11. Centrioles

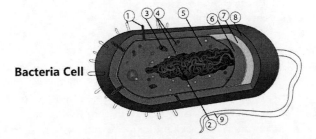

Bacteria Cell

1. Pili
2. Nucleus (ADN circular)
3. Plasmid
4. Ribosomes
5. Cytoplasm
6. Plasma Membrane
7. Cell Wall
8. Capsule
9. Flagella

Fig. 6.1 Types of cells: Animal, plant, and bacterial cells.

6.3 Cell Cycle

According to the cell theory, all cells originate from preexisting cells and this is done by the process of cell division. Cells divide and produce another cell. Although cell division happens in all types of cells, the overall process is different for prokaryotes and eukaryotes. Cell division can take place through mitosis and meiosis. In eukaryotic cells, mitosis produces two daughter cells when the parent cell transfers its genetic material to each of them. Both daughter cells then

Questions to ponder over

1. What is the cell theory?
2. What is the cell membrane made of? What are its main functions?
3. Which part of the cell is called the power house of the cell and why?
4. Which part of the cell provides support to the cell?
5. How do cells communicate with their microenvironment?

have same genetic material. Meiosis on the other hand, is the basis of producing sexually reproducing organs. We will focus on mitosis of eukaryotes in this chapter. Fission yeast, a single celled eukaryote, is mostly used for investigating the regulatory network which regulates the progression of events during the entire cell cycle (Figure 6.2).

In 2001, Leland H. Hartwell, Sir Richard T. Hunt, and Sir Paul M. Nurse shared the Nobel Prize "for their discoveries of key regulators of the cell cycle." In their later careers, all three scientists proceeded to conduct pioneering work in the scientific understanding of cancer.

Leland H. Hartwell, an American scientist., began his career as a faculty at University of California, Irvine in 1965 after receiving his PhD from Massachusetts Institute of Technology in 1964, where he began eukaryotic cell model studies. In the late 1960's he started using baker's yeast to examine the behavior of cells in growth and cell division. He identified more than 100 genes (cell-division-cycle or CDC genes) involved in cell-cycle regulation, including the CDC28, "start gene", that regulates the first growth stage. He also found out from his experiments that there are several check points which provide time to repair any DNA damage.

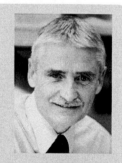

Sir Richard Timothy Hunt is a Nobel Prize winner in medicine and renowned British biochemist and molecular physiologist. Following his PhD., he worked in New York where his team discovered that tiny amounts of oxidized glutathione are extremely inhibitory to the protein synthesis in reticulocytes. Later with another collaborator, he also found out that even tinier amounts of dsRNA (double-stranded RNA) can kill protein synthesis. Even after he returned to Cambridge, he spent his summers in Massachusetts at Woods Hole for its advanced summer courses for scientists interested in the phenomenon of mitosis. It was at Woods

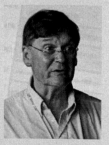

Hole that he discovered cyclins using sea urchin eggs as model organisms. He concluded that the proteins underwent specific proteolysis during the early development of the fertilized eggs leading to the discovery of the synthesis of cyclins during cell division. He also discovered that cyclins can regulate cell cycle. He demonstrated that cyclin can bind and activate protein kinases (cyclin-dependent kinases) and regulate cell cycle. Cyclins are present in vertebrate cells and Hunt and others showed that they bind and activate a family of protein kinases, now called the cyclin-dependent kinases, one of which had been later identified as a crucial cell cycle regulator.

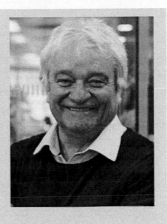

Sir Paul Maxime Nurse, earned his PhD in 1973 and was a professor at Oxford from 1987 to 1993. He began his research using yeast as his model organism. Beginning in 1976, he had identified the gene *cdc2* in fission yeast (*Schizosaccharomyces pombe*) as a controlling switch, regulating the timing of cell-cycle events such as the progression of the cell cycle from G1 phase to S phase and the transition from G2 phase to mitosis. In 1987, he isolated the corresponding gene in humans which was named cyclin dependent kinase (cdk1). The gene encodes a protein that belongs to a family of key enzymes, the cyclin dependent kinases (CDK's), which participate in many cell functions. By 2001, he had identified half a dozen other CDKs in humans.

There are two phases of cell cycle (Figure 6.2), mitosis phase (the M phase) and the interphase (G1, S and G2 phase). The M phase includes (1) mitosis, in which the chromosome is replicated and distributed equally into two nuclei and (2) cytokinesis, where the cells divide into two daughter cells. The M phase lasts for about an hour.

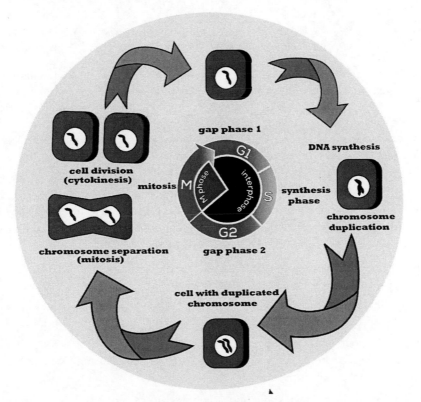

Fig. 6.2 The cell cycle.

6.3.1 Mitosis

Mitosis is a stage where the cell focuses all its energy into one activity, i.e., chromosomal segregation. At this stage the cell becomes relatively unresponsive to external stimuli. It can be further be divided into 5 stages, each starting with a characteristic event (Figure 6.3).

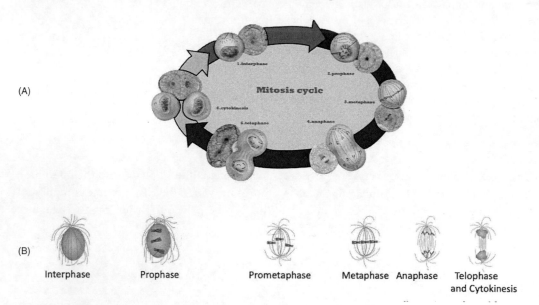

(A)

(B)

Interphase   Prophase   Prometaphase   Metaphase   Anaphase   Telophase
and Cytokinesis

Fig. 6.3 (A) The different phases of mitosis. (B) Structure of mitotic spindle. In interphase, most of the chromatin condenses into nucleus, and microtubules are organized in radial array from the chromosome. During prophase, the highly condensed chromosome and centrosome begin to separate. During prometaphase, chromosomes start moving to the center. Alignment of chromosomes at the center, spindle equator, defines metaphase. In anaphase, the chromosomes move towards the pole. DNA begins to condense during telophase and proceeds for division of cytoplasm which begins the cytokinesis phase (Adapted from Walczak et al., 2010).

Prophase: Chromosomal material condenses to two identical chromatids both attached by a structure called the centromere. This step includes disassembling of cytoskeleton, assembling of mitotic spindle, and disappearance of golgi and endoplasmic reticulum (ER).

Prometaphase: In this step, microtubules are attached to the kinetochore. All the chromosomes are assembled at the equator.

Metaphase: In this phase, after alignment at the metaphase plate chromosomes are attached to the microtubules. The microtubules can be differentiated into three types at this stage: (1) Astral microtubule – radiate outward from the centromere, (2) Chromosomal or Kinetochore microtubule – extend between the centrosome and kinetochore of the microtubule, and (3) Polar microtubule - extend from the centrosome past the chromosome.

Anaphase: Replicated chromosomes split and daughter chromatids moved to both poles.

Telophase: Clustering and dispersing of chromosomes at both poles. Formation of a nuclear envelope around the clusters Followed by the reformation of golgi and ER.

Cytokinesis: Is a process by which two daughter cells are formed by parent cells. Once the DNA has been segregated into two daughter nuclei by mitosis, cytokinesis begins by indenting the cell surface in the anaphase step, and progresses to forming a furrow. Furrows are long narrow trenches in the same plane where chromosomes assembled in the metaphase. In the later stages the furrow deepens to form midbody, forming a bridge between the two daughter cells known as cytoplasmic bridge. Abscission is the final step of cytokinesis when the surface of the cleavage furrow fuses with another, splitting the cells into two. The idea of the contractile ring theory was proposed by Douglas Marsland in 1950. He hypothesizes that the cortex, which contains a large amount of actin filament, generates the required force to cleave the cell. The unbranched actin filaments are assembled together by the action of the protein formin. Short, bipolar myosin filaments are scattered over these actin filaments. The assembly of the actin-myosin complex is brought about by the G protein called RhoA. RhoA, in GTP bound state, initiates the pathway which leads to activation of actin filaments and myosin's motor activity. Actin filaments pull the cortex towards the center of equatorial region and attach the plasma membrane. In the anaphase, mitotic spindle determine the position of the cleavage furrow, which leads to the activation of RhoA. There are two different mechanisms that are believed to be at play for the generation of the signals. Some results demonstrate that the site of actin myosin filament assembly and the plane of cytokinesis is determined by the signals emanating from the spindle poles and moves through the astral microtubules. Some believe that the signal originates at the central part rather than the poles. However, the simplest explanation might be that the (1) different signals emanate from different cell type; (2) both mechanisms operate in the same cell.

The interphase of a cell cycle is divided into three phases; G1, S, and G2 phases. In the G1 phase, cells grow and function normally as centers for protein synthesis and metabolic activities. Depending on the cell type and their condition, cells can stay in this phase ranging from days to weeks or longer.

Questions to ponder over

1. What is the cell cycle?
2. What are the stages of cell cycle?
3. What is meant by cell cycle checkpoints?
4. What is the role of cyclins?
5. What are some of the activities of kinetochore during mitosis?
6. Describe the mechanism of Cytokinesis.

Points for Reflection

- **What are the number of cells in a human body and the number of bacterial cells in one's palm?**
  An average human body contains 37.2 trillion cells. 1500 bacteria live on each cm^2 of skin on our hands.
- **What is the range of cell size in nature?**
  Eukaryotic cells normally range from 1–100 μm in diameter and prokaryotic cells range from 0.1–5 μm in diameter.
- **What are the variations in the number of chromosomes in different kinds of cells?**
  Aneuploidy (when one or more of a normal set of chromosome is missing or present), **monoploidy** (loss of an entire set of chromosomes) and **euploidy** (the entire set is duplicated once or several times) are the variations that can occur with the changing of chromosome number.

The G2 phase is a gap period between the S and M phases. G2 stands for second gap, in which a cell resumes its growth and prepares itself for division. In this phase mitochondria divide (in plants, chloroplasts also divide). DNA replication and chromosome duplication occur during the S phase of the cycle. It is the period when the cell synthesizes additional histones, which are required for the packaging of chromosomes into nucleosomes. The duration of the S phase depends on the percentage of cells involved in the activity of the S-phase (directly proportional). The duration of the M-phase is determined by the percentage of cells involved in mitosis and cytokinesis. Upon adding the periods S+M+G2, an additional period was observed that was unaccounted for. This came to be known as the G1 phase or gap one.

Cell systems have several check points that act as a surveillance mechanism to halt the progression of DNA replication: (1) in cases of DNA chromosomal damage, and (2) during replication in the S phase or incomplete chromosomal alignment in the M phase. Check points make sure that the events of the cell cycle occur properly. Several checkpoint events or pathways are only activated in case of abnormality; otherwise, they remain dormant. Check points are generally activated through internal signals which recognize any defect in DNA or their alignment. When a signal is activated after detection of an abnormality, it triggers a response which arrests the cells in the cell cycle progression. The cell uses this delay to repair the damage or carry out realignment. The cells proceed to the next phase only when it has cleared the checkpoints. If the cells cannot repair the DNA damage, the checkpoint mechanism triggers a series of responses that either lead the cell to (1) cell death or (2) senescence, when the cells stops dividing.

In fact, the progression of the cell cycle depends on other factors as well. The initiation of the M phase is mainly controlled by MPF (maturation promoting factor). MPF consists of two parts: the kinase subunit which transfers phosphate to serine, threonine unit from ATP to specific proteins, and cyclin, which is a regulatory subunit. During stages of the cell cycle, cyclin concentration increases or decreases. High concentration of cyclin activates the kinase subunit, whereas in cases of low concentration the kinase subunits are in inactive state. Activation of kinase subunits allow cells to enter into the M-phase. The progression of the cell cycle through the interphase involves two checkpoints. One regulation occurs near the end of G1 phase, called the START, and the other near the end of G2 phase. At these points the cell becomes committed to either begining DNA replication or entering mitosis, respectively. Once START has been initiated, it begins DNA replication. Passage from the G2 phase to the mitotic phase is initiated by MPF as mentioned previously. Cells may make a third transition at the middle of mitosis to determine if the cell will progress into another cycle of the G1 phase after the completion of this cycle.

The quiescent state of cells is known as G0 phase (referred to as the G zero phase). This phase is also considered either an extension of G1 phase or a different stage outside the cell cycle. Cells such as neuronal and heart muscle, stay in the G0 phase when they are fully differentiated. However they continue to perform their regular functions till the life of the cells or organism. Lack of growth factors or nutrients allow cells to stay in this phase and they continue to be in this state until there is a reason for them to divide. In this phase, cyclins and cyclin-dependent kinases disappear. Some cells enter this phase semi-permanently, and proceed further with the cell cycle only under specific circumstances. Examples of these cells are parenchymal cells such as of the liver and kidney.

6.4   Cell Microenvironment

Cells are cultured in isolation in physiochemical environments that resemble the physiological environment of their origin. Various environmental factors can affect the different stages of cell culture.

Substrate: Most commonly used substrates for cell proliferation and differentiation are plastic and glass. Cells mostly grow in monolayers by adhering to the surface of the substrate or in cell suspension in desired media. In some cases, the surface properties of the substrate are enhanced by treating the surface with collagen, matrigel, or poly-L-lysine (PLL) to provide an extracellular like matrix structure for supporting cell adhesion.

pH: Optimal pH range for cellular grow this between 7.0 and 7.4. However, this can vary with respect to treatment, such as transformation.

CO_2: Equilibrium with HCO_3^- ions is an important factor and dissolved CO_2 can decrease the pH. Although, bicarbonates have low buffering capacity, they are preferred choice as a buffer for cell culture because of their low toxicity and nutritional benefits.

Temperature: The body temperature of the species (animal, plants, bacteria, fungi) in its natural environment determines the optimal temperature of the cellular environment, which is usually maintained at 37°C as recommended for most warm-blooded animals.

O_2: Oxygen is required for cell respiration. An appropriate supply of O_2 is necessary for optimal function and continual survival as it plays a crucial role in many cellular processes ranging from metabolism to signaling.

Osmolarity: Osmolarity is one of the important parameter for homeostasis. In practice, the osmolarities between 260mOsm/kg and 320mOsm/kg are acceptable and tolerable for most cells.

Ions and glucose: Culture media consists of several ions including Na^+, K^+, Mg^{2+}, Ca^{2+}, Cl^-, SO_4^{2-}, PO_4^{3-}, and HCO_3^-. These ions provide optimum buffering and contribute to the osmolarity of the culture medium. The major energy and carbon source in cell culture medium is glucose.

Amino acids/vitamins: Essential amino acids and vitamins are other important additives required in cell culture medium. All cell types have their own requirements of amino acids. Vitamins additives are choline, folic acid, inositol, and nicotinamide.

Organic supplements: A variety of substances like proteins, peptides, nucleotides can be added to the media. The addition of these complexes reduces the use of serum and promotes cell differentiation and organ development.

Hormones and growth factors: Generally, hormones and growth factors are added in the serum-free media. General additives are fibroblastic growth factor, epidermal growth factor, vascular endothelial growth factor, insulin-like growth factor, insulin, and hydrocortisone.

Antibiotics and antifungal: They are used to reduce the frequency of contamination and provide an aseptic environment to prevent microbial growth by bacteria and fungi.

> **Questions to ponder over**
>
> 1. What is the need for culturing cells?
> 2. What are the suitable conditions for cell culturing?

Serum: Serum is added to the medium to provide growth factors, adhesion factors, and antitrypsin activity. It also provides lipids, nutrients, minerals, and proteins. Cow, calf, horse, fetal, and humans are sources of serum.

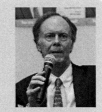

William G. Kaelin is an American scientist, who is a professor of medicine at Harvard University and the Dana Farber Cancer Institute. After receiving his MD from Duke University in 1982, he did his residency in internal medicine at John Hopkins University and oncology fellowship at Dana Farber Cancer Institute. His research at Dana Farber has focused on understanding the role of mutations in tumor suppressor genes in cancer development. His major work has been on retinoblastoma, von Hippel-Lindau and p53 tumor suppressor genes.

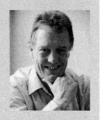

Peter J. Ratcliffe grew up in North Lancashire and won an open scholarship to study medicine at Gonville and Caius College, Cambridge. He undertook clinical training at St. Bartholomew's Hospital, London, and after a series of positions held at the London postgraduate hospitals, moved to Oxford to train in nephrology. In 1990 he obtained a Welcome Trust Senior Fellowship to work on cellular responses to hypoxia, retrained in molecular biology and founded a new laboratory working on hypoxia biology in cancer and circulatory diseases. It was here that the team discovered the widespread system of direct oxygen sensing in the form of cell signaling involving post-translational hydroxylation of specific amino acids.

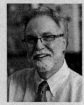

Gregg L. Semenza is a professor at Jon Hopkins University School of Medicine. His area of expertise is molecular mechanism of oxygen regulation. Dr. Semenza has led the field in uncovering how cells adapt to changing oxygen levels. He is best known for his ground-breaking discovery of the HIF-1 (hypoxia-inducible factor 1) protein, which controls genes in response to changes in oxygen availability.

In 2019, the **Nobel Prize** was jointly awarded to **William G. Kaelin, Jr., Sir Peter J. Ratcliffe** and **Gregg L. Semenza** for their ground breaking work in the response of how the "cells sense and adapt to oxygen availability."

Taken from nobelprize.org

6.5 Primary Explantation versus Disaggregation

Primary cultures are the cell cultures obtained directly from donor tissues, but before the first subculture. Such cultures are called the **primary explant** and the migration of cells from the explant is called **outgrowth**. Outgrowth cells are selected and processed further. Normally, primary cells have several differentiated cells including fibroblasts, lymphocytes, macrophages, and epithelial cells. For efficient development of primary cultures, the following characteristics are taken into consideration.

1. Embryonic tissues are preferred because they are easier to disaggregate and so lead to better viability of recovered cells which can proliferate faster.
2. The quantity of primary cells should be higher as their cell survival rate is low.
3. While processing tissue care must be taken so that there is minimum damage to the cells.

4. It is essential to use nutrient rich medium for growth, preferentially fetal bovine serum instead of calf or horse serum.
5. Enzymes used for disaggregation need to be removed.

There are three basic techniques used for primary cells culture (Figure 6.4):

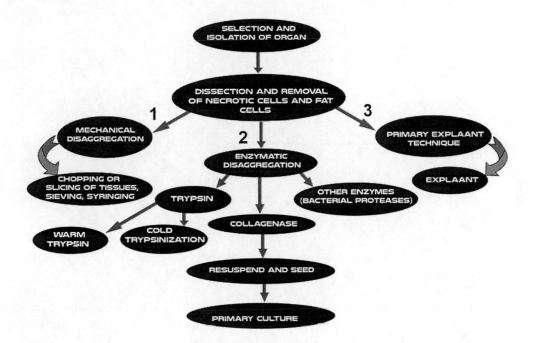

Fig. 6.4   Different techniques used for primary explant and setting up primary cell culture.

1. **Mechanical disaggregation**: This technique involves cutting tissues into several pieces which allows outgrowth of cells. Outgrowth cells are processed further and collected. The cells are collected by either passing the tissue through the syringe and needle or passing it through a series of sieves, with a reduction in sieve size. The primary disadvantage of this technique is cell damage and low cell viability of cells. This technique is usually used for soft tissues like brain, spleen, liver, and such.

2. **Enzymatic disaggregation**: To detach cells from the tissue, requires enzymes such as trypsin and collagenase. Collagenase, a fibrous protein, is the most abundant structural protein present in the extracellular matrix. It is the major component of connective tissue which consist of several kinds of tissues. Therefore, enzyme collagenase can be used for the disaggregation of cells in tissues which are sensitive to trypsin. This technique is very efficient in producing high yield of viable cells. Collagenase disaggregation is very effective in producing primary cells for brain, lung and other epithelial tissues, tumors, and other animal tissues. In combination with hyaluronidase and neuraminidase, collagenase is also very effective in dissociating animal tissues.

Trypsinization can be used as a cold treatment or warm treatment (Figure 6.5).

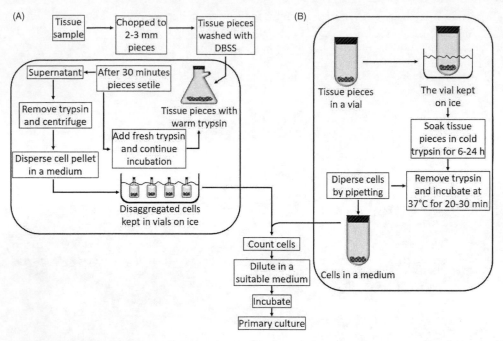

Fig. 6.5 Preparation of primary cell culture by trypsin disaggregation: (A) warm trypsinization, (B) cold trypsinization (DBSS – Dissection basal salt solution) (Taken from biologydiscussion.com).

A. **Warm trypsinization**: One of the widely used methods for disintegration of cells from tissue. The slashed tissues are washed with dissection basal salt solution (DBSS). After washing, the tissues are dissociated into cells by using warm trypsin (37°C). Trypsin is removed after dissociation and the cells dispersed in a suitable medium; then counted, diluted and stored properly till further use.

B. **Cold trypsinization:** Warm trypsinization techniques may harm some cells because prolonged exposure of trypsin at 37°C (in warm trypsinization) can damage these cells. To avoid this risk, cold trypsin is used to disintegrate cells. First, the tissue is soaked with cold trypsin for 6–24 hours. Pieces of tissue are then incubated at 37°C for 20–30 minutes. Dispersion of cells is done by repeated pipetting. Finally, the dissociated cells are counted, diluted and used or stored properly. The advantages of this technique include higher yield of viable cells, improved survival, and being simpler. The major disadvantages include inability to handle large volumes of cells; damage to some cell types and ineffectivity with others.

Apart from trypsin and collagenase, certain bacterial proteases such as pronase and dispase are also used.

3. **Primary explant technique**: This technique is useful for smaller samples of tissues. This has the lowest risk of losing any cells. First, the tissue is sliced in basal salt solution and washed before insertion into a proper medium that promotes the growth and dispersion of cells. Cells are allowed to grow for 3–5 days. Finally, after substantial outgrowth, the explants are removed and transferred into another flask (Figure 6.5).

When a tissue sample is disaggregated, the suspension of cells generated contains a certain population of cells that can attach to the solid support of the culture flask creating a monolayer of individual cells. This becomes the first subculture (Figure 6.6), which ultimately generates a cell line. In general, tissue disintegration is preferred for generating larger cultures. However, explant culture may still be better where only small fragments of tissue are available for creating a cell line.

> **Questions to ponder over**
> 1. What is the difference between primary explantation and disaggregation?
> 2. What are different methods of disaggregation?

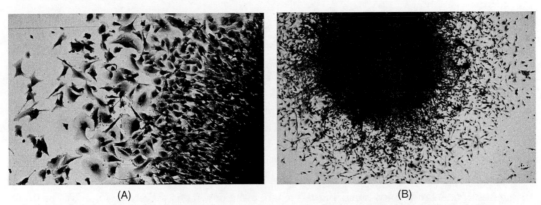

(A)   (B)

Fig. 6.6 Primary explant and outgrowth thereof. Microphotographs of a Giemsa-stained primary explant from human non-small cell lung carcinoma. (A) Low-power (4× objective) photograph of explant (top left) and radial outgrowth. (B) Higher-power detail (10× objective) showing the center of the explant to the right and the outgrowth to the left (Adopted from Freshney, 2006).

6.6   Proliferation versus Differentiation

Cell culture is a technique in which the cells are removed from the host body and placed in a fluid medium. The cells can live and grow under proper conditions. The growth of the cells is characterized by proliferation (cell division) or differentiation (where the cells change their functional or phenotypic type)

6.6.1   Proliferation

Cell proliferation is a biological process which allows cells to increase in cell number by active cellular replication and division over time. This process is necessary for experimentation as well as creating stocks of cell for future use. It refers to the growth of cell population by division of cells where a mother cell divides into two daughter cells (as been explained previously in the cell cycle). In other words, cell proliferation is a process for normal cell development, regeneration and renewal. For better cell proliferation, adequate number of fully functional viable cells, proper nutrients, fully integrated membranes and their structures, and proper waste disposal is required. If any of the above parameters are not properly maintained, the cells will not proliferate or their stability and viability suffers. Proliferation is regulated by signals from internal and external environment. The different factors that influence cell growth are as follows: (1) the substrate, (2) the degree of contact (closeness with the neighboring cells) with other cells, (3) the media composition, (4) the constitution of gas phase (humidity and CO_2), (5) the incubation temperature, and (6) the growth factor concentration. Any deviation from proliferation may lead to cancer or other disease pathology.

> **Questions to ponder over**
>
> 1. What is the importance of cell differentiation?
> 2. What is the difference between cell differentiation and proliferation?
> 3. What are the different kinds of stem cells? What are their differences and similarities?

6.6.2 Differentiation

A process that leads to a functionally mature cell of specific phenotypic properties is called differentiation. In this process a cell undergoes some specific changes by which the cell changes from less specialized type to more specialized type. The properties required for cell differentiation are cell–cell and cell–matrix interaction, cell density, and the presence or absence of several growth factors forcing the cell to become more specific in its properties. Expression of differentiated phenotypes can be maintained by appropriate selective medium usually in the absence of serum. Transcription factor is the key to differentiation. There are two main pathways for cellular differentiation. In constantly renewing tissues, like the epidermis the precursor cells proliferate and move towards terminal differential on demand that will not further divide. There are tissues that do not turn over, but have the capacity to regrow in conditions of trauma and injury. In these cases, the mature cells show little proliferation but retain the ability to divide. When the tissue regains cell density, cell proliferation stops and differentiation is induced.

Stem cells have the property to differentiate to specific cell types in the body during the early phase of cell cycle. They are unspecialized cells that are capable of dividing into either their own type or become another cell type with a more specialized function. They can constantly divide for repairing or replenishing other cells. Stem cells have become a basic research tool for understanding the development of an organism from a single cell and how a healthy cell replaces a damaged cell by differentiation and factors affecting it to become specialized cell bodies. It is also used for screening of drugs in abnormal conditions.

According to the stem cell theory, the more primitive a stem cell, the greater is its potency. Unipotent stem cells differentiate into just a single type of cell. Multipotent stem cells will generate more than two lineages e.g., bone, muscle, cartilage, and fat cell, whereas the pluripotent types give rise to neural cells, blood cells, cardiac cells from different germ layers, and totipotent ones give rise to all cell types e.g., the embryonic cell (ES). It has now been shown that mature cells from a differentiated compartment, such as fibroblasts from the dermis, may be reprogrammed to produce what have been called induced pluripotent stem cells (iPScells). iPS cells can differentiate into several different lineages. Though both multipotent and pluripotent have the same meaning, here there is a slight difference in usage. Multipotent as a term is reserved for progenitor cells within a lineage e.g. neuronal cells, which can differentiate into neurons and astrocytes. Pluripotent cells are capable of differentiating into several different lineages like ectoderm, mesoderm, and endoderm like the embryonic stem cell.

6.7   Organotypic Culture

Mammalian cells are challenging to study due to the inaccessibility of the organs for experimental manipulation. An organotypic culture system (OCS) creates a cellular system that allows recombination of previously prepared cell lines. Therefore, OCS is a combination of cells from different cell lines and mimics organ structure and functioning, exhibiting differentiation characteristic of the parent organ. It is a synthetic approach where the cells are regenerated from different origins and recombined to study the interactions and their responses to external stimuli. Earlier OCS facilitated histological characterization, but later it was developed to model organs because certain phenotypic expression are only possible when different cells are maintained in close proximity (Figure 6.7). The OCS has its own advantages and limitations.

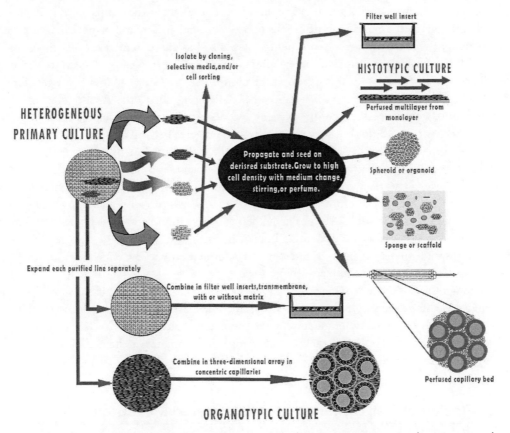

Fig. 6.7   Organotypic culture: the cells can be recombined in many ways to simulate tissue, such as perfusing a monolayer, porous matrices, highly perfused membranes, or concentric microcapillary beds.

In OCS, cells are organized into 3D stratified space similar to in vivo. It gives overall control of the microenvironment isolating cells and conditions and provides further insights in growth, development and disease which is not adequately clear in animal model and tissue culture environments, due to the large number of cells and morphological heterogeneity of developing organs. Once the basic culture has been established, its behavior can be used to study and compare response to various disease like conditions.

OCS has gained its popularity in studying various organs such as skin and epidermis, helping to validate disease and therapeutic potential of drugs for preclinical trials. When mouse models are employed in

Questions to ponder over o

1. What are the pros and cons of using OCS?
2. How is OCS culture beneficial?

the study of human diseases, they are selected because of the similarity in terms of genetics, anatomy, and physiology. Moreover, the animal models are also selected for experimental purposes because of unlimited supply. Even though the animal model is considered the best model, closely related with the human model, it has its limitations, e.g., the growth rate of cells in animals is different from that in humans. Also, the response to various growth factors and hormones varies between animals and humans. Despite the genomic similarities to humans, most animals do not contract the same disease as humans and drugs might not have the same effect in the human body as in animals. Slight variations in the genetic modifications between animal and mouse model can lead to major functional changes between the two systems. OCS also has the potential for real time imaging of the cells for prolonged periods of time giving us more insight into the cell–cell interaction and possible pathways leading towards development and disease, focusing on possible targets for drug development. Gas and nutrient exchange become challenging due to the absence of a vasculature system in OCS. In normal cell culture systems, although the gaseous exchange takes place from the periphery through diffusion, survival of cells in aggregates becomes difficult beyond a certain point due to the unavailability of gaseous exchange through diffusion. To alleviate this problem, organ cultures are grown between the interface of liquid and gaseous phase. This facilitates the gas exchange as well as nutrient uptake. This is why the preferred positioning of the explant is either in a filter well insert or on a raft or gel exposed to the air. However, an explant anchored to a solid substrate could also be possible by exposing it alternately to a liquid and a gas phase by rocking the culture. Due to the density limitations and physical restriction by organ culture geometry OCS may not grow adequately. If they do, proliferation is limited only to the outside cells, the cells can undergo differentiation in a conducive environment.

Although OCS is a powerful research tool, by modeling organ systems, it has some limitations which includes its complexity, propagation issues, labor intensity, it is susceptible to variations, and lack of a properly validated system. For example, engineered epidermal OCSs lacks the complexity of skin, the ability for signaling feedback, and a proper inflammatory system. This is why they are not suitable for experimentation related to wound healing.

6.8   Basics of Cell Culturing and Associated Measurements

Cells, the fundamental unit of life, are remarkable scientific tools in biological and biochemical research. Cellular models are often used for understanding physiological processes, biochemical production, antibody production, vaccine production, cancer research, along with a multitude of other uses. Additionally, they are useful in understanding the mechanism of signal transduction, protein synthesis, drug actions (pharmacology and toxicology), drug metabolism, cell–cell interactions, and genetics. Furthermore, cell culture also provides future avenues for medical treatment. Human cells particularly exploit the opportunities in cell-based therapy and regenerative medicine. These are the reasons why in vitro propagation of cells becomes a necessity for every biochemical lab. This technology provides a user-friendly and relatively cheap tool to examine biological issues. This technology can circumvent several ethical, legal, and moral questions otherwise associated with in vivo studies. To do so, the cells (here) are cultured in an environment which is outside their physiological environment. In brief, cell culture involves isolation, growth, experimentation, maintenance, and storage of the cells isolated from tissues or organs, under precise conditions.

Wilhelm Roux was a German zoologist who studied in Berlin and Strasbourg. He was an assistant at the Institute of Hygiene in Leipzig (1879–86) and a professor at the universities of Breslau (1886–89), Innsbruck, Austria (1889) and Halle (1895–1921). He believed that mitotic cell division of the fertilized egg is the mechanism by which future parts of a developing organism are determined. The first cell culture protocol was developed by him in 1885. He became the founder of experimental embryology through his research in finding how organs and tissues are assigned their structural form and function. He was able to maintain a section of medullary plate of an embryonic chicken in warm saline solution for 13 days.

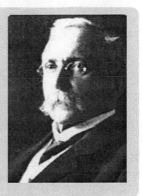

Cells are isolated from animals, microbes or plants. Once isolated, all cells require aseptic conditions for viable growth and proliferation. Generally, cell sensitivity is influenced by several factors (external or internal), so, it is very important that cells should be exposed to an optimal environment for proper growth. Cellular growth demands variety of nutrient (sugars, amino acids, mineral, growth factors, metal ion, salts, buffers, etc.).

The requirements of a cell line have been mentioned earlier in Section 6.1. Each cell line is distinguished by several characteristics such as growth pattern, morphological appearance, biological markers (protein markers, chromosome markers, specific surface markers, etc.), and dividing capacity. In general, there are two types of cell cultures: adherent and suspension (Table 6.2).

Table 6.2 Difference between adherent and suspension cultures.

Adherent Culture	Suspension Culture
Appropriate for most cell types, including primary cell cultures. Cells grow in a single layer attached to a tissue culture dish.	Appropriate for cells that are non-adhesive and suspension cells. Cells are suspended in a liquid or as free-floating clumps of a few cells.
Require periodic passaging; and may be seen only under a microscope.	Easier for passage, but require daily cell counts and viability determination.
Cells can be dissociated enzymatically.	Do not require enzymatic or mechanical dissociation.
Require tissue-culture treated vessel coated with extracellular matrices.	No need for tissue culture treated vessel but require agitation for adequate gas exchange.
Growth is limited by the surface area of the vessel which limits the yields.	Growth is limited by concentration of cells in the medium, which allows scale-up.

6.8.1   Types of Cell Culture

6.8.1.1   *Primary Cell Cultures*

As mentioned earlier (in Section 6.5), primary cell culture is obtained by dissociating and disaggregating cells from the tissues mechanically or enzymatically, maintaining the growth in controlled environmental conditions in plastic or glass containers (Figures 6.4 and 6.5). The primary cells contain the same karyotype (number of chromosomes) as those of the original cells. Primary cell cultures have a limited life span. Although their growth depends on the proximity of cells, increasing the number of cells will not be beneficial as this leads to depletion of substrate and nutrients. Also, greater cellular activity generates more toxic metabolites in the external and internal media, which further hampers cellular growth.

The primary cell culture is classified into (i) adherent or anchorage dependent, requiring the attachment of cells for growth, and (ii) suspension and anchorage independence where the cells do not attach to the vessel for growth.

There are four steps involving the initiation of primary cell culture: (1) procuring organs, (2) tissue isolation, (3) disaggregation, and (4) optimization of culture condition after seeding into the culture vessel. Once the tissue has been obtained, the cells can be detached mechanically or enzymatically (described in Section 6.5) to produce a suspension of cells, some of which attach to the culture vessel. Some of the enzymes used for disaggregation are trypsin, accutase, collagenase, DNase, elastase, dispase, and so on. Crude enzymes are more effective as they contain more proteases as contaminants, whereas the purified enzyme complexes are comparatively less toxic and specificity is higher. Trypsin and pronase are the most preferred enzymes for disaggregation but could be harmful to the cells. Collagenase and dispase, in contrast, are comparatively less harmful, but mostly result in incomplete disaggregation. For digesting extracellular matrices, hyaluronidase is used along with collagenase. To disperse DNA from the lysed cell, DNase is used to disperse DNA because DNA can inhibit proteolysis and promote reaggregation. Care should be taken when combining enzymes as some may inactivate others. For example, DNase should be added after trypsin has been removed, as the trypsin may degrade the DNase.

Each tissue requires a unique set of conditions, but certain requirements are necessary for all of them; such as:

(a) Dissection: for fat and necrotic tissues
(b) Tissues finely chopped
(c) Centrifugation
(d) Higher concentration of cells
(e) Nutrient rich medium

Embryonic tissues disaggregate more easily yielding more viable cells and their proliferation rate is better than those of adult tissue.

As described above, once either of the substrates are occupied (in case of adherent cultures) or the capacity of the medium is exhausted (in case of suspension cultures), cell proliferation rates either drop or completely stop. Therefore, maintaining optimal cell density is very important for proliferation. This is done by subculturing the primary cells by a process known as secondary cell culture.

6.8.1.2 *Secondary Cell Culture*

During a secondary cell culture, the cells from the primary cell culture are removed from the original vessel and seeded in a separate vessel with fresh media providing fresh nutrients and more space, thereby promoting proliferation and so increasing the number of cells. This also allows for the long term maintenance of cells from a more heterogeneous culture, and a more homogenous cell line emerges. The practical significance is that not only can it be optimally propagated, characterized, and stored, but it also opens up several different experimental possibilities.

6.8.1.3 *Cell Line*

Once the primary culture is subcultured, it is known as the cell line, and generally denoted by the term passage number. The number of times subculturing is done is called passage. An interval between consecutive division of cells is called the cell culture generation time. Doubling of cells depends on species, cell types, cell lineage, and culture conditions. Finite cell lines have a limited life span.

Continuous cell lines are obtained from surviving cells from the primary cell culture. When a cell line escapes senescence control then it becomes a continuous cell line, hence the generation number is not of much significance. More important is the passage number calculated from storage through each subculture. A continuous cell line is generally easier to maintain, has a faster growth rate, and generates high yield.

While choosing a cell line, various other characteristics should be taken into consideration such as species, growth characteristics, fulfilling functionality, availability, phenotypic expression, validation, and stability. Once the culture has been initiated, the cells need to be maintained periodically by changing media, both in case of proliferation as well as differentiation. The cells start to lose their viability when the pH of the media drops from 7 to 6.5. Change in the media color is indicative of changing pH. Depending on the cell type, its growth rate, the media should be changed accordingly. For a slow growing culture, the media can be changed every 4 to 7 days depending on the concentration of cell seeded.

6.8.1.4 *Stem Cell Cultures*

Stem cells are undifferentiated cells that can be introduced into a specific tissue or cells with special function. Two important characteristics of stem cells are, (a) they can renew themselves after long periods of inactivity, and (b) they can be induced for specific cell lineage. Mammalian stem cells can be derived from embryonic cells (ESC), to induce (genetically modified) pluripotent adult stem cells (iPSC). In some organs, stem cells divide regularly to repair the damaged tissues (such as the gut and bone), whereas in some cells they divide under special circumstances (such as in the pancreas and the heart).

ESC can be grown in cultures as cell lines. ESC isolated from the umbilical cord of a mammalian embryo is pluripotent, meaning that they have the unique ability to differentiate into the three layers: ectoderm, mesoderm, and endoderm. Adult stem cells are derived from adult somatic tissues (mesenchymal cells), which are normally formed in conditions of damage or injury. The adult stem cells are multipotent and can develop into more than one cell type but are more limited than pluripotent (Figure 6.8).

Most widely used ESCs have been derived from mice but human derived ESC has also been isolated and is extensively being used in research for disease progression and drug therapeutics. These cell lines are capable of differentiating into a number of cells and have emerged as a powerful tool in tissue engineering. ESC can be derived from both early stage and late stage embryos.

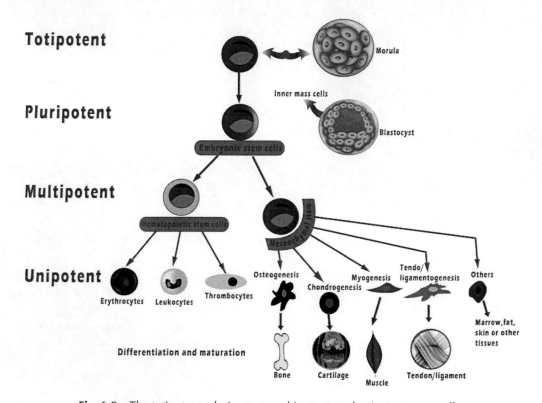

Fig. 6.8 The totipotent, pluripotent, multipotent, and unipotent stem cells.

6.8.1.5 *Subcultures*

Subculture is the process of transferring the original culture form a previous culture to a fresh growth medium and thus giving it more space for growth (Figure 6.9). This is also termed as passaging. It is used to prolong the life of the cells, while simultaneously increasing their number. Primary cell culture is the first step in isolating cells from sample tissues. It is heterogenous in nature. Subculturing the cells develops a more homogenous cell system.

Subculturing should be done mechanically. Chelation of Ca^{2+} and degradation of extracellular matrices are required for subculturing cells and, even the extracellular domains of some cell adhesion molecules. Before designing an experiment, standardization of the culture condition is essential for maintaining phenotypic stability, which should remain constant throughout the entire protocol.

1. *Choice of cell line*: cells should be chosen depending upon the experimental requirement, e.g., choosing between a primacy cell or selecting an immortalized cell line from a renowned cell bank. The passage number must be diligently recorded.

2. *Media*: the choice of media will determine the phenotype expression. Once the culture has been standardized, the vendor should also remain the same.

3. *Serum*: most serums contain the basic growth factors required for the cells to flourish, but switch of serums could give rise to variations in the culture. In order to minimize this, serum free media could be used, containing various supplements to compensate for the lack of growth essentials for the cells.

4. *Antibiotics*: most cell cultures require doses of antibiotics in order to avoid microbial contamination in the culture medium.

5. *Substrate*: plastic substrate is most widely used for the subculturing. In order to minimize the slightest variation, the type of flask or dish and the supplier should remain exactly the same.

6. *ECM (extracellular matrix)*: this condition is determined by the cell type. Some cells adhere to plastic while some need the ECM for proliferation and differentiation. Most commonly used matrix coatings are collagen and matrigel.

7. *Dissociation agent*: the most commonly used dissociating agents are trypsin and accutase. In order to maximize cell viability, the dissociation time should be standardized as low as possible. The effect of the trypsin can be neutralized by adding FBS or PBS.

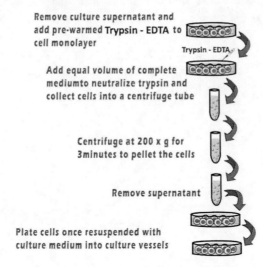

Remove culture supernatant and add pre-warmed **Trypsin - EDTA** to cell monolayer

Trypsin - EDTA

Add equal volume of complete medium to neutralize trypsin and collect cells into a centrifuge tube

Centrifuge at 200 x g for 3 minutes to pellet the cells

Remove supernatant

Plate cells once resuspended with culture medium into culture vessels

Fig. 6.9 Schematics of subculturing cells.

Knowing When to Subculture

8. *Cell Density*: cells should be cultured as soon as they reach levels of confluency (% of the surface of the culture dish that is covered by adherent cells) greater than 80–90%. The time taken to reach optimum confluency depends upon the cell type and the initial seeding density. Some endothelial cells can be grown beyond confluence as they can grow on top of the monolayer forming a secondary layer, but media needs to be constantly changed in order for the cells to survive. In some cases, the cells need to be subcultured before the cells reach optimum confluency (Figure 6.9). Although the cells will continue to proliferate, they may start to deteriorate or not survive adequately long.

9. *Medium*: while culturing, the medium should be changed intermittently, as the nutrients get depleted. Change in color of the media is indicative of the need for such change. Basically a rapid drop in pH is the indicator that change in medium is required.

10. *Time*: for continuous subculturing, it is important to determine a constant time for the cells to reach confluency. The time required is based on the seeding density.

11. *Other requirements*: subculturing can also be done to prepare the stock for future use or to change the vessel or medium as required by the experiment.

6.8.1.6 *Growth Cycle*

The growth of the cell follows a specific pattern and it can be assessed as a sigmoid curve. The period right after seeding is called the lag phase (Figure 6.10). After this lag phase there is an exponential growth of cells, called the log phase, where the cells divide. When the cell concentration reaches optimum confluency or when no more substrate is available, it reaches a plateau phase where the concentration of the cells exceeds the capacity of the media. The best time to subculture is right before the growth reaches the plateau, in order to maximize the number of viable cells.

The growth cycle of normal cells are defined in four phases: (a) *Lag phase*: during this phase cells do not divide, they just adapt to culture conditions and are dependent on the cell line and the seeding density. (b) *Logarithmic (log phase)*: in this phase, cells actively proliferate, viability is very high. (c) *Stationary (plateau) phase*: in this phase, proliferation of cells slow down and cells are more susceptible to injury. (d) *Death phase*: in this phase, cell starts dying; there is significant reduction of viable cells even lesser than stationary phase.

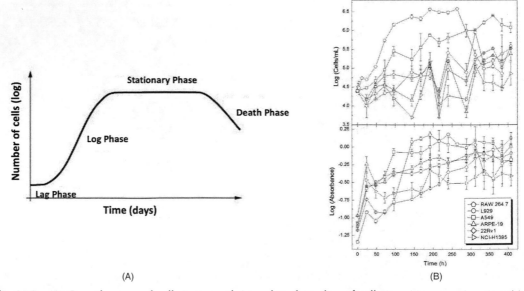

(A)   (B)

Fig. 6.10 (A) Growth curve of cells in general. Log plot of number of cells (y-axis) versus time (x-axis) from a subculture, showing the lag phase, exponential phase, plateau, and death phase. (B) Cell growth curves of a few cell lines (Adopted from Assanga et al., 2013).

6.8.1.7 *Serial Subculture*

When the cell culture has been standardized and the culture is optimally sustained, during the propagation, the repetition of the growth cycle is called serial subculture for each cell line. The subculture is useful in controlling the seeding concentration, the duration of growth (before subculture), the experimental parameters, and appropriate sampling time for precise and consistent experimental findings.

Questions to ponder over

1. Why do we need a cell culturing platform?
2. What are the basic conditions for cell culture?
3. What are the different types of cell culture; which would you consider?
4. What is the meaning of growth cycle?

6.9 Propagation, Population Doubling and Passage Number

An important factor to consider is the proliferation phases of the cells. As described earlier, there are four phases: lag, log, stationary, and decline. The determination of these will allow for fixes on growth time, passaging duration, storage time, and appropriate time for experimentation. The lag phase is the appropriate one for seeding, allowing cells to enter into the log phase in fresh medium.

One of the parameters to evaluate is population doubling. This parameter is defined as the total time required for the cells in a culture condition to double its population. Population doubling is calculated through the following formula:

$$\text{Log}^{10} (N/N_o) \times 3.33$$

where N is the number of cells in the culture vessel at the end of a certain time interval, and N_o is the original number of cells placed in the vessel.

6.10 Cell Viability

Cell-based assays are becoming quite relevant for many biochemical experiments, such as drug discovery, cell proliferation assays, cytotoxicity assays, or genetic profiling. All these experiments require cell manipulation and often require downstream analysis.

6.10.1 Common Assays for Cell Viability

It is very important to optimize the condition in which cells survive better or viability is more. In some experiments obtaining a sufficient number of cells may be a rate-limiting step.

In general, there are three main assay platforms: fluorometric, colorimetric, and radiometric. Each assay requires a different set of conditions and instrumentation. Other possible methods could be based on determination of total protein/culture, total DNA/culture, nuclear counts, lactate dehydrogenase or alkaline phosphatase enzyme measurement, packed cell volume, ATP consumption, caspase assay, extra cellular release of proteins, immunological methods, and many others. Technological platforms available for measuring the cell viability include luminometer, fluorimeter, immunoblotting, flow cytometer, impedance reader, microscopy, absorbance, and radiological assay.

(a) In the fluoremtric assay, a probe, calcein-acetoxymethyl (AM) is made to permeate the intact cell membrane. Calcein-AM is a hydrophobic compound, which passes easily through cell membranes into live cells and is used for estimating cell viability. The non-fluorescent calcein AM dye is hydrolyzed by cellular esterase to give free calcein which is fluorescent and is retained in the cytoplasm. Finally, a fluorescence plate reader will be used to measure the output signal, after the incubation period, after setting the appropriate excitation and emission wavelength.

(b) The most commonly used assay for cell viability is the MTT assay developed by Tim Mosmann in 1983. The MTT [3-(4,5-dimethylthiazolyl)-2-5-diphenyltetrazolium bromide] assay is a colorimetric assay. Reduction of MTT by live cells to an insoluble precipitate (in an otherwise aqueous solution) is a measure of cellular activity. This cellular activity can be directly translated to cell viability, being dependent on the number of live cells. NADPH-dependent oxidoreductase enzymes in the viable cells reduce the MTT reagent to an insoluble product, formazan. The dark purple colored precipitate of formazan is then dissolved with a suitable reagent and absorbance can be measured by a standard absorbance plate reader.

(c) In viable cells, DNA replication (or repair) happens frequently during cellular growth and division. Radiometric assays use this as a measurement of viability of cells. By using radiolabeled [3H] Thymidine, a radio probe can be incorporated into DNA during nuclear replication (or repair). This labeled DNA can be precipitated by trichloroacetic acid (TCA). Radio signals and the incorporated counts are then measured by a scintillation counter. This otherwise quantitatively satisfactory assay is generally avoided due to the involvement of radioactive material.

In any of these assays it is important to note that there are several factors that can influence the outcome, such as growth time, media, number of cells, etc. So care must be taken to ascertain the consistency of validated protocol to get the precise experimental outcome.

6.11   Cryopreservation

Preservation of cells is an important step in proper cell culture protocol. In a cell culture lab, freezing of cells (cryopreservation) is done regularly for purposes of maintaining cell stocks, to preserve cell cultures when not in use, to save cost of materials, prevent finite cells from reaching senescence, and avoid any genetic drift/instability in long term cultures.

Freezing Cells

Whether it is a suspension culture or adherent culture, the first step is to prepare a cell pellet. In case of suspension cells, cells are spun down in a centrifuge and collected as a pellet and dissolved in cryopreservation media. In case of adherent cells, they are first removed from the flask using trypsin (just as in the case of subcultures). Pelleted cells are then re-suspended in cryopreservation media. These cells are normally, persevered in liquid nitrogen (Figure 6.11). Then temperature of the resuspended cells is lowered gradually. During the cooling process, the loss of water increases the concentration of solutes. Also rapid cooling produces ice crystals which can damage the cells. To preserve the cell viability and prevent the damage due to cooling, cryoprotectant agents such as dimethyl sulphoxide (DMSO) or glycerol are added to the cryopreservation media. Serum is frequently added in the media as well.

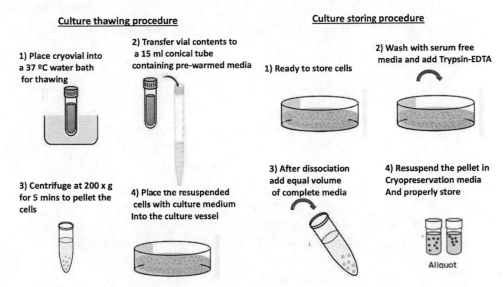

Fig. 6.11 Thawing and storing procedures for cells.

6.12 Characterization and Validation

6.12.1 Characterization

To determine their long-term pluripotency, cells must be characterized by their morphology, expression of markers, telomerase activity, karyotype and pluripotency both in vitro and in vivo. Some of the techniques used to characterize the cells are as follows. The morphology of the cells can be qualitatively and quantitatively assessed by membrane staining observed under a microscope. The cells' biochemical and functional characteristics can be examined by immunofluorescent staining, immunocytochemistry, or immunohistochemistry using suitable markers.

6.12.2 Cross Contamination

When more than one cell line is maintained by a laboratory there are chances of accidental cross contamination, should one cell line be accidentally introduced into the other. If the proliferation rate of the contaminant is faster it overgrows, replacing the original cell line. Cross contamination can occur during propagation and cryopreservation and from mislabeling or poor inventory control. Various steps can be taken to prevent cross contamination:

1. Obtain appropriate validated cell lines.
2. Do not culture more than one cell line at one point of time.
3. Keep media and reagents separate for each cell line.
4. Never use the consumables for different cell lines.
5. After using any consumable in a cell culture flask, never touch the original stock of media or reagent.

6. Always add the media and reagents first and then the cells.
7. Monitor the cell culture flask regularly for any change in morphology, growth rate, or other phenotypic properties.
8. Follow an aseptic protocol.

6.12.3 Microbial Contamination

Microbiological contamination generally refers to the introduction of microbes such as yeast, bacteria, fungi, and protozoa. Changes due to contamination can be observed by change in pH, sedimentation, peculiar smell, etc. The following precautions should be adopted to prevent microbial contamination:

1. Aseptic conditions should be followed to prevent microbial contamination.
2. Biosafety hood should be sprayed with 70% ethanol before and after use.
3. Incubator should be autoclaved once a month.
4. Antibiotics like penicillin should be added to the media to prevent bacterial growth.
5. Contaminated sample should be immediately disposed off.
6. Water in the water-bath should be constantly recycled by deionized, autoclaved water.
7. Any spills in the incubator should be immediately cleaned.
8. All the items used in the cell culture should be sterilized and autoclaved.

Control of microbial growth is necessary to prevent the growth of microorganisms. There are two basic methods to control microbial growth: (1) by killing microorganisms, or (2) by preventing the growth of microorganisms.

This is done either by using physical or chemical agents. Cidal agents such as bactericides and fungicides kill cells. Static agents such as antibiotics inhibit the growth of cells (without killing them).

> **Questions to ponder over**
>
> 1. What are the types of contamination?
> 2. How can cross contamination be avoided?
> 3. Is microbial contamination a usual occurrence? Can it be avoided?

6.13 Microscopy

Microscopes are devices employed to see objects that are so small as to be invisible to the naked eye. A microscope enlarges the objects and allows focusing on the minor details. Because of the small size of the cells, their visual examination has to rely on new instruments and technology to collect relevant data. Robert Hook (1665) is known as the pioneer of microscopy. His microscope had a separate objective, eye piece, and a source of light and could see small objects like fungi. Antony Von Leuwenhoek came up with a simple microscope which could magnify many micro-organisms and cells, including blood cells and muscle fibers, thereby revolutionizing microscopy.

The discovery of capillaries in the dried lungs of the frog, by Marcello Malpighi in 1625, was known as the first *truly scientific finding of the microscope*. Robert Hook's book *Micrographia*, of 1665, confirmed the importance of the new technology with the illustrations of the tiny things. With improvements in the microscope, scientists were able to make discoveries in cellular biology and thus gain understanding of the systems and then conceptualize pathways to follow in dealing with issues connected with health and diseases.

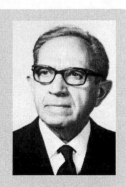

Albert Claude was a Belgian–American cell biologist and a medical doctor. Upon obtaining his M.D. at Liège University, Belgium, in 1928, Claude began research at the Rockefeller Institute for Medical Research (now Rockefeller University) in New York City. He started isolating the cellular components by centrifugation; the heavier particles settled at the bottom of the test tube and lighter particles in the layers above. For comparison, he began centrifuging normal cells. This centrifugal separation of the cell components made it possible for their biochemical analysis that confirmed that the separated particles consisted of distinct organelles. Such analysis enabled Claude to discover the endoplasmic reticulum (a membranous network within cells) and to clarify the function of the mitochondria as the centers of respiratory activity. He developed the principal methods for separating and analyzing components of the living cell. In 1942, Claude turned to the electron microscope — an instrument that had not been used in biological research — looking first at separated components, then at whole cells. His demonstration of the instrument's usefulness in this regard eventually helped scientists to correlate the biological activity of each cellular component with its structure and its place in the cell.

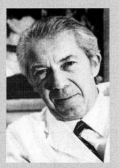

Christian de Duve was a Belgian cytologist and biochemist who discovered lysosomes (the digestive organelle of the cell) and peroxisomes (organelles that are the sites of metabolic processes involving hydrogen peroxide). De Duve's discovery of lysosomes arose out of his research on the enzymes involved in the metabolism of carbohydrates by the liver. While using Claude's technique of separating the components of cells by spinning them in a centrifuge, he noticed that the cells' release of an enzyme called acid phosphatase increased in proportion to the amount of damage done to the cells during centrifugation. De Duve reasoned that the acid phosphatase was enclosed within the cell in some kind of membranous envelope that formed a self-contained organelle. He calculated the probable size of this organelle, christened it the lysosome, and later identified it in electron microscope pictures.

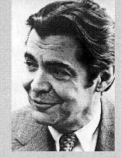

George E. Palade, Romanian born American was a cell biologist. He developed tissue-preparation methods, advanced centrifuging techniques and conducted electron microscopy that resulted in the discovery of several cellular structures like mitochondria, chloroplast, Golgi bodies, and others. His most important discovery were ribosomes which were initially thought to be parts of endoplasmic reticulum

In 1974 **Albert Claude** along with his students, **Christian de Duve** and **George E. Palade** received a joint Nobel Prize award for the discoveries related to the structural and functional organization of the cell.

Taken from nobelprize.org

6.13.1 The Light Microscope

One of the widely used compound microscopes in the cell culture laboratory; it consists of an internal or external light source for illuminating the specimen. The diffused light is gathered by a substage condenser lens which focusses it on the small part of the specimen. The objective lens of the microscope collects the light rays. Now there are two light rays, one that has been altered by the specimen and one that has not been altered. The rays that have not been altered become the background light while the altered light is seen as the image of the specimen. Enlarging the image formed by the objective lens is done by using the ocular lens. The relative distance of the specimen can change focusing the image on the retina, and is adjusted by moving the stage. The product of the magnification produced by the objective lens and the ocular lens provides the total magnification (Figure 6.12).

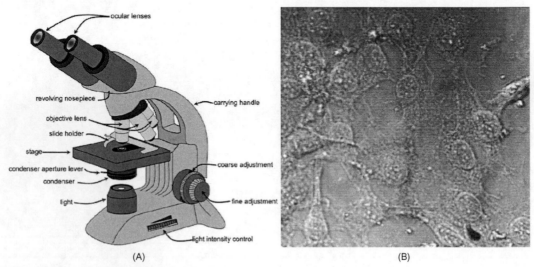

Fig. 6.12 (A) Schematic of a light microscope. (B) Bright field image of a neuron-astrocyte co-culture taken from a light microscope.

6.13.2 Fluorescence Microscopy

Over the last few decades, the light microscope has been transformed for studying minute details by using fluorescence light signals. It can be used to study fluorochromes as well as those cells that do not fluoresce, by tagging the proteins with different antibodies conjugated with fluorophores like fluorescein, rhodamine, or cy5. This technique has enabled live cell imaging. Fluorophores absorb ultraviolet light and release a portion of the energy with longer wavelengths in uv/visible range, through fluorescence (Chapter 4). The light source of the fluorescence microscope travels through a filter that blocks all the wavelengths of light except ultraviolet which is capable of exciting the particular fluorophore (Figure 6.13). The specimen is focused by a beam of monochromatic light, and the collected emitted light is at a visible wavelength. This emitted light is now focused by an objective lens to get the image of the specimen. The image obtained by the fluorescence microscope appears bright against the black background, providing very high contrast. Fluorophores can be used to locate cell membrane, nucleus, membrane proteins, DNA or RNA molecule, amount of Ca^{2+} expression, and such. In some cases the DNA can be genetically modified to produce GFP tagged proteins which can be observed under fluorescence microscope, but the fluorescence intensity reduces slightly with every passage.

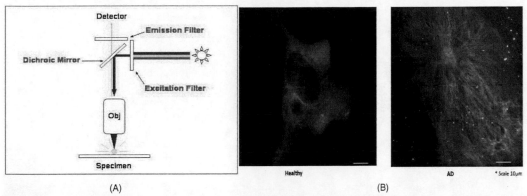

Fig. 6.13   (A) Schematic diagram of a fluorescence microscope. (B) Fluorescent image of nonactivated and activated astrocyte in healthy and AD (Alzheimer disease) model. Protein was tagged with Alexa fluor 488 dye (green) and nucleus was tagged with DAPI (4′,6-diamidino-2-phenylindole; blue). [See color plates]

6.13.3   Confocal Microscopy

As one of the most extensively used techniques in scientific and industrial communities, it overcomes some of the limitations of a fluorescence microscope, by capturing 2D pictures at different depths and hence iterating a 3D image. It consists of two pinholes. The specimen is stimulated uniformly with a light source. It uses two pin holes, one located before the specimen (excitation aperture) and the other right before the photodetector (emission pinhole), hence the term confocal (Figure 6.14). Much of the light is blocked due to the pin hole, hence long exposure time is required, which leads to the possibility of quenching of the signal in case of prolonged exposures. Successive slices make up a Z-stack and a variety of software can be used to stitch a 3D image from the 2D slices obtained. Biological samples are often treated with fluorophores to make the object of interest visible with a contrasting black background. The pinhole at the detector helps in removing the out-of-focus signals, giving a sharp image.

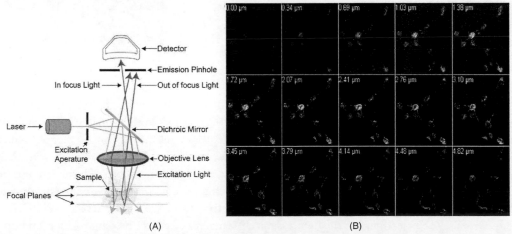

Fig. 6.14   (A) Diagram of a confocal microscope. (B) Z-stack image of SHSY-5Y cell demonstrating internalization of a protein (green). Z-stack feature of confocal microscopy provides images of a cell at different depths (one end to the other) (Adopted from Kumar et al., 2012). [See color plates]

6.13.4　Electron Microscope

This excellent tool uses an electron beam to present microscopic images. The resolution power of the electron microscope is very high and very useful in getting the information about minute objects (Figure 6.15). Types of electron microscope: TEM (Transmission electron microscope) and SEM (Scanning electron microscope). Tables 6.3 and 6.4 describe the difference between light and electron microscopy, and TEM and SEM, respectively.

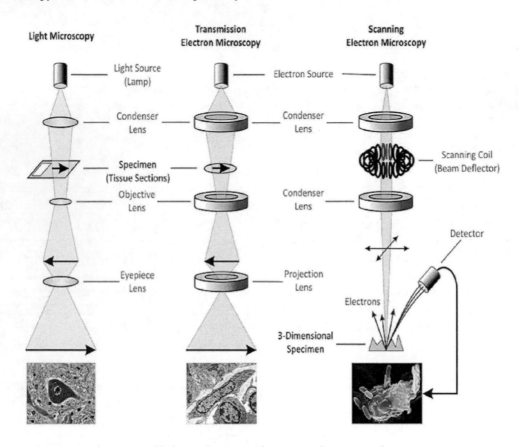

Fig. 6.15　Schematics of light, transmission electron, and scanning electron microscopy.

TEM uses a high voltage beam from an electron gun for illuminating the specimen. The electrostatic and electromagnetic lenses are used to focus the accelerated electron beam. The emitted electron beam is then magnified by an objective lens. To focus the electron beam on the specimen a condenser is placed between the electron lens and the specimen. The objective provided by the lens is only magnified 100 times but shows more details than the light microscope. The electron beam moves in horizontal lines forward and backwards across the sample. Depending on the height size and shape black, grey, and white dots are obtained creating an image on the screen. White color results when all the electrons hit the detector; black, when no electrons hit the detector; and grey is in-between. Cells or tissue are fixed and stained with solution of heavy metals, such as gold and palladium. Metal staining is used to increase electron scattering by selectively binding to the organelles inside the cell. The bound part of the cell will reduce the distance electrons will have to travel.

After passing through the specimen, electrons hit the photographic plate to produce an image. The image can also be captured on a video camera. While TEM has been utilized to observe the structure inside the cell, SEM is the technique used to study the surface properties of the cell. For sample preparation, the specimen is fixed and passed through a series of alcohol solutions and then dried using a process known as critical point drying. The density of the vapor and the density of the liquid is equal at critical temperature and pressure, and at this point there is no surface tension between the two phases. Taking advantage of this fact, the solvent inside the cell is systematically replaced by a liquid transitional fluid (CO_2) in vaporized form. Finally, the specimen is ready for EM once a thin coating of metal has been applied.

Questions to ponder over
1. What is the importance of Microscopy?
2. What may perhaps be missing in microscopy of biological specimens?
3. What is the basic concept of microscopy?
4. What are the differences between confocal microscope and SEM?
5. Which microscope do you think is better? Why?

Table 6.3 Comparison of light microscopy with electron microscopy.

Light Microscopy	Electron Microscopy
Illuminating source is light.	Illuminating source is the beam of electron.
Live and dead specimens can both be seen.	Only dead or dried specimen can be used and so, seen.
Low resolution power (0.25 μm to 0.3 μm).	High resolving power (0.001 μm).
About 500 -1500 X magnification is possible.	About 100,000 – 300,000 X magnification is possible
Image can be colored as well as in black and white.	Only black and white.
No need of high voltage electricity, therefore no cooling system is required.	High electric current is required, therefore need of cooling system.
Specimen can be stained with dyes.	Specimens need to be coated with heavy metals to reflect electrons.
Image can be seen by eyes.	Image is produced using either a fluorescent screen or photographic plate.
Used for the study of overall internal structure of the cell.	Used in the study of external surface, organelles and other structures inside the cell, and very small organisms.

Table 6.4 Differences between TEM and SEM.

Transmission Electron Microscopy (TEM)	Scanning Electron Microscopy (SEM)
Appropriate for studying structure inside the cell.	Suits studies of surface properties of the cell, processes, extracellular material.
Electron beam focuses on the condenser lens to hit the whole specimen.	Electrons are accelerated as fine beam that hit the specimen.
The electron beam passes through the specimen to form image.	Image is reflected back from the specimen to form the image.
Water removed by dehydration in alcohol or frozen specimens used for non-fixed specimen.	Fluid removed by critical point drying.
Tissue spaces are filled with epoxy resins.	Solvent replaced by CO_2.
Focus approximately 100 times more than light microscopy.	Focus approximately 500 times more than light microscopy.
Metal binds to macromolecules.	Target coated with thin layer of metal.
Image formation is direct.	Image formation is indirect.

6.13.5 Atomic Force Microscopy

Measuring the mechanical properties of cells and extracellular matrix is very important while examining phenomena like differentiation, tumor formation, and wound healing. Cell stiffness is an important parameter to evaluate the status of cell. Micro-indentation techniques are used to measure the stiffness of cells and tissues and this technique is called atomic force microscopy (AFM). AFM allows 3-D imaging and measurements of biological samples in air or fluid in a single scan, and it is capable of providing details of the surface topography. This technology allows measurement of surface stiffness or elasticity in living cells and membranes and height information enabling determination of changes in surface levels.

Stiffness of living cells is an index while examining cytoskeletal structure, myosin activity, force generation by cell movement, adhesion measurements, surface structures, cell-to-cell or cell-to-surface structures, exocytosis or endocytosis, and many other cellular processes. In AFM, a micro-tip indents a cell and measures the applied force from bending of the AFM cantilever. Force indentation curves thus generated, provide the quantitative measurements of material stiffness (Figure 6.16). Both surface and mechanical data of cells can be obtained by AFM (Figure 6.17). This technique does not require tedious fixing, staining or labeling processes. Combined with optical microscopy and fluorescence microscopy, AFM techniques provide immense possibilities for cell microscopy. AFM can provide mechanical measurement and florescence can be used for an optical analysis. Combined measurement will be used to interpret overall biochemical responses of the cell to external or internal stimulating factors.

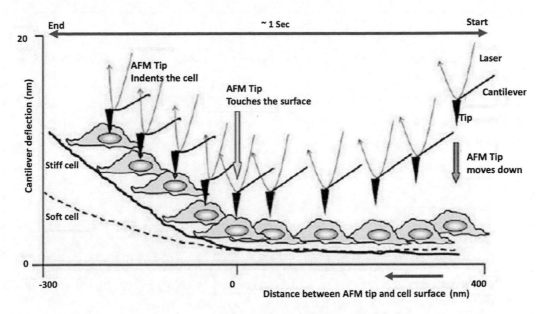

Fig. 6.16 A specimen atomic force microscopy curve. At the longer distance between the tip and surface, overall force felt by the tip is almost zero (start of the plot). As the tip approaches the surface, atoms between the probe and the surface begin experiencing attractive Van der Waals forces (Adopted from Morton and Baker, 2014).

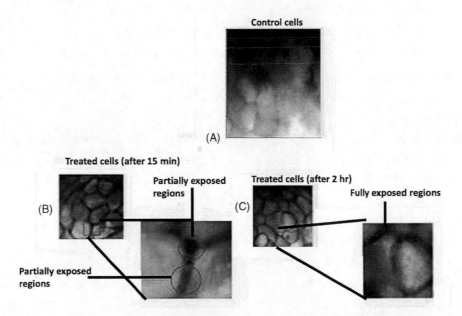

Fig. 6.17 AFM images of HT-29 cells carried out in the non-contact mode using a cantilever of 0.01N/m spring constant. (A) 50μm x 50 μm area of the untreated HT-29 cells; (B) 50 μm x 50 μm section of HT-29 cell monolayer after 15 min treatment; inset 20 μm x 20 μm area of the same sample; (C) 50 μm x 50 μm section of HT-29 cell monolayer after 2 hour treatment; inset 20 μm x 20 μm area of the same sample.

Terminology

The vocabulary of cell culture is unique. Some common terms which are used regularly in literature on cell culture are given below:

Adherent cells: Cells that are able to adhere to their culture vessel.

Suspension culture: The type of culture where cells multiply while suspended in a liquid medium.

Cell culture: The entire process of growth, maintenance, and storage of cells in vitro.

Cell line: The set of subcultures (generation upon generation) that follow after the development of a primary cell line.

Cell strain: A population of cells that have undergone some genetic change from the initiating cells of the parent cell line. This can happen both naturally or by design. Strains generally retain many of the characteristics of the originating cells.

Primary culture: Starting a culture directly from an organ.

Organotypic: Culture in three-dimensional form, resembling an organ both structurally and/or functionally.

Cell viability: Defined as the number of healthy cells in a sample; it is the quantification of the number of live cells in the culture versus those in the control and denoted by percentage.

Apoptosis: Programed cell death of multicellular organisms.

Necrosis: Death of cells or tissues due to injury, radiation, or chemicals.

Finite cell culture: A cell culture which is capable of only limited numbers of subculture.

Immortalization: Cells that can proliferate continuously generation after generation.

Passage: The procedure of transferring cells from one culture vessel to another.

Attachment efficiency: Within a fixed time, the percentage of cells that attach to the surface of the culture vessel.

Aseptic technique: Technique to prevent contamination of cell culture. Prevent sepsis.

Cryopreservation: The procedure of storage of cells, tissues, embryos, or seeds at very low temperatures.

Differentiated: Cells with a specialized structure and function.

Diploid: All cells with a pair of chromosomes. Only reproductive cells such as gametes, eggs, and sperm cells have a single chromosome and are called haploid.

Explant: Process of growth and maintenance of tissue outside their original environment.

General Protocol for Cell Culture and Immunostaining of Neurons

- Coat the plates (24 well) with the desired ECM, at 200 µl per well. Incubate at 37°C for 30 min.
- Detach the cells in the T-75 flask by adding trypsin (4–5) µl for not more than 7 min at 37°C.
- Observe the cells under the microscope to see that the cells are completely detached.
- Pipette the cell solution in a 15 ml tube. Add equal amount of PBS 1x.
- Spin the cells at appropriate speed (speed is specific for each cell type).
- After centrifugation, a thick palette is seen at the bottom.
- Aspirate the supernatant.
- Resuspend the cells in 1 ml media.
- Count the cells by hemocytometer.
- Dilute the cell suspension to the appropriate seeding concentration (for 24 well plate, number of neuronal cells = 10^5 cells per well). Total vol. per well = 500 µl.
- The cells can differentiate in 7–21 days depending on the type of neuronal cells.
- Media is changed every week.
- The cells are fixed with 4% PFA for 15 min, Vol = 200 µl per well.
- Wash with 1x PBS/ PBST, 3x with 5 min interval between each wash, Vol = 500 µl per well.
- Cells are permeabilized with PBSTT for 5 min, Vol = 200 µl per well.
- Wash with PBS for 5 min X2, Vol = 500 µl per well.
- Block with 3% BSA for 30 min at RT or overnight at 4°C, Vol = 500 µl per well.
- 1' ab (anti-TUJ1; host type = mouse), 1:100), overnight 4°C, Vol = 200 µl per well.
- Wash with PBS for 5 min X3, Vol = 500 µl per well.
- 2' ab (anti-mouse, 1:100) for 3 hrs at RT or overnight at 4°C.
- + Counterstaining with DAPI (1:1000).
- Wash with PBS for 15 min X5, vol = 500 µl per well.
- Depending on the flurofore used for secondary antibody, the microscope setting can be adjusted to FITC/TRITC or Cy5.
- Magnification can be adjusted to 4x–60x, depending on the experiment requirement.
- Time of exposure should be minimal, typically limited to minutes, to avoid photo-bleaching and false results.

Protocol for Cell Culture

Subculture Monolayers

- Prepare the hood for subculturing.
- Warm the medium and trypsin.
- Take out the flask that needs to be subcultured and examine for any contamination.
- Detach the cells by adding trypsin for not more than 7 min at 37°C.
- Observe the cells under the microscope to check that the cells are completely detached.
- Pipette the cell solution in a 15 ml tube. Add equal amount of PBS 1x.
- Spin the cells at appropriate speed (speed is specific for each cell type).
- After centrifugation, a thick palette is seen at the bottom.
- Aspirate the supernatant.
- Resuspend the cells in media.
- Count the cells by hemocytometer.
- Dilute the cell suspension to the appropriate seeding concentration.
- Add the appropriate volume to the flask in premeasured volume of media in flask.

Subculture Suspension Cell

- Take a small sample and count the samples.
- Decide if the subculture is required.
- Mix the cell suspension and disperse any clumps by pipetting the cell suspension up and down.
- Add medium to the stirrer flask to a maximum depth of 5 cm. If a greater volume of medium is required, CO_2 must be supplied via a sparging tube.
- Add a sufficient number of cells to give a final concentration of 1×10^5 cells/mL for slow-growing cells (36–48 hrs doubling time) or 2×10^4/ mL for rapidly growing cells (12–24 hrs doubling time).
- Gas the airspace of the stirrer flask with 5% CO_2.
- Cap the stirrer flask and place on magnetic stirrers set at 60 to 100 rpm, in an incubator or hot room at 37°C.

Protocol for Immunostaining

Cell Membrane

Cell membrane staining on live cell culture:
- Treat trypsin 0.25 for 3 min in 1ml PBS.
- Spin down
- Wash with PBS 1x
- Spin down
- Prepare diluent 1ml with 4 µl dye
- Mix well
- Incubate at R.T. for 5 min
- Stop reaction by adding 1% BSA in PBS
- Add 2 ml media
- Spin down
- Add 2 ml media
- Spin down
- Plate the surface after cell counting

Nucleus

Both live cells and fixed cells can be stained for nucleus using DAPI or Hoescst stain:
- For live cell staining, follow above mentioned protocol when the cells have to be plated.
- For live cell staining in flask, prepare the stain 1:1000, add it to the coated flask for 5 min.
- Wash with PBS/HBSS.

Transmembrane Protein

Fixing the cells is required for transmembrane staining.
- Wash the cells to be stained in PBS 1x
- Fix the cell using paraformaldehyde. Add the amount depending upon the plate size. Incubate at R.T. for 15 min.
- Wash cells with PBS 1x, 3 times at 5 min interval
- Permeabilize the cells using PBS 1x with 1% Tween and 0.1% Triton for 15 min at R.T.
- Wash the cells using PBS 1x, 3 times at 5 min interval.
- For blocking the cells, add 3% (w/v) BSA in PBS.
- For best result, leave it overnight at 4°C.

Protocol for Cell Viability (MTT Assay)

- Plate 1,000–100,000 cells per well in a 96-well plate and treat as appropriate.
- Remove the medium and wash with PBS.
- Ass MTT to a final concentration of 0.5 mg/ml.
- Incubate for 30 minutes to 4 hrs at 37°C, until purple color formazan is visible.
- Remove MTT and add solubilizing solution.
- Incubate at room temperature or 37°C for 30 mins to 2 hrs.
- Measure the absorbance at 570 nm.

Protocol for Counting the Number of Cells

Some microscope can also be used for counting the number of cells but the most common and widely accepted method of counting the cells is by using hemocytometer. In general, the hemocytometer is of "H" shape. The total volume required to load the hematocytometer is 10 µl.

To distinguish between dead and viable cells, the sample is often diluted with a particular stain, such as Trypan blue. This staining method, also known as dye exclusion staining, uses a diazo dye that selectively penetrates cell membranes of dead cells, coloring them blue, whereas it is not absorbed by membranes of live cells, thus excluding live cells from staining.

The area of the middle (Figure B) and each corner square is 1 mm × 1 mm = 1 mm^2: the depth of each square is 0.1 mm. The final volume of each square at that depth is 100 nl.

For large cells, we can count total number of cells in the outside four corners or include the middle along with the outer corners, as specified in Figure B.

Once the number of cells has been counted the cell total number of cells/ml can then be calculated by the following formula:

Total # cells/ ml = (total cell counted/ total # of squares) × dilution factor × 10,000 cells/ml.

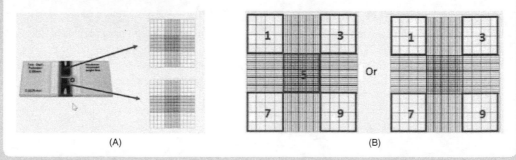

(A)   (B)

Questions

1. What is the need of a cell culture model?
2. What are the checkpoints in mitosis?

3. What is the significance of cell morphology?
4. What are the criteria for a subculture model?
5. How does the cell behave when DNA synthesis is compromised?
6. What is differentiation? What are the major pathways of differentiation?
7. What is the difference between cold and warm trypsinization?
8. What are 3-D cultures? What are the limitations of organ culture?
9. Explain the roles of a matrix in cell culture?
10. Which matrix materials are generally used?
11. What aspects should be put into consideration while selecting a cell line?
12. How do we determine what kind of imaging is required for the experiment?
13. What are the different kinds of contamination and how can we overcome such contamination?

References

Assanga, I. and Lujan, L. (2013). Cell growth curves for different cell lines and their relationship with biological activities. *International Journal of Biotechnology and Molecular Biology Research*, 4(4), 60–70.

Freshney, R. I. (2006). Basic principles of cell culture. In Gordana Vunjak-Novakovic and R. Ian Freshney, eds., *Culture of Cells for Tissue Engineering*. New Jersey: John Wiley & Sons. pp. 3–22.

Heins, N., Englund, M. C., Sjöblom, C., et al. (2004). Derivation, characterization, and differentiation of human embryonic stem cells. *Stem Cells*, 22(3), 367–376.

Kumar, R., Zhou, Y., Ghosal, K., Cai, S. and Singh, B. R. (2012). Anti-apoptotic activity of hemagglutinin-33 and botulinum neurotoxin and its implications to therapeutic and countermeasure issues. *Biochemical and Biophysical Research Communications*, 417(2), 726–731.

Morton, K. C. and Baker, L. A. (2014). Atomic force microscopy-based bioanalysis for the study of disease. *Analytical Methods*, 6(14), 4932–4955.

Oh, J. W., Hsi, T. C., Guerrero-Juarez, C. F., Ramos, R. and Plikus, M. V. (2013). Organotypic skin culture. *The Journal of Investigative Dermatology*, 133(11), 14.

Rodríguez–Hernández, C. O., Torres–Garcia, S. E., Olvera–Sandoval, C., et al. (2014). Cell culture: history, development and prospects. *International Journal of Current Research and Academic*, 2(12), 188–200.

Settembre, C., Fraldi, A., Medina, D. L. and Ballabio, A. (2013). Signals from the lysosome: a control centre for cellular clearance and energy metabolism. *Nature Reviews Molecular Cell Biology*, 14(5), 283–296.

Zhang, L., Hu, J. and Athanasiou, K.A. (2009). The role of tissue engineering in articular cartilage repair and regeneration. *Critical Reviews in Biomedical Engineering*, 37(1–2).

Antibody Technology*

7.1 Introduction to Immunochemical Techniques

Life on the earth has an abundance of pathogenic and non-pathogenic microbes, which apart from mutual symbiotic and survival connections contain several toxic and allergenic molecules that bring about imbalance in homeostasis. These substances have a variety of mechanisms to disturb the functioning of their host. To counter these threats, mammals developed a complex and evolutionary matured array of immune and defensive mechanisms to check or annihilate these substances without damaging their own tissues. In general, there are two mechanisms which permit recognition and destruction of microbial, toxic, or allergenic substances: 1) **Innate response**: This is the first line of defense against the invading pathogen or toxin, and 2) **Adaptive response**: The second line of defense. Although the adaptive responses are temporary, they leave a memory associated with this process and for a specific antigen. The organism resorts to the same defense mechanism when it encounters the same antigen again. The adaptive response has the capability to regulate immune memory, and create an effective and specific host response against invading pathogens, even decades after the first encounter.

For identification of foreign material, immunoglobulins (IgG) and antibodies are integral parts of adaptive immune response in mammals. IgGs are present in the tissues and fluids of all vertebrates. Research related to antibodies started way back in 1890, when Emil von Behring and Shibasabura Kitasato began to immunize infected animals against diptheria. According to the side-chain theory, proposed by Paul Ehrlich in 1900, the pathogens bind to their side-chain receptors. Then, the modern era of antibody research and discovery started with examination at the atomic level of details of its structure (in 1973) and invention of monoclonal antibodies (in 1975).

The formation of an antigen–antibody complex, is due to a very specific interaction between antibody and its antigen, and is the basis of all immunochemical based technology. An antigen in general, is an exogenous substance that elicits an immune response and is recognized by very specific antibodies produced by the immunological responses to counter the invading antigen. They are usually either proteins or polysaccharides of high molecular weight. However, small molecules can also function as antigens, such as polypeptides, lipids, and nucleic acids. These small molecules (haptens) may generate immune response by coupling themselves to a larger "carrier protein", such as bovine serum albumin or hemocyanin or other synthetic matrices.

---

* Ghuncha Ambrin, co-authored this chapter, contributing significantly to the writing of this book.

Immunochemical techniques are simple, highly specific, and sensitive methods of analysis. The basis of these techniques is highly specific interaction of an antigen and its antibody. The specificity and sensitivity of an assay depends on the type of antibody and its affinity for the antigen. Based on the assay format, the immunoassay can be either qualitative or quantitative.

Paul Ehrlich, the German medical scientist who pioneered work in hematology, immunology, and chemotherapy is famous for his discovery of the first effective treatment of syphilis. He received the Nobel Prize for Medicine in 1908 jointly with Elie Metchikoff. He was the proponent of the side-chain theory of antibody that sought to describe how these proteins are produced by the immune system and react with other substances. In this theory, Ehrlich postulated that on the surface of each cell there are many side chains that function by attaching with specific nutrient molecules. These side chains interact irreversibly with toxins as well and result in toxin-side chain blocks. Toxins trigger the body into, then, producing these side chains in overwhelming amounts. Since not all of these molecules can fit on the limited surface of the cell, most are secreted into the body's circulatory system. These circulating molecules are termed as antibodies. Although this much-debated theory was ultimately proven wrong it had a profound influence on the further conceptualization of how immune systems work.

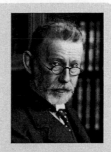

7.2 Antibodies

Antibodies or immunoglobulins are proteins that are produced by the immune system, mainly by the plasma cells, in response to foreign molecules (antigens) that invade the body. After production, antibodies keep circulating throughout the blood and the lymph system where they identify and bind to their specific antigen. Binding of antibody to an antigen neutralizes the antigen and the resultant waste is processed further to be cleared from circulation.

There are various features, which are unique to antibodies: (a) very high specificity for recognition and binding, usually with a dissociation constant (K_D) in the nM and pM range, (b) they are characterized by a well-defined and uniform protein structure, and (c) they have a memory associated with their production and recognition. These features are useful for various detection and diagnostic purposes, where, the specific interaction between an antigen and its antibody can be utilized.

Characteristics required of effective antibodies are: (a) randomness of structure, (b) ability to be metabolized, (c) exposed immunogenic regions which can be utilized in the antibody formation mechanism, (d) structural elements that are significantly different from the host, and (e) molecular weight ranging from 8,000–10,000 daltons (although haptens are as low as 200 Da).

Structurally, antibodies are visualized as Y-shaped molecules, each containing four polypeptide chains—consisting of heavy chains and light chains (Figure 7.1). In general, there are five classes of antibodies: IgG, IgM, IgA, IgE, and IgD. These classifications are based on the number of Y-like units and the type of heavy-chain polypeptide (γ, μ, α, ϵ, and δ). IgG is the most abundant antibody found in serum and it contains two identical Fab fragments that form the arms of the Y. Each Fab region consists of a unique site which can recognize and bind to an antigen (antigen binding site). The third domain, often termed as the "tail", is a complement-binding Fc fragment which forms the base of the Y. It serves as a control unit for manipulating antibodies during the immunochemical reaction, response, and regulation. All the three domains (two Fab domains and one Fc domain) of an antibody can be separated by the proteolytic enzyme papain; or into two parts (one $F(ab)_2$ and one Fc) by the proteolytic enzyme pepsin. The interactive forces between antigens and antibodies are primarily non-covalent interactions such as hydrogen bonds, hydrophobic, electrostatic, and Van der Waals forces. Although these interactive forces are weak, binding between antigen and antibody can be quite strong mainly due to high specificity of the interaction between antigen and its antibody. The binding of an antibody to the antigen is dependent on reversible, non-covalent interactions, and the complex is in equilibrium with the free components. All antigen–antibody binding is reversible and follows the basic thermodynamic principle:

$$K_A = [\text{Ab-Ag}]/[\text{Ab}]^*[\text{Ag}]$$

$$K_D = I/K_A = [\text{Ab}]^*[\text{Ab}]/[\text{Ab-Ag}]$$

where, K_A is the affinity constant, Ab and Ag are the molar concentrations of free antibody, antigen, respectively. Ab-Ag is the molar concentration of the antibody–antigen complex. The binding site of an antibody comprises of a packet which can accommodate about 6–10 amino acids. Strength of Ab–Ag interaction can be affected by even a slight change in the antigen structure. The binding strength of an Ab-Ag complex is measured by their affinity and is usually represented by their dissociation constant, K_D (ranging from micro (10^{-6}) to pico (10^{-12}) molar). Higher affinity levels for an antibody results in a quicker rate and more stable binding. This is why higher-affinity antibodies are preferable in immunochemical techniques.

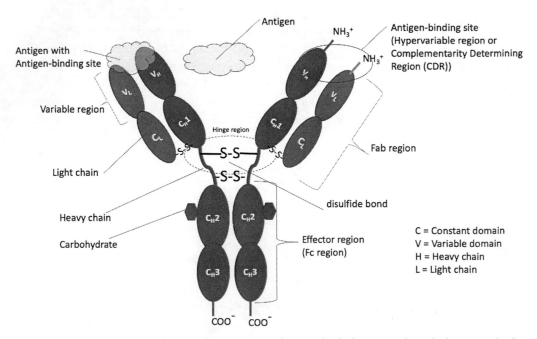

Fig. 7.1 A model of a Y-shaped antibody structure with Fc and Fab domains. The Fab domain is further divided into two regions: a constant and a variable region. Variable region is the part which identifies the antigen.

In general, two molecular parameters are used in classifying Ab-Ag binding. 1) *Affinity*, which measures the attractive or repulsive forces between the individual epitope and individual binding site. High affinity values reflect strong interaction between an epitope and antibody binding site. It is easier to measure this in monoclonal antibodies as they have only one epitope and are homogenous. For polyclonal antibodies, due to their heterogenous nature, the rate is calculated as an average of the affinity values with the different antigenic epitopes. 2) *Avidity*, which is related to the antibody–antigen binding reaction. It is a measure of binding strength of all interactions between a multivalent antigen and a multivalent antibody. In addition, it determines the overall stability of the complex, Ab-Ag, the number of binding sites per antibody molecule, and the required geometric arrangement of the interacting components (Figure 7.2). Successful outcome of any immunological technique is determined by the factors involved in the binding reactions and avidity takes into account all these factors. Although, the specificity of an Ab-Ag interaction may be high, there could be a possibility of some cross-reactivities to the similar epitopes on other molecules.

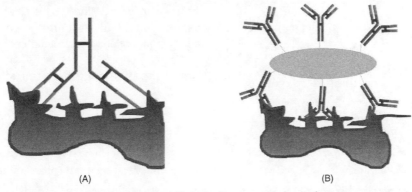

(A)   (B)

Fig. 7.2   (A) Schematics for defining affinity: Affinity is the strength of a single antigen–antibody interaction. Binding site on the antibody has high affinity for its target. (B) Schematics of avidity: Avidity is the combination of strength of all the interactions. The IgG may have low affinity, but due to higher concentration its avidity could be high.

Quality of antibodies is very important consideration in any immunological assay and its sensitivity. From an immunological point-of-view, antibodies can be either polyclonal or monoclonal. Monoclonal antibodies are produced by cloned immune cells, and specifically bind to only one type of antigen. Being designed to identify only one epitope, these antibodies are homogeneous in their specificity and affinity. Polyclonal antibodies are produced by injecting animals with peptide/ protein antigens. Large amounts of antigens are produced by the animals in response to the injection. Antibodies are then isolated from the whole serum. These antibodies are heterogeneous and can identify several epitopes. When the antigens have multiple epitopes, they result in the production of multiple antibodies, and this grouping is called polyclonal antibody.

> **Epitope:** it is an area or part of an antigen of the foreign molecule to which an antibody binds non-covalently.

There are several ways to design an assay based on an antibody–antigen interaction. In an in vitro assay, when both antibodies and antigens are present in a solution, a large precipitation may be observed in the test tube. Some of the techniques of antigen–antibody binding are precipitin reaction, Ouchterlony assay and radial immune-diffusion assay (explained in Section 7.9).

Precipitin reaction: A precipitin reaction involves the addition of soluble antigens to a test tube containing solution of antibodies. The two arms of antibody can bind to an epitope. A lattice is formed as more and more antibodies bind to corresponding antigens together, resulting in precipitin. Most tests use polyclonal antiserum, because then they can bind to multiple epitopes creating a more visible lattice. Precipitin formation is visible only when there is an optimal ratio of antibody to the antigen. Antigen is slowly added to the solution containing antibodies to obtain an optimal ratio. Initially, when the antigen concentration is low, there is no visible formation of precipitin. This is called the zone of antibody excess. Increase in concentration of antigen now results in lattice formation. This is called the equivalence zone. Here in the equivalence zone, the optimal antibody–antigen interaction with maximum precipitation, occurs. Addition of more antigen causes a drop in the amount of precipitation. This is the zone of antigen excess.

7.3   Epitope Mapping

An "epitope" is a region of an antigen which is recognized by an antibody. This region is also known as the immune-determinant region. Such regions are usually present on the surface of an antigen and one to six monosaccharide or aminoacid residues long. Epitopes are

> **Questions to ponder over**
>
> 1. What is an antibody? What are the different types?
> 2. Describe a typical structure of an antibody elaborating functions of various domains?
> 3. What is an epitope?
> 4. What is the difference between affinity and avidity?

of two types (Figure 7.3): (a) *conformational epitopes*, that have a specific three-dimensional antigenic conformation, and (b) *linear epitopes*, that have a simple specific primary sequence region and identifiable 2D conformation. Specific recognition of the conformational state of an antigen provides for greater selectivity and affinity because linear epitopes can be masked by conformational folding.

Epitope mapping is a helpful tool in therapeutics, disease and vaccine development. It can also aid in knowing the mechanism of an antigen binding to an antibody. It is commonly performed with the purpose of structural analysis or for the identification and characterization of antibody-binding properties.

Characteristics of an Epitope

1. Epitopes that occur naturally are relatively small (either amino acids or sugar residues).
2. Specific epitope should fit the recognition site present on antibody (antigen–antibody site).
3. The shape of the antibody of an antigen–antibody combining site is cave pocket shaped to match the convex shape with the epitope.
4. Small antigens are mono-epitope, large proteins can express either different or identical repeating epitopes.
5. Forces responsible for binding are Van der Waals forces or hydrophobic ones. Electrostatic forces may also be in play but they act at a distance.
6. Formation of stable immune complexes occur when the epitope and paratope fit "Jigsaw Fashion."
7. For inducing an immune response not only is the position on the epitope important, but also the position of each subunit within the epitope.
8. Any amino acid can contribute to a protein epitope. The residues that are not a part of the

epitope might not bind to an antibody but might influence antigen conformation and thus affect epitope binding.

9. The antigen, however, may contain other epitopes in addition to the one initially recognized.

The several techniques for epitope mapping include X-ray crystallography, NMR, hydrogen-deuterium exchange coupled to mass spectrometry, peptide-based approaches and mutagenesis.

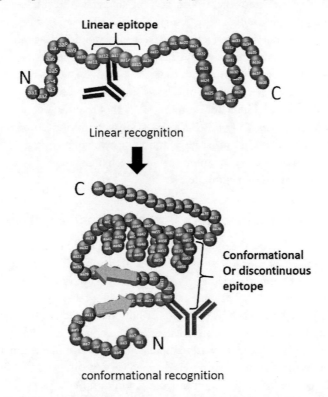

Fig. 7.3 Representation of linear and conformational epitopes.

7.4 Immunoassay

In the last 50 years, immunoassays have been extensively used in hospitals, industry, and research labs. Information gained from immunoassays have shortened hospital stays, led to proper diagnosis, improved understanding of biological systems, and detected contaminants in food and water. An immunoassay is a *biochemical* assay that uses an antibody or an antigen to determine the *concentration* of a bio*molecule* or a small molecule in a solution. These assays are routinely used in the quantitative measurement of drugs or biomarkers in biological fluids like serum, plasma, or urine. These assays are quick and reliable and based on the inherent ability of an antibody to bind to the specific structure of the antigen molecule. As mentioned before, two types of antibodies are used for immunoassay: monoclonal and polyclonal. Monoclonal antibodies are mostly used as they bind to only to one site of a specific molecule, whereas polyclonal antibodies have multiple binding sites.

The selected antibodies should have a high affinity for the antigen. For the quantitative assessment, the fluids (serum, urine, etc.) should be run against the standards of known concentrations. The quantity of the specimen is determined by plotting the standard curve. The antibody or antigen concentration can be determined by different methods such as ELISA, immunohistochemistry, and immunoblotting. Immunoassays can be divided into two types: assays with labeled reagents (fluorogenic, radioactive, or electro chemi-luminescent) and assays involving non-labeled reagents. The label-free format directly produces the observable detection signal, whereas the labeled format requires signal producing molecules attached to the immunological reagents, such as the antigen or antibody, which produces detectable analytical signals. Labeled reagents can be further divided into homogenous and heterogenous immunoassays. In heterogenous assay it is required to remove the unbound antibody or antigen from the site. This step is not required in a homogenous assay.

Heterogeneous immunoassay: These are immunoassays that require separation of bound and free antibodies prior to measurement, e.g. ELISA (enzyme linked immunosorbent assay).

Homogeneous immunoassay: Immunoassays that do not involve much examination of bound and free fractions. They are simpler assays but require more mechanical steps to be conducted, e.g. EMIT (enzyme multiplied immunoassay technique).

7.4.1   Heterogenous Immunoassays Can Be Competitive or Noncompetitive

(i)   *In a competitive immunoassay*, the unlabeled antigen (in the sample under examination) competes with a labeled antigen for the same antibody. The unlabeled analyte displaces the bound labeled analyte, and the remaining labeled analyte is measured by using proper detection platform. The unlabeled and the labeled antigens are then mixed together. After equilibration is reached for this reaction (displacement), the amount of bound, labeled Ab-Ag complex is measured. In this method, the amount of bound labeled Ab-Ag complex is inversely proportional to the concentration of antigen present in the sample being assayed. The competitive assay requires only a a small amount of antibody and so is deemed very specific and highly sensitive. They are often slow and require long incubation times, e.g. radioimmunoassays (RIA).

(ii) *Noncompetitive immunoassays*, also referred to as "sandwich assays" require large amounts of labeled antibody against the analyte (antigen) in the specimen. In this assay two antibodies are employed, one labeled and another unlabeled. The antigen in the specimen sample is bound to the antibody site which is immobilized on a solid surface. After incubation with the sample containing the antigen, the labeled antibody is allowed to bind to the antigen. The amount of labeled antibody on the site is then measured. The amount of labeled antibody is directly proportional to the concentration of the analyte present in the sample. One of the formats of ELISA is based on this immunoassay technique. Noncompetitive immunoassays are very specific and less time consuming than competitive immunoassay. However, they consume large amounts of pure specific antibodies. This limitation has been overcome by the development of monoclonal antibodies.

7.5   ELISA

ELISA, stands for *Enzyme Linked ImmunoSorbent Assay*, is a plate-based technique designed for detecting and quantifying peptides, proteins, amino acids, and such. Enzyme immunoassays (EIA) also work on the same principle. ELISAs are quick, easy to carry out and large samples can be handled in parallel. This method is frequently used for detection, diagnostics, immunological, and biochemical research. In general, ELISA is a multi-step procedure, as follows: (1) the microtiter plate wells are coated with antigen, (2) all unbound sites are blocked to prevent false positive results, (3) a primary antibody (IgG) is applied to the antigen in the wells, (4) a secondary antibody (IgG, against the primary antibody) conjugated to an enzyme is then added to the wells, and (5) finally, a substrate is then added to the wells which reacts with the conjugated enzyme to produce color which can be measured by a spectrophotometer, spectrofluorometer, or other optical/electrochemical device.

The presence of antigens or antibodies can both be detected by ELISA. On a solid support, such as polystyrene microtiter plate, latex bead, or magnetic bead, either antigen or antibody is immobilized. Using the solid matrix allows separation of unbound antibodies or antigens through repeated washing to minimize nonspecific binding. The antibodies can be labeled with biotin, alkaline phosphatase, horseradish peroxidase, or β-galactosidase.

There are mainly three different types of ELISA:

(a) Direct
(b) Indirect
(c) Competitive

7.5.1 Direct ELISA

In this method, antigen coated wells of microtiter plates are allowed to bind with the labeled antibody directly. Antigens are quantified by using colorimetric, chemi-luminescent, or fluorescent signals as an end-point (Figure 7.4). Resultant signal is directly proportional to the antigen present.

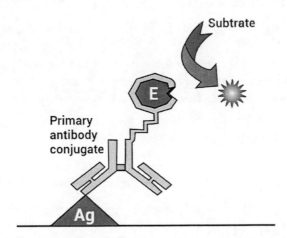

Fig. 7.4   Schematics of direct ELISA. Ag stands for antigen and E stands for enzyme.

Advantages of Direct ELISA

(a) Faster than other formats of ELISA due to fewer steps.
(b) Less prone to error.

Disadvantages of Direct ELISA

The main disadvantage of the direct ELISA is higher background noise, lack of signal amplification and reduced sensitivity.

Protocol for Direct ELISA

1. Immobilize the sample of known antigen on surfaces of the wells of a plate.
2. The microtiter plate is then coated with a blocking buffer to prevent the non-specific binding to the surface of the plate.
3. The enzyme–antibody conjugate is incubated and allowed to react with the bound antigen. The condition of incubation will vary depending upon the experimental design and would need to be optimized. Unbound enzyme–antibody conjugate is washed off, leaving only antigen bound enzyme–antibody conjugate.
4. The substrate solution is added to the wells and allowed to react with the attached enzyme which produces a colored product. The intensity of the color from this enzyme-substrate determines the amount of antigen present in the sample.

7.5.2   Indirect ELISA

Indirect ELISA involves a two-step binding process, in which a primary antibody is used to bind to the antigen and a secondary antibody is used for detection (Figure 7.5).

Advantages of Indirect ELISA

(a) Enhanced sensitivity, as more than one labeled secondary antibody is bound per primary antibody.
(b) Possibility of using different primary antibodies for a single labeled secondary antibody allows greater flexibility in optimization of experimental protocol.
(c) Cost effective, since fewer labeled secondary antibodies are required.

Disadvantage of Indirect ELISA

The main disadvantage of the indirect ELISA is the possibility of background noise due to cross reactivity of the secondary antibody. Secondly, it takes longer than direct ELISA.

Protocol for Indirect ELISA

1. Incubate antigens in the wells of microtiter plates; to be followed by washing off and blocking.
2. Primary antibody is added to wells, followed by incubation.
3. Unbound antibody is washed off after incubation.
4. Add enzyme linked secondary antibody, and wash off the unbound antibody.
5. An appropriate substrate solution is added to generate chromogenic or fluorescent signals.

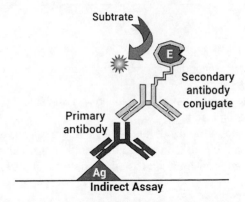

Fig. 7.5   Schematics of the indirect ELISA. Ag stands for antigen and E stands for enzyme.

7.5.3   Sandwich ELISA

Sandwich ELISAs require two antibodies: a capture antibody and a detection antibody. Both antibodies have specific and different epitopes for the antigen so that they will be able to recognize the antigen at different sites, without inhibiting each other. The capture antibody binds to the surface of the ELISA plate and binds the antigen. Then the detection antibody with an attached enzyme binds to the antigen which can be identified by using a suitable reagent (Figure 7.6).

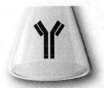 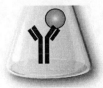 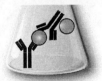

Fig. 7.6   Overview of direct sandwich ELISA. Capture antibody is in red while detection antibody is in blue, with antigen in the middle (sandwiched between the two antibodies). [See color plates]

Sandwich ELISA is mainly employed for analysis of complex samples.

Advantages of Sandwich ELISA

(a) High sensitivity and specificity.
(b) Flexibility, both direct and indirect detection can be used.
(c) Antigen does not need prior purification, as specific capture antibodies capture only the antigen, discarding other contaminants.

Disadvantage of Sandwich ELISA

Optimization for coating concentration of antibody, its capture and detection in the sandwich ELISA is difficult to achieve. It may also need considerable fine-tuning of the washing step and blocking solution.

Protocol for Sandwich ELISA

1. First; the well of an ELISA plate should be coated with a capture antibody.
2. The space between two antibodies should be blocked by blocking reagent (3 or 5% BSA, non-fat dry milk, or casein).
3. After washing (usually three times) with a suitable washing solution, add the antigen sample and incubate for an optimized time.
4. After washing the unbound analytes and other contamination, add enzyme conjugated secondary antibody to the plate and incubate for an optimized time.
5. After washing the unbound antibody, add an appropriate substrate to produce a chromogenic or fluorescent signal.

7.5.4   Competitive/Inhibition ELISA

Another form of ELISA is through competitive binding, and so, is called competitive ELISA (Figure 7.7). It is one of the most complex ELISA techniques; however, each of the above assays can be used in a competitive format.

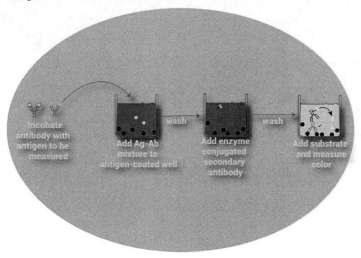

Fig. 7.7   Schematics of competitive ELISA. Ag: antigen; Ab: antibody.

Advantages of Competitive ELISA

(a) Major advantage is that this method can deal with crude or impure samples.
(b) High specificity: as two antibodies are used on the antigen/analyte complex for capture and detection.
(c) Antigen purification is not required for measurement; therefore rendering this method even more suitable for complex and impure samples.
(d) Flexibility and sensitive.

Questions to ponder over

1. What is an immunoassay?
2. What are the different types of ELISA? Which one is better?
3. How many antigens can each antibody bind to?

Protocol for Competitive ELISA

1. Incubate unlabeled antibody with a titrated amount of its antigen.
2. Add bound antibody/antigen complexes to an antigen-coated well.
3. Wash the wells of the plate to remove the unbound antibody (if more antigen is added to the sample in Step 1, less amount of antibody will be able to bind to the antigen in the well, hence "competition").
4. Incubate with the secondary antibody which is specific to the primary antibody. This second antibody is conjugated with an enzyme.
5. Add an appropriate substrate, which is capable of eliciting a chromogenic or fluorescent signal.

Typical Working Protocol for ELISA

- Antigen preparation: Antigen is diluted in 1 x PBS or bicarbonate buffer ranging in concentration from 1:10 to $1:10^8$. The 96 well plate (100 µl per well) is coated with the diluted antigen in triplicate. Buffer pH of 7.6–8.0 should be optimal for most proteins, although some procedures recommend pH of 9.0. A similar dilution should be made for the primary antibody.
- Coated plate is incubated 12–18 hrs at 2–8°C.
- Wash: The excess antigen is removed by washing (5x) with PBST (0.1% Tween 20 in 1x PBS).
- Blocking: Nonspecific bindings are reduced by coating the cells with 3% BSA in PBST. Milk casein or albumin, or a combination of both, are also used. 100 µl per well incubated at room temperature for 30–60 min.
- Wash: Similar to what has been mentioned above.
- Sample: The plates are further incubated 1–3 hrs after adding 100 µl of the sample solution with repeated gentle shaking.
- Wash: Similar to what has been mentioned above.
- Primary antibody: 100 µl of working dilution concentrations of the primary antibody to be incubated at room temperature for 30–60 min.
- Wash: Similar to what has been mentioned above.
- Secondary antibody: 100 µl of diluted concentration per well to be incubated at room temperature for 30–60 min.
- Wash: Similar to what has been mentioned above.
- Chromophore generation: Addition of HRP substrate (100 µl incubated for 30 min at room temperature with continual shaking) for indirect detection of bound protein.
- Wash as above.
- STOP: Add 100 µl stopping solution to each well.
- Measure absorbance at 490 nm within 30 min of adding STOP solution.

   * HRP substrate: 0.04% o-Phenylenediamine dihydrochloride and 0.012% H_2O_2 in phosphate citrate buffer, pH 5.0 (25.7 ml 0.2 M dibasic sodium phosphate, 24.3 ml 0.1 citric acid, and 50 ml deionized water)
   * STOP solution 2M H_2SO_4

7.6 Immunofluorescence

In 1944, Albert Coons established this technique by demonstrating fluorescence analysis on a labeled antibody. This technique uses the antibodies labeled with fluorescent dyes, which attach to the specific antigens (targets) within the cell. An image of the target molecule inside the cell will be captured when fluorescent molecules emit light after excitation with a suitable wavelength. Most commonly used fluorescence compounds are fluorescein (at 490 nm excitation onwards; it emits an intense yellow-green fluorescence at 517 nm), rhodamine (at 515 nm excitation onwards; it emits deep red signal at 546 nm) and cy5 (excitation at 640 nm onwards; it emits deep yellow fluorescence at 660 nm). However, other fluorescent substances like polyerythrin (fluorescent pigment from algae) are also used. Polyerythrin absorbs light ~ 30-fold higher than fluorescein and emits a brilliant red fluorescence.

There are two different ways of fluorescent immunostaining: direct and indirect (Figure 7.8 and Table 7.1), as given below.

Table 7.1 Advantages and disadvantages of direct and indirect immunofluorescence.

Types of Immunofluorescence	Technique	Advantages	Disadvantages
Direct	• Primary antibody is conjugated with fluorescent dye	• Saves time	• Expensive • Degrades faster
Indirect	• Unlabeled primary antibody • Detected with additional fluorochrome labeled reagent (secondary antibody)	• Primary antibody does not need to be conjugated with a fluorochrome • Less loss of primary during conjugation • More sensitive • Cost effective	• Takes more time • More washing steps required

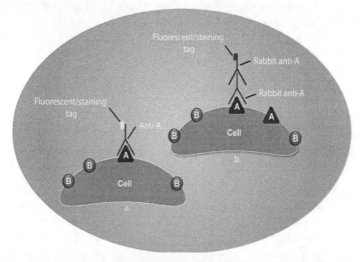

Fig. 7.8 Schematics of (a) direct and (b) indirect immunofluorescence.

Protocol for Immunostaining

Slide preparation

1. Coat coverslips with polyethyleneimine or poly-L-lysine for 1 hr at room temperature.
2. Rinse coverslips well with sterile H_2O (three times 1 hr each).
3. Allow coverslips to dry completely and sterilize them under UV light for at least 4 hr.
4. Grow cells on glass coverslips or prepare cytospin or smear preparation.
5. Rinse briefly in phosphate-buffered saline (PBS).

Fixation

1. Incubate the cells in 100% methanol (chilled at $-20°C$) at room temperature for 5 min.

or

2. Using 4% paraformaldehyde (PFA) in PBS pH 7.4 for 10–20 min at room temperature.

** The cells should be washed three times with ice-cold PBS.

Permeabilization

If the target protein is intracellular, it is very important to permeabilize the cells. Methanol fixed samples do not require permeabilization.

1. Incubate the samples for 10 min with PBS containing 0.1–0.25% Triton X-100 (or 100 µM digitonin or 0.5% saponin). Triton X-100 is the most popular detergent for improving penetration of the antibody. However, it is not appropriate for membrane-associated antigens since it destroys membranes.
2. The optimal percentage of Triton X-100 should be determined for each protein of interest.
3. Wash cells in PBS three times for 5 min.

Blocking and immunostaining

1. Incubate cells with 1% BSA, 22.52 mg/mL glycine in PBST (PBS + 0.1% Tween 20) for 30 min to block unspecific binding of the antibodies (alternative blocking solutions are 1% gelatin or 10% serum (goat serum or donkey serum).
2. Incubate cells in the diluted antibody in 1% BSA in PBST in a humidified chamber for 1 hr at room temperature or overnight at 4°C.
3. Decant the solution and wash the cells three times in PBS, 5 min each wash.
4. Incubate cells with the secondary antibody in 1% BSA for 1 hr at room temperature in the dark.
5. Decant the secondary antibody solution and wash three times with PBS for 5 min each in the dark.

* Incubation time should be optimized.
** For wash buffer 1x PBS 0.1% Tween 20.

Fluorescence microscopy is a powerful tool for examining the molecular architecture of tissues and cells to their overall macroscopic anatomy and physiology in plasticity, homeostasis, and disease. With the help of immunofluorescence techniques, it is possible to map the actual location of target antigens.

Question

1. A researcher wants to use immunofluorescence to stain proteins called actin and Trem 2. Trem 2 is located on the surface of the cells whereas actin is located inside the cells. Which reagents must he use to make sure that the proteins are stained? Describe your protocol?

7.7 Immunoblotting

Immunoblotting is a technique used for analysis of individual proteins in a mixture of proteins (e.g., as in cell lysate). Three blotting techniques are used routinely for immunoblotting: the DNA Southern blot, the RNA Northern blot, and the Western blot for protein. Towbin et al., in 1979 introduced the Western blotting technique which is now a standard technique for protein analysis. Western blotting employs the use of an antibody to specifically detect its antigen. Procedures for Southern and Northern blots are similar to that of Western blot.

In Western blot, the protein mixture is first, separated by using a gel electrophoresis (SDS-PAGE) to sort the proteins by size, charge, or other differences in individual protein bands. After separation of proteins in SDA-PAGE, the protein bands are transferred to a membrane made of nitrocellulose, nylon, or PVDF (polyvinylidene fluoride). The membrane is placed over the gel in a sandwich format, along with transfer pad (Figure 7.9). During transfer, the protein partially regains its 2D and 3D structure due to removal of SDS in the process. Transfer is achieved by application of voltage which causes the proteins to travel perpendicular to the direction of gel and get transferred onto the membrane. This transfer of protein bands to the membrane is what is known as blotting. The pattern of protein on the membrane is the same as in case of SDS-PAGE. When the membrane is exposed to a specific antibody, then it binds to the target protein, and this can be detected by following a protocol similar to the direct or indirect ELISA. The detection antibodies could be either fluorescent

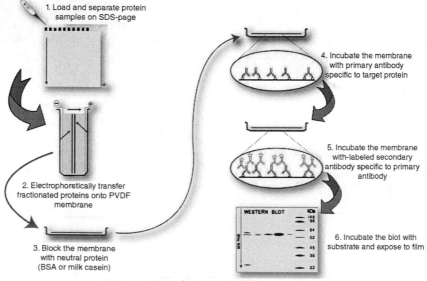

Western Blotting Procedure

Fig. 7.9 Schematics of the Western blot.

or radioactive or enzymes (horseradish peroxidase and alkaline phosphatase) labeled. The light produced by the detection antibody enables detection of target protein. Depending on the experimental criteria, different methods of gel electrophoresis for the separation of proteins can be used. Commonly used electrophoretic methods are: Sodium dodecyl sulphate polyacrylamide gel electrophoresis (SDS-PAGE), native-PAGE, and isoelectric focusing. Although the procedure is time consuming and optimization is required, there are several advantages including determination of the size of target protein, determining the expression pattern of a specific protein, multiple target detection, and examination of macromolecular interactions.

> **Questions to ponder over**
>
> 1. What do the band intensities indicate on a Coomassie blue stained SDS-PAGE gel?
> 2. Which step is a prerequisite for Western blotting?

7.8 Immunoprecipitation Reaction

One of the most widely used techniques for detection and identification of biomolecules is immunoprecipitation (IP). Immunoprecipitation (IP) is a technique used to separate proteins from the rest of a sample by binding to the target protein a specific antibody that is immobilized to a solid support. Additionally, it enables the separation and purification of an antibody from different serum samples.

7.8.1 How does IP work?

As name suggests, immunoprecipitation employs precipitation technique by forming an Ag-Ab complex. While immunoprecipitation is similar to affinity chromatography, it follows different protocols for incubation of sample, washing, and elution solutions. In affinity chromatography, the sample passes through a immobilized target-specific antibody column that is packed with porous resin (typically beaded agarose). Immunoprecipitation involves the use of antibodies incubated with the cell extract instead of using a packed column, enabling the antibody to bind to the targeted protein (Figures 7.10 and 7.11). The Ab-Ag complex is then extracted out of the sample using protein A/G- (genetically engineered protein with IgG binding domains for both protein A and G) coupled to agarose beads at the end of incubation step. The beads are then pelleted to the bottom of the tube by centrifugation (or a magnet) and the protein of interest is eluted from the bead by using a suitable elution buffer. Pelleting of antibody–antigen complex is done by using either magnetic beads or agarose beads (Table 7.2).

There are two general methods for immunoprecipitation, direct and indirect.

1. **Direct:** Super paramagnetic microbeads or microscopic agarose (non-magnetic) are used as a solid-phase substrate, where the antibodies that are specific for a particular protein (or group of proteins) are immobilized. These beads are then added to the protein mixture or cell extract. The targeted proteins are then captured by the immobilized antibodies on the beads and are thus immunoprecipitated.
2. **Indirect:** This is the free antibody approach. The target specific antibodies are free and not attached to the beads as in the direct method. The immune complexes (Ab-Ag complexes)

are first formed in the cell extract or cell lysate. The antibodies are free to float around the protein mixture and bind to their targets. With the passage of time, the beads coated with protein A/G are added to the mixture. The Ab-Ag complex that is through binding to the protein A/G gets precipitated.

Table 7.2 Differences between use of agarose and magnetic beads in immunoprecipitation.

Magnetic Beads	Agarose Resin
Solid and spherical (1–4 μm in diameter)	Sponge like structures (50–150 μm in diameter)
Avoids centrifugation. The magnetic beads are aligned on the side wall of the incubation tubes using magnets to enable easy aspiration of the cell lysate.	Centrifugation is required for separation of beads from sample.
Non-porous and antibody binding is limited to the surface of beads.	Porous center to increase the antibody binding capacity due to large surface to volume ratio.
The antibodies bound to the surface are less likely to be washed away in the washing step.	Due to its porosity, the immobilized target antibody may not always be accessible to the target protein and hence lost in washing.
All the beads are uniform in size and all interaction occurs on the outer smooth surface; pre-clearing is not necessary. Moreover, it provides higher reproducibility and purity.	Requires longer incubation time to enable diffusion of solutions and removal of non-specific binding.

Indirect methods are more frequently used when the target protein is low in concentration or when the affinity of the antibody for the protein is weak.

7.8.2   Types of Immunoprecipitation (IP)

1. **Individual protein IP:** This technique is based on the basic principle of immunoprecipitation which involves isolation of a particular protein from a complex matrix, such as biological fluids, crude lysate of a plant or animal tissue, and other samples of biological origin.

2. **Co-immunoprecipitation (Co-IP):** The Co-immunoprecipitation assay (Co-IP) is also based on the same methodology as immunoprecipitation involving capture and purification an antigen of interest. However, this technique is useful for identifying additional molecules bound to the target protein and determining the physiological relevance of protein–protein (or other factors) interaction. These interacting proteins or other molecules could be complex partners, structural proteins, co-factors, or signaling molecules. This technique involves specific antibodies to capture proteins that are bound to a specific target protein. Protein complexes are then analyzed using techniques for identifying new binding partners, binding affinities, kinetics of binding, receptors, and the mechanism of the target protein function.

3. **Chromatin immunoprecipitation (ChIP):** This is a technique to identify the location of DNA binding sites on the genome for a protein of interest. It gives detailed information on the DNA-protein interaction, transcription factors on promoters, defining cistromes, transcription co-factors, DNA repair proteins, and DNA replication factors that incur inside the nucleus

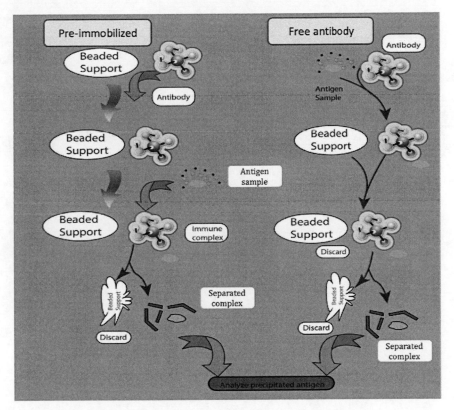

Fig. 7.10   Schematics of immunoprecipitation (IP).

of living cells or tissues. This variant of IP involves a process which determines whether the identified protein binds to, or is localized to a specific DNA. It is a powerful technique to probe protein–DNA interaction within the chromatin. There are two different ways in which this assay can be used: (i) to identify multiple proteins associated with a specific region of chromatin, and (ii) to identify different regions of the chromatin associated with a particular protein. Additionally, this assay can be used to determine the spatial and temporal relationship of a protein–DNA interaction. Alternatively, combination of ChIP assay with micro-array (ChIP on chip) enables the examination of the genome wide protein–DNA interactions and histone modifications.

Immunoprecipitation of the protein–DNA complex out of cell lysate can be done by using a specific antibody which binds to the DNA-binding protein. Generally, ChIP assay is done in four steps: (i) Cells are fixed with formaldehyde which is also a reversible protein–DNA cross-linking agent. Formaldehyde is used with DTBP (dimethyl 3,3' dithiobispropionimidate) for cross-linking. The cross-linkers permeate directly into the cells to form protein–DNA complexes together, allowing transient complexes to be trapped and stabilized for analysis. (ii) Lysed cells harvest the chromatin and extract the protein–DNA complexes from cells or tissues into the solution. The integral membrane proteins are solubilized by dissolving the cell membrane with a detergent based solvent. This helps in reducing the cell background and increasing the

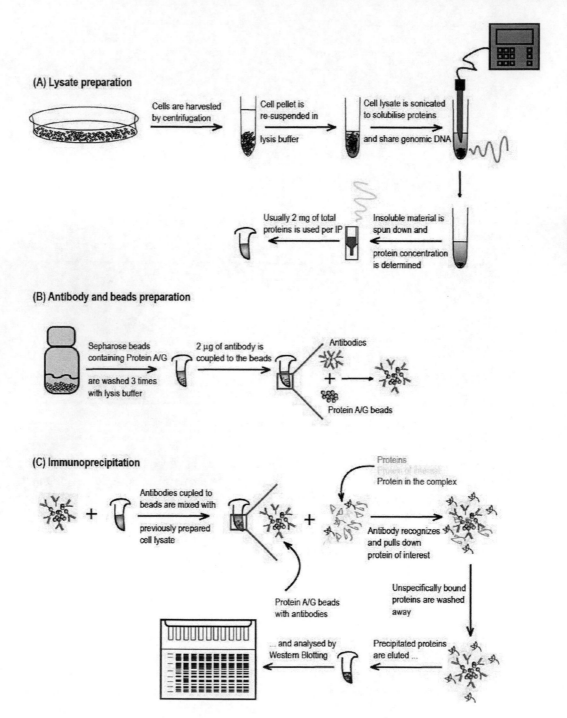

Fig. 7.11 Steps for immunoprecipitation: Cell lysate is prepared by cell lysis in the IP buffer of choice. The cell lysate is also soniciated to shear the DNA and solubilize the proteins.

sensitivity. The protein–DNA complex is not affected by detergents or salts. (iii) In order to examine the protein-binding complexes, the extracted genomic DNA is shredded into smaller pieces, using either enzymatic digestion (micrococcal nuclease (MNase)) or sonication. (iv) Immunoprecipitation of chromatin is achieved by using antibody specific to the target protein or histone modification. The immuno-selection process selects all the DNA sequences which are associated with the target protein or histone modification will co-precipitate. This will enrich the DNA further. Purification is achieved by using an antibody-binding resin such as immobilized protein A, protein G, or protein A/G. For biotinylated antibodies, immobilized streptavidin or avidin is used. (v) After IP, purified DNA can be enriched and detected by PCR-based techniques.

There are several limitations with ChIP, including, (1) maintaining temperature during the soniciation step, (2) only randomized DNA fragments from sonication, (3) variability in DNA digestion due to change in enzyme activity.

4. **RNP immunoprecipitation:** Ribonucleoprotein (RNP) is a complex of RNA and RNA binding protein that drives the regulation of post-translational gene expression. A detailed understanding of RNPs not only provides valuable information about a pathway, but RNPs are useful for identifying marker and potential therapeutic markers. This technique is very similar to chromatin immunoprecipitation (ChIP). Protein associated RNAs are immunoprecipitated using a protein specific antibody. The steps involve lysis of live cells followed by the immunoprecipitation of the target protein and associated RNA using an antibody targeting the protein of interest. RNA extraction can be done to separate the purified RNA-protein complexes. The RNA can then be identified by cDNA (complementary DNA) or RT-PCR. Some variants of RIP (RNA immunoprecipitation), such as PAR-CLIP (photoactivatable ribonucleoside-enhanced cross-linking and immunoprecipitation) include cross-linking steps, and make do with less careful lysis conditions.

IP follows two routes: either through pre-immobilized antibodies or free antibodies. Each step involves incubation, followed by the collection of bead (by centrifugation or magnetic) and final removal of the solution. Elution during the last step is typically done by heating the beads in the elution buffer containing urea, glycine solution, or low pH buffer. Elution processes in the mentioned conditions generally denature the proteins (including the antibody) and cause irreversible damage to the beads, which are then discarded. In the first condition (left), an antibody (monoclonal or polyclonal), specific for a target protein, is immobilized onto an insoluble support, such as agarose or magnetic beads. It is then incubated with a cell lysate containing the target protein. The immobilized Ab-Ag complexes are then collected from the lysate by centrifugation, eluted, and analyzed by SDS-PAGE and Western blot. In the second condition (right), free, unbound antibody is allowed to form Ab-Ag complexes in the lysate and the complexes are then retrieved by the beads. Pre-immobilized antibody approach is more commonly used for IP, whereas free antibody immune complexes can also be used when the target protein is present in low concentrations.

For antibody bead preparation, the beads are washed three times with lysis buffer to remove bead storage solution. Washed beads are mixed with antibodies. After coupling, the cells beads are mixed with the cell lysate. The solution is now ready for immunoprecipitation. After precipitation, the combination of beads, antibodies and protein of interest, is washed with lysis buffer to remove unspecific binding. Lastly, the precipitated proteins are eluted and analyzed by Western blotting.

Protocol for Immunoprecipitation

- Lyse the cells.
- Remove non-specific bindings by passing the sample over the beads alone or bound to an irrelevant antibody.
- Incubate solution with antibody against the protein of interest to allow the antigen–antibody complexes to form. Antibody can be attached to solid support before this step (direct method) or after this step (indirect method).
- Precipitate the complex of interest by removing it from bulk solution.
- Wash precipitated complex several times. Spin between washes when using agarose beads or place tube on magnet when using super-paramagnetic beads. After the final wash, remove as much supernatant as possible.
- Elute proteins from the solid support using low-pH or SDS sample loading buffer.
- Analyze complexes or antigens of interest. This can be done in a variety of ways: SDS page and Western blotting, or enzyme activity.

** Perform all IP steps using micro-centrifuge tubes on ice unless noted otherwise.

7.9 Immunodiffusion

Generally, antigens are detected by using antibodies, but sometimes their roles are reversed. In immunodiffusion techniques, detection and measurement of antibodies, antigens or both is done by their precipitation when diffused together through gel or another medium. Both the antibody and antigen interact with each other through diffusion and form a white precipitate, which is visible to the naked eye. The precipitate is formed in a zone called zone of equivalence. This zone of equivalence is used to determine the concentration or titer of both the antigen and antibody. The movement can be linear or radial. It is often used for quantitative and qualitative analysis of serum proteins. In most cases, this technique has been replaced by ELISA.

There are several techniques for immunodiffusion:

1. The antibody or the antigen remains fixed, and the other reactants move.
2. Both the antigen and the antibody are free to move towards each other.

Based on the approach, the immunodiffusion techniques can be:

7.9.1 Radial Immunodiffusion (RID)

Radial immunodiffusion has several other names, such as the Mancini method, Mancini immunodiffusion, or single radial immunodiffusion assay. In this technique, an appropriate ratio of antibody and antigen is used to form a cross-linked precipitate complex. It is an immunodiffusion technique used to determine the concentration of an antigen or antibody in a sample. The antibody or antigen is incorporated in molten agarose and allowed to solidify forming a uniform layer. Once solidified, circular holes are punched into the agarose and a known concentration of antigen (or antibody when antigen is incorporated in molten agarose) is poured into the wells. The sample containing the antibody or antigen (as desired) is also loaded. The antigens diffuse through the agar in all directions and react with the antibody to form a visible precipitate in form of a ring called precipitin ring. The diffusion occurs until the formation of a stable ring due to the antigen–antibody precipitation (Figure 7.12). Ring shaped bands of precipitates form around the well indicating reaction and lines of precipitation form where maximum Ab-Ag complexes are deposited. The amount of antigen in the solution can be determined by the endpoint of the precipitation ring. By comparing the standards (plot of standard curve of diameter against the antibody or antigen) to the unknown, the amount of antibody (or antigens) can be determined.

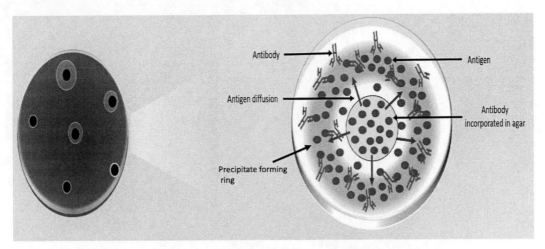

Fig. 7.12   Schematics of radial immunodiffusion.

7.9.2   Ouchterlony Double Immunodiffusion (ODI)

In RID either one of antigen or antibody diffuse through the agarose medium, whereas in ODI diffusion of both the antigen and antibody takes place through the agarose (Table 7.3). It is a passive double immunodiffusion and helpful in the measurement and quantification of antibodies and antigens. Molten agar is allowed to solidify in a petri dish without antibody or antigen. A few small wells are punched a few mm apart. Antigen and corresponding antibody solutions are dropped in the wells. The petri dish is incubated in a moist chamber for 18–24 hrs. The antigen–antibody complex moves through the agar to form the precipitated complex. When the edges of circular diffusion meet at the zone of equivalence it forms a linear pattern of precipitation. For double diffusion, the wells can be placed at different angles for comparative purposes. It is widely used for the detection, identification, and quantification of antibodies/antigens and fungal antigens.

For the ODI double diffusion, three possible patterns can occur (Figure 7.13).

Reaction to full identity (a continuous line or an arc): If the precipitin lines are due to identical antigenic determinants of antigens, the precipitin line of antigen well and antibody well stop at their point of intersection forming an arc.

Reaction to non–identity (the two lines cross completely): If the precipitin lines at the precipitation zone cross, due to non-identical antigenic determinants of antigens, then it may be inferred as unrelated antigens which share no common epitopes.

Reaction of partial identity (a continuous line with a spur at one end): If the precipitation zone of one well stops at the intersection point of two separate precipitin lines, whereas the other line continues past it, it may be inferred that both the antigenic determinants (epitopes) have some similarity but not all.

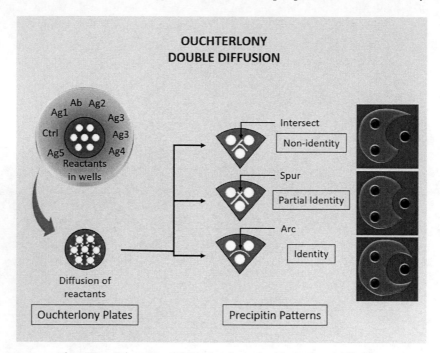

Fig. 7.13   Schematics of Ouchterlony double immunodiffusion.

Table 7.3   Comparison of radial and Ouchterlony double diffusion techniques.

	Radial	**Ouchterlony Double**
Limitations	• Long reaction time • Either antigen or antibody diffuse • Replaced by other assays	• Long reaction time • Distance between the wells
Advantages	• Specific and sensitive result • Properties of two different antigens can be compared • The purity of antigen can be determined • Used for disease diagnosis • No major equipment is needed	• High sensitivity • Early diagnosis of disease • Both antigen and antibody diffuse simultaneously. • No major equipment needed

7.10   Radioimmunoassay (RIA)

All the immunoassay techniques use extremely specific antibodies to target molecules of interest and determine their concentration in samples. The first immunoassay was developed by Yalow and Berson in 1959. By using radio labeled insulin they were able to assess the concentration of insulin in human plasma. The first immunoassay developed was radioimmunoassay (RIA) (Figure 7.14).

This technique is used for the quantification of minute amounts of ligands in samples of biological fluids. The method offers a technique to assay materials that are otherwise difficult to detect. The competition between labeled and unlabeled antigen for specific antibody sites, forming antigen–antibody complexes, is the basis of this technique. The reaction is described by the expression:

$$\text{Antigen} + \text{Specific antibody} \leftrightarrow \text{Antigen} - \text{Antibody complex}$$

$$\text{Radioactive antigen} + \text{Specific antibody} \leftrightarrow \text{Radioactive antigen} - \text{Antibody complex}$$

A known quantity of antigen is made radioactive. The radioisotope that is usually tagged is iodine-125 or iodine-131. At equilibrium, the radioactive complex (bound-B) is separated from radioactive antigen (free -F). Comparison of the B/F ratio of unknown to the B/F ratios obtained by incubating varying amounts of known nonradioactive antigen with the same amount of antibody as in the unknown sample, under similar assay conditions, will determine the antigen concentration in the unknown sample. The radio labeled antigen competes with the sample antigen and displaces it from the antibody. The more antigen present in the sample, the less radio labeled antigen binds to the antibody. The separation of bound antigens from the unbound ones is achieved by using a secondary antibody, which binds to the primary antibody, causing the separation of primary antibody from the solution, and the radioactivity of the unbound fraction is measured. With new emerging techniques like immunofluorescence, RIA is being used less because of the cost of reagents and instrument, short half-life of radio-labeled compound, safety and disposal requirements of radioactive material. However, it is most useful when applied to cases where the antigens and antibodies in the serum are present in minute quantities.

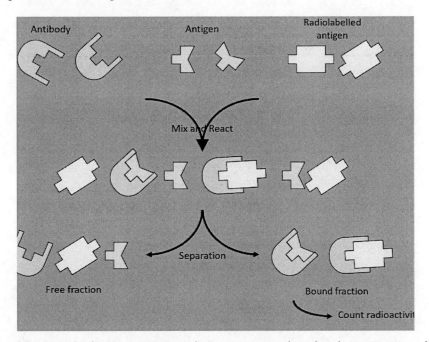

Fig. 7.14 Schematics of radioimmunoassay. Radioimmunoassay is based on the competition of unlabeled with labeled antigen for antibody binding.

7.11   Immunoelectrophoresis

It is a variation of the Ouchterlony double diffusion and a gel-based technique, which is based on precipitation in agar under an electric field. Immunoelectrophoresis involves two distinct and separate operations: immune-diffusion and electrophoresis. When an electric current is passed through the gel, the antigen mixture is separated into individual antigen components. Following separation by electrophoresis, the antigens will react with specific antibody placed in troughs parallel to the electrophoretic migration and antibody diffusion then occurs resulting in a formation of precipitin lines; each line indicating a reaction between individual proteins with their antibody. Precipitates are deposited as arcs between the antibody trough and the antigen track. The buffers used in the gel have an influence on electrophoretic mobility and on the position of the immunoprecipitate. The pH of the buffer must be chosen with the isoelectric point of the antigen in mind; it is desirable usually to work at a pH slightly above the isoelectric point so that the proteins have a negative charge and do not react with the agar. Two basic methods are available: the original macro technique and the micro technique on microscope slides. The macro technique is time-consuming. The separating power of micro-immunoelectrophoresis is enhanced by carrying out the electrophoresis below light petroleum ether. In immunoelectrophoresis of different samples, it is possible to evaluate the amount of an antigen semi-quantitatively by measurement of the distances of a certain precipitation arc from the antibody trough. This technique is widely used in diagnosis of various diseases by detecting abnormal proteins, evaluation of the therapeutic response in disease states affecting the immune system, and in identification of a single antigen in a mixture of antigens.

Protocol for Immunoelectrophoresis

- Prepare agrose gel on a glass slide.
- Place the gel in an electrophoresis chamber with the samples on the cathodic side, and run for 20 minutes at 100 volts.
- After completion of electrophoresis, add antisera or antibody in the troughs in a moist chamber and incubate for 18–20 hours at room temperature.
- Dry the agarose gel with blotter sheets.
- Soak the gel in saline solution for 10 minutes and repeat the drying and washing step for three times.
- Dry the gel at a temperature less than 70°C and stain.
- After decolorizing the stain dry the gel and evaluate the result.

There are three more variants of immunoelectrophoresis, as under:

a. **Crossed immunoelectrophoresis:** Also known as two-dimensional electrophoresis, this is particularly useful for the quantification of mixtures of proteins and the analysis of the composition of protein mixtures. It is also useful in examining the association/dissociation phenomena, hereditary polymorphism, micro-heterogenicity, and fragmentation.

In brief, this is done in two steps. In Step 1, the antigens are separated by electrophoresis in an agarose gel. In Step 2, the separated antigens are applied into a freshly prepared layer of agarose containing predetermined amount of antibody (Figure 7.15).

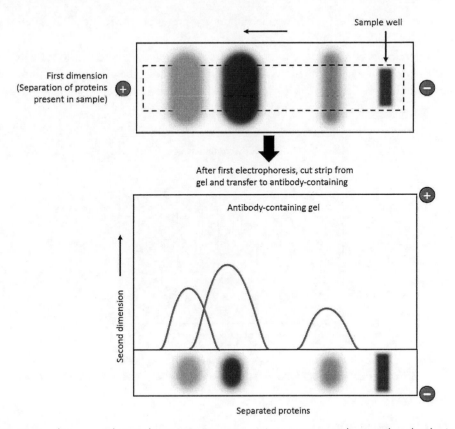

Fig. 7.15 Crossed immunoelectrophoresis: In Step 1, proteins are separated on a gel under the influence of an applied field. In Step 2, liquid agarose is allowed to fuse with the gel and after solidification an electric field is applied. Precipitation occurs when the protein and antibodies interact.

b. **Rocket immunoelectrophoresis:** This is a modified technique of radial immunodiffusion. A rocket shaped pattern is generated upon migration of the antigen towards the anode, hence the name rocket immunoelectrophoresis (Figure 7.16). In this method, the antibody in the gel is incorporated at a specific pH in which the antibody remains essentially immobile. As antigen is electrophoresed through the gel, it combines with the immobile antibody in the gel to form an immune complex. Initially, there is more antigen than antibody and no visible precipitation occurs. However, further migration of the antigen through the agarose gel allows more antigen–antibody interaction which results in a precipitin line that is conical in shape resembling a rocket. A graph is plotted between the rocket height (on Y-axis) and concentration of antigen (on X- axis) and concentration of the unknown is determined. This method is primarily used in the quantification of an antigen in the serum. Additionally, it is being used in the determination of protease activity, enzyme activity and concentration of a specific protein in the mixture of protein.

c. **Immunofixation electrophoresis (IEF):** When the proteins in body fluids are separated by electrophoresis, they form a very distinct pattern, reflecting the mix of proteins present. The pattern consists of five fractions: albumin, alpha 1, alpha 2, beta, and gamma. Immunofixation electrophoresis is used to detect the abnormal bands seen in the body fluids in order to determine which antibody is present and how much albumin is present in the fluids. This is done by either conventional zone electrophoresis or isoelectric focusing.

The antibodies are applied to the surface of a gel after electrophoresis, and at the equivalence point they form large precipitates with their counterparts in the gel. Upon washing, only the bound immunoprecipitate remains in the gel and can be identified by staining or any other techniques.

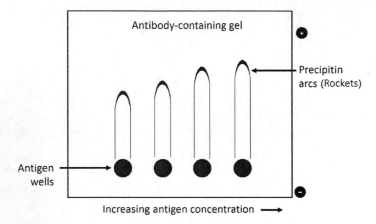

Fig. 7.16 Rocket electrophoresis: Antigen is electrophoresed through the gel containing antibodies. The distance of the arc of the resultant rocket pattern from the well is related to the concentration of the antigen.

7.12   Immunosensors

The immune system recognizes and identifies foreign molecules (antigens) and cells (healthy or infected) as part of the body defense system. For this they use antibodies, which can be used to develop sensors.

Designing an immunosensor requires the following: (a) quick identification of antigens, (b) reproducibility with acceptable accuracy, (c) stable immunocomplex (robust identification), and (d) ability to detect antigens in complex matrices. In principle, immunoassays can be in competitive, noncompetitive, direct, indirect, or sandwich ELISA format and all these formats can be applicable in the development of immunosensor. Immunosensors have following constituents (Figure 7.17):

  (a) An Analyte: A component to be detected.
  (b) A Bioreceptor: A bioreceptor is the molecule which will recognize the antigen molecule. They can be enzymes, cells, or antibodies. In the process of bio-recognition, interaction of bioreceptor and analyte generate signals in the form of heat, charge, change in mass, pH, and so on.
  (c) A Transducer: It is the part of biosensor which collects the bio-recognition signal and converts it into a measurable signal. The generated signal can be displayed in the form of graphs, numbers, or images. Several types of transducers are available, such as electrochemical (measure electrical signal generated by chemical reaction between bioreceptor and analyte), optical (employ chemiluminescence, light absorbance, fluorescence, phosphorescence, light polarization or rotation, and total internal reflection), piezoelectric (using mass sensitivity of piezoelectric quartz crystals), and thermometric (using either release or absorption of heat).

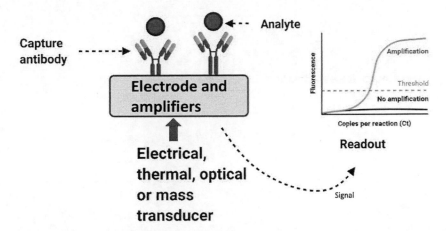

Fig. 7.17   Schematics of an immunosensor.

7.12.1   Surface Plasmon Resonance (SPR)

One of the most popular applications of immunosensor technology is surface plasmon resonance technology. This technology is very useful for estimating binding kinetics, biomolecular interactions, and to determine nucleic acid hybridization. A SPR immunosensor consists of these parts: a light source, a prism, a transduction surface (usually gold film), a biomolecule (antibody or antigen), a flow system and a detector. SPR detects excites and collective oscillation of surface electrons (that is why it is called surface plasmon). At a fixed angle these plasmons resonate with light resulting in absorption of light. In a SPR immunosensor, within thin inert metal (typically gold) filament, antibodies are immobilized and the targeted ligand is introduced through a flow cell. Polarized light through a prism is beamed on this metal film. The metal film reflects this light but with a shift in SPR angle when ligands bind to the immobilized antibodies. The extent of this shift depends on the concentration of the target. Signal outputs are in terms of a resonance angle or a refractive index value (Figure 7.18).

7.13   Immunotherapy

Many proteins are known to be highly modulated (up regulated or down regulated) in terms of expression or biological function. In the pathological states, these proteins could be used as biomarkers for diagnosis or treatment. They are generally identified by using immunohistochemistry and are considered as potential candidates for therapies utilizing monoclonal antibodies. These antibodies can be engineered for their specificity to their potential therapeutic biomarkers. Once bound to the target, they can activate, repress, or modulate endogenous immune responses to specific cells or molecules. Due to their binding specificity and affinity, antibody-based drugs are widely considered as a possible treatment option for various diseases including cancer, inflammatory and autoimmune disease, and many other such. There are three notable aspects to the power of immunotherapy.

(a) The immune system is precise. If properly engineered for the specific biomarkers, then it can exclusively target the diseased cell/tissue while sparing healthy cells.

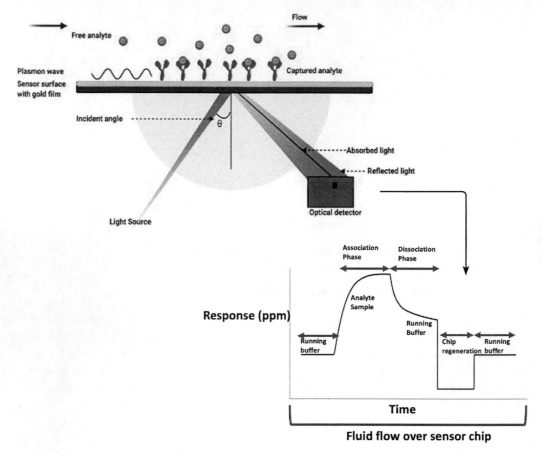

Fig. 7.18 Schematics of SPR and description of the plot obtained in an SPR experiment.

(b) The immune system is adaptive. It can re-evaluate the changes in diseased state and modify its attack accordingly.

(c) The immune system memory allows it to remember previous targets and thereby eliminate the reoccurrence of disease.

The first use of immunotherapy was demonstrated by William Coley, MD, a New York surgeon, when he found that picking up an infection after surgery helps some cancer patients. Since then scientists and doctors have learned a great deal about immune systems and its therapeutic potential. Immunotherapy primarily works in three different ways.

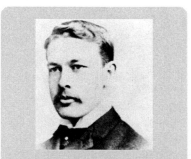

Dr. William Colley, considered as a "Father of Immunotherapy". He used immunotherapy to save a patient with an inoperable cancer.
Image credit: Cancer Research Institute, NY, USA.

1. Boosting the immune system of the body.
2. Helps to train the immune system to attack diseased cells specifically.
3. Provides immune system components, such as engineered immune system proteins.

Several types of molecules have been identified for immunotherapy, including monoclonal antibodies, vaccines, engineered antibodies, and non-specific immunotherapy. As mentioned, the basic molecules of immune-base therapy are antibodies. Most antibodies which are produced by a number of distinct B lymphocytes, as part of normal immune response, are polyclonal and they have different specificity towards their antigens. However, it is possible to produce large amounts of an antibody from a single B-cell (monoclonal antibody, mAbs). More than 100 monoclonal antibodies (mAbs) have been in use as drugs. They are mainly used in the treatment of immunological diseases, reversal of drug effects, and cancer therapy. The nomenclature of these therapeutic antibodies is governed by the rules from the International Nonproprietary Name (INN) expert group of the World Health Organization (WHO). The name of the therapeutic mAb includes certain distinct features such as proposed target, original host, modifications, and conjugation to the other molecules.

Rule 1: The prefix is referred to as "random" and intended to give a unique name for the drug.

Rule 2: The substems or infixes designate the target. For example: "ci" for cardiovascular, "so" for bone, and "tu" for tumor.

Rule 3: The source in which the antibody was originally produced is another infix. For example: "u" for human, and "o" for mouse. Also, "xi" for chimeric and "zu" for humanized. This subsystem was introduced in 2017 and all the names after 2017 apply this change.

Rule 4: The suffix for all mAbs in "mab."

mAbs are homogeneous preparations from a single clone, in which every antibody is expected to recognize the same antigen with identical affinity and specificity. There are several approaches for creating antibodies that react to a desired target: (a) Immunize an animal – this was the most popular method in the early days. Risk of an allergic reaction and/or reduced bioavailability limits their clinical use. Thus mice have been engineered with human immunoglobulin loci (transgenic mice) in place of the endogenous mouse sequences, thus regenerating human antibodies in mice. (b) Obtain an existing antibody and multiply the same – this is generally isolated from the patient and mainly use in cancer therapeutics. (c) Screen a library – a library of antibodies can be screened in vitro for binding to a target antigen.

Once a desired mAb is selected, it must be produced in a large quantity for therapeutic use. This is done by creating a hybridoma in which the antibody producing cell is fused with an immortalized partner cell (usually a malignant B cell) (Figure 7.19). The fused and unfused cells are transferred to a medium which allows

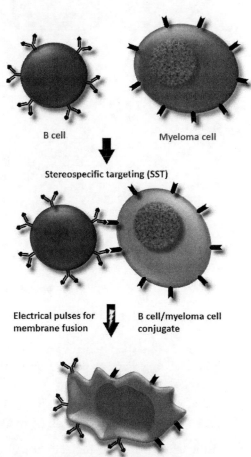

Fig. 7.19 Fusion of B-cell to myeloma cell to create hybridoma.

only hybridoma cells to grow. The most widely used selection system involves adding antibiotic aminopterin (a synthetic derivative of pterin) to the growth medium. Aminopterin is a competitive inhibitor of enzyme dihydrofolate reductase which is involved in catalyzing the reduction of dihydrofolate into tetrahydrofolate. Tetrahydrofolate is required by normal cells for de novo synthesis of DNA. For screening, the fused myeloma cell line is engineered to be deficient in the enzyme hypoxanthine-guanine phosphoribosyltransferase (HGPRT) which permits a cell to use xanthine and guanine as nucleotide precursors rather than synthesizing them de novo. After fusion of lymphocytes with HGPRT negative myeloma cells, the aminopterin-containing medium is supplemented with hypoxanthine and thymine (HAT medium: Hypoxanthine, Aminopterin, Thymidine). This kills myeloma cells but allows hybridomas to survive, as they have inherited HGPRT from the lymphocyte parent. Final screening of optimized hybridomas for better antibody production can be done using an immunoassay on the cell supernatant for binding to the target antigen (Figure 7.20).

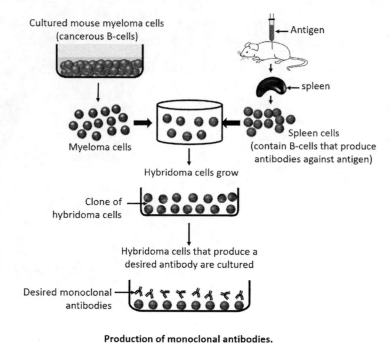

Production of monoclonal antibodies.

Fig. 7.20   Steps to produce monoclonal antibodies. [See color plates]

There are some alternative assays available for immortalization such as transfection with an immortalizing virus or production in an immortal cell culture such as Chinese hamster ovary (CHO) cells or phage display.

7.13.1   General Principles of mAb Activity

Although all mAbs are similar in structural details, they may have unique mechanisms of action. The key distinguishing attribute is their affinity for the target antigen, but it could be either monovalent or bivalent. Generally, their affinity is in the range of 10^5 to 10^{11} L/mol. Their affinity is determined by the variable region or complementarity-determining region (CDR). Another factor of mAbs which distinguishes them from other antibodies is their ability to recruit other immune cells and molecules. Fc portion of the antibody mediates this recruitment. For therapeutic purpose, most of the approved antibodies are chimeric or humanized. Chimeras are created by fusing murine/mouse variable domains. These chimeric antibodies are 70–90% human and possess a fully human Fc portion. Having a human Fc portion in chimeric antibodies serves two purposes: (i) the engineered antibody is less immunogenic to humans, and (ii) it allows them to interact with human cells and complement cascades. In a humanized mAbs, on the other hand, only the CDRs are of murine origin.

7.13.2   Targets of Therapeutic Antibodies

Based on their affinity and purpose there are several targets for therapeutic mAbs (Figure 7.21).

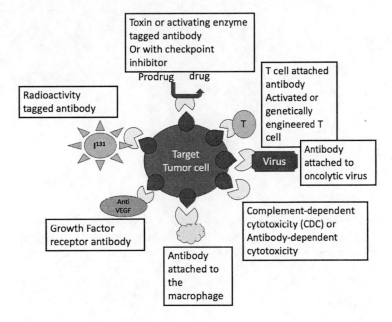

Fig. 7.21   Different mechanism of mAbs action for attacking a tumor cell.

Cell surface antigen: By targeting the cell surface antigen, mAbs either block the functioning of the cell or kill the target cells. Blocking of cellular function is achieved by binding to the receptor, thus interfering with the receptor function and in turn affecting the cell proliferation and survival. Whereas, to kill cells mAbs may involve in the recruitment of complement proteins, phagocytes, or natural killer cells, which can then initiate immune-mediated destruction of the cells.

Recruitment of immune modulators is achieved through interaction with the Fc portion of the mAb. This can modulate the cell, killing either by antibody-dependent cellular cytotoxicity (ADCC) or antibody-mediated phagocytosis by monocytes/macrophages. Fc regions can also kill cells through complement-dependent cytotoxicity (CDC) by activation of the complement cascade. Some antibodies can do both (ADCC and CDC). Both antagonistic and agonistic effects of CDC and ADCC are possible but it may be unclear which will dominate in the elimination of the tumor cells.

Plasma protein or drugs: In this, a mAb is directed against a soluble molecule such as a plasma protein such as TNF (tumor necrosis factor) and VEGF (vascular endothelial growth factor) or a medication (such as dibigatran and digoxin) to sequester them from their normal binding partners. A chimeric fusion of single chain variable fragment (scFv) and an enzyme, convert a nontoxic prodrug to becoming a toxic drug in the vicinity of the targeted cells.

An infectious organism: Potential use of this includes prevention and targeting specific infections. Most mAbs target proteins on the surface of a virus, thus neutralizing the virus from entering the cells. Antibodies against bacteria can act both prophylactically and therapeutically. However, mAbs directed against pathogens are unlikely to be used routinely due to their high cost and requirements for administration. However, they can be used for certain emerging infections such as Ebola or Zika virus.

The Nobel Prize in Physiology or Medicine 1984

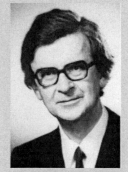
Niels K. Jerne

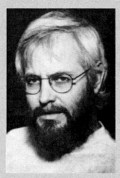
Georges J. F. Köhler

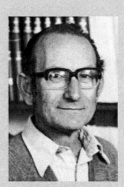
César Milstein

The Nobel Prize in Physiology or Medicine 1984 was awarded jointly to Niels K. Jerne, Georges J.F. Köhler, and César Milstein "for theories concerning the specificity in development and control of the immune system and the discovery of the principle for production of monoclonal antibodies."

7.13.3 Modifications

Selectivity of tumor cells over healthy cells is of utmost importance for treatment of diseases such as cancer. Antibodies directed against the antigens, is the most common method of targeting. With the development of monoclonal antibodies, and advancement of protein and molecular biology technologies, we can now engineer mAbs, which includes optimizing the Fab portion, prepare a chimeric or humanized mAbs (Figure 7.22). With technological advancement, it is now possible to produce various antibody fragments that retain binding characteristics similar to the full-length molecule and use these modified molecules for certain specific applications.

Antibody fragments: Due to their small size, antibody fragments can be used to enhance pharmacokinetic properties and/or increase the efficiency of penetration into cells or tumor masses instead of full length antibodies. However, using antibody fragments will decrease the half-life of the molecule. Fragments usually have a single binding site for the antigen, rather than multiple binding sites that are typical characteristics of full-length antibodies. The types of different fragments of antibody which are used for various therapeutic purposes, are given below:

- **Fragment antigen binding (Fab):** Fab fragments consist of an antigen binding site but are monovalent and without any Fc portion.
- **Bispecific (Fab')$_2$:** (Fab')$_2$ fragments have two antigen-binding sites, linked by a di-sulfide bond. This fragment retains the portion of hinge region. It does not have an Fc domain. When (Fab')$_2$ is reduced, it produces two monovalent Fab' fragments, which have a sulfhydryl group that is useful for conjugation to the other molecule.
- **Single-chain variable fragment (scFv):** scFv is not a fragment of an antibody, it is a fusion protein. It consists of a light chain and heavy chain variable region joined by a linker peptide (~ 25 amino acids).
- **Single-domain antibody (sdAb):** An sdAb is an antibody fragment consisting of a light chain variable region or a heavy chain variable region
- **Fragment crystallization region (Fc):** This is the tail region of an antibody which interacts with the cell surface receptors called Fc receptors and some proteins of the complement system.
- **Heavy chain only antibody (HcAb):** Also known as $V_H H$ antibody. They are naturally produced by camelids and sharks.
- **Bispecific antibody (BsAbs):** These are the antibodies containing two different antigen-binding sites in one molecule.
- **Tandem scFv:** It is a bispecific antibody fragment. Two or more moieties of scFv string together to form tandem scFv.
- **Diabody:** This is either a noncovalent dimer of scFv fragments or covalently linked two scFv fragments.
- **Minibody:** Minibodies are scFv-CH$_3$ fusion proteins.
- **Variable fragment (Fv):** This fragment has the antigen-binding site made of the V_H and V_L regions held together by non-covalent interactions, but they lack the constant region.

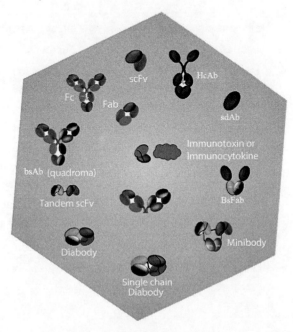

Fig. 7.22 Antibody fragments with therapeutic potential. [See color plates]

- **Immunotoxin or immunocytokine:** These are engineered protein molecules in which the toxin or cytokine molecules are attached to the antibody. Protein is taken inside the cell through endocytosis, after cell surface binding, and the attached toxin or cytokine molecule kills the targeted cell.

Other potential modifications: With the help of protein engineering, it is now possible to optimize the antibody function with a modified Fc region. Such s Fc region elicits immune reaction by binding to the receptors. There are two ways to increase the therapeutic effectiveness of antibodies: either by increasing the mAbs binding to the activating receptors (FcγRI, FcγRIIa and FcγRIIIa) or by decreasing their interaction with inhibitory receptors (FcγRIIb).

To allow the antibody to access the inner compartments of the cells, its design requires special alterations, using the in-frame incorporation of some intracellular peptidic trafficking signals. Such types of antibodies are called intrabodies. Intrabodies can be developed against various target antigens present at different location of the cells, such as cytosol, nucleus, endoplasmic reticulum, mitochondria, peroxisomes, and the plasma membrane. Because of their specificity to the target inside the cell, they have the potential to interfere with biosynthetic pathways, and this characteristic is widely used for developing therapeutic solutions in cancer, viral diseases, and neurological disorders. Recent developments involve the delivery of intrabody genes using recombinant adenovirus and vaccinia virus vectors or immunoliposomes.

Table 7.4   List of therapeutic antibodies approved by the US FDA.

USFDA Approved Therapeutic Antibodies	Disease	Target
Abciximab (Reopro)	Blockage in blood vessels	Prevents platelets to stick to each other
Adalimumab (Humira)	Rheumatoid arthritis	Inhibits structural damage
Alefacept (Amevive)	Psoriasis	Suppresses immune system
Alemtuzumab (Campath)	Lukemia	Attaches to protein CD52, activating immune system to kill lymphocytes
Basiliximab (Simulect)	Transplants	Prevents organ rejection
Certolizumab, Golimumab, infliximab	Crohn's disease, rheumatoid arthritis	Binds to TNFα
Omalizumab	Asthama	Prevents allergic reactions and inflammations
Tocilizumab	Rheumatoid arthritis	Block the effect of IL-6
Brentuximab vedotin	Hodgkin lymphoma	CD30 antigen binding
Emicizumab (BsAb-2017)	Heamophilia A	Coagulation factor IX xFX

Questions to ponder over

1. Where are the antigen binding sites of an immunoglobulin located?
2. What are the different types of bonds between the heavy chain and the light chain fragment in the Fab?
3. What is the location of majority disulphide bonds in, and what do they bind?
4. Why self-reactive antibodies are not found in significant concentration in normal serum?
5. What is chromatin immunoprecipitation?
6. Which is the best method to quantify serum insulin, radioimmunoassay (RIA) or ELISA?
7. What are the different types of biological analysis where ELISA can be used?
8. What are the advantages and disadvantages of immunotherapy? Can you think of an example where it can be used?

Questions

1. How does immunotherapy work?
2. Specifically, what part of the immune system does immunotherapy primarily use?

References

Chames, P., Van Regenmortel, M., Weiss, E. and Baty, D. (2009). Therapeutic antibodies: successes, limitations and hopes for the future. *British Journal of Pharmacology*, 157(2), 220–233.

Goldsmith, S. J. (1975). Radioimmunoassay: Review of basic principles. *Seminars in Nuclear Medicine*, 5(2), 125–152.

Koivunen, M. E. and Krogsrud, R. L. (2006). Principles of immunochemical techniques used in clinical laboratories. *Laboratory Medicine*, 37(8), 490–497.

Lim, S. A., and Ahmed, M. U. (2019). Introduction to Immunosensors. In *Immunosensors*. Royal Society of Chemistry. pp. 1–20.

Milstein, C. U. and Cuello, A. C. (1983). Hybrid hybridomas and their use in immunohistochemistry. *Nature*, 305(5934), 537–540.

Neuberger, M. S., Williams, G. T., Mitchell, E. B., Jouhal, S. S., Flanagan, J. G. and Rabbitts, T. H. (1985). A hapten-specific chimaeric IgE antibody with human physiological effector function. *Nature*, 314(6008), 268–270.

Nisonoff, A., Wissler, F. C. and Lipman, L. N. (1960). Properties of the major component of a peptic digest of rabbit antibody. *Science*, 132(3441), 1770–1771.

van Weemen, B. and Schuurs, A. H. W. M. (1971). Immunoassay using antigen–enzyme conjugates. *FEBS Letters*, 15(3), 232–236.

Appendices

Appendix 1   Troubleshooting: Cell Culture

Appendix 1.1   *Problems and Solutions*

Problem	Reason	Solution
No/insufficient viable cells after thawing stock	Cells stored incorrectly	Store in liquid nitrogen until thawing
	Frozen stock is not viable	Freeze cells at recommended density
		Use low passage cells for freezing stocks
		Follow protocol exactly recommended by the supplier
		Obtain new stock
	Cells thawed incorrectly	Follow protocol exactly as recommended by the supplier
		Make sure to dilute the frozen cells quickly by adding media to increase cell viability
	Thawing media is not correct	Prewarm media
		Follow protocol
	Cells are too dilute	Plate cells recommended by the supplier
	Cells not handled gently	Freezing and thawing procedures are stressful to most cells. Do not vortex, bang the flasks to dislodge the cells, or centrifuge the cells at high speeds.
	Glycerol used in the freezing medium was stored in light (if applicable)	If stored in light, glycerol gets converted to acrolein, which is toxic to cells. Obtain new stock

Contd.

Appendix 1.1 *contd.*

Problem	Reason	Solution
Slow cell growth	Growth medium is not correct	Use prewarmed growth medium as recommended by the supplier
	Serum in the growth medium is of poor quality	Use serum from a different lot
	Cells have been passaged too many times	Use healthy, low passage-number cells
	Cells were allowed to grow beyond confluency	Passage mammalian cells when they are in the log phase before they reach confluence
	Culture is contaminated with mycoplasma	Discard cells, media, and reagents. Obtain new stock of cells and use them with fresh media and reagents.

The matter given below lists some potential problems and offers possible solutions that may help you troubleshoot your cell culture experiments. Note that the list given below includes only the most commonly encountered problems in cell culture and provides guidelines to solutions only.

Appendix 1.2   Equipment for Cell Culture

- *Laboratory refrigerator/freezer combination.* Separation of refrigerator from the freezer unit for tissue culture media and ingredients is recommended to minimize contamination.
- *Two-stage vacuum trap for aspiration.* Construct an aspirator for the culture hood using two Buchner or Erlenmeyer flasks, two 1-hole or 2-hole rubber stoppers, glass Pasteur pipettes or glass tubes, and Tygon® tubing. Use a 1000 ml or larger flask for the first stage trap. Connect the second stage to a vacuum supply or pump through a vacuum filter to protect the pump from residual water vapor.
- *Stainless steel pipette sterilization boxes.* Obtain at least two sterilization boxes and keep one autoclaved box of pipettes in the culture hood at all times (suggested model: Fisher scientific 03-475-5 rectangular box for 9 inch Pasteur pipettes).
- *Set of pipettes for flow hood.* Keep a separate set of autoclavable 2–20 µl, 20–200 µl, and 100–1000 µl pipettes to be used only for cell culture. Autoclave the pipettes according to the manufacturer's instructions. Autoclave repeatedly every one to two months or in case of contamination.
- *Tissue culture microscope.* An inverted, phase contrast microscope with 10x, 20x, and 40x phase-contrast objectives and a long working distance condenser should be used for observing the extent of cell extraction, for counting cells, and for cell maintenance.
- *Clinical centrifuge.* A fixed-angle or swinging bucket centrifuge for 15 ml conical tubes with a maximum speed of 1,300 g can be used for pelleting nematodes and floating eggs on sucrose (suggested model: Fisher scientific 228 benchtop centrifuge).

- *Portable serological Pipet–Aid® (Drummond Scientific) for flow hood.* An electric Pipet-Aid with aspiration and dispensing buttons and a sterile inlet filter. This Pipet-Aid should be used only for cell culture. Keep a supply of spare filters to replace wetted or contaminated filters.
- *Hemocytometer.* Obtain a standard, four-quadrant glass hemocytometer slide for counting cells. Note that hemocytometers use non-standard, 0.5 mm thick coverslips. These thick coverslips do not bend under liquid surface tension and ensure a consistent volume for cell counting. Hemocytometer coverslips can be rinsed and reused indefinitely but keep at least one extra coverslip at hand in case of breakage.
- *Glass bottles.* Cell culture glassware should be kept separate from other laboratory glassware to limit contamination from residual detergents, salts, lipids, and proteins. Fill the bottle with deionized water and autoclave on a liquid cycle with the tops loose. Wash and rinse bottles once more. Fill with deionized water, and autoclave again. Thereafter, do not use detergents in tissue culture glassware or limit their use.

Appendix 1.3   *Disposable Supplies for Cell Culture*

- *Serological pipettes (10 ml, 5 ml).* Sterile, graduated, plastic pipettes for tissue culture come individually wrapped and have a cotton plug at one end to prevent wetting of the Pipet-Aid filter. Keep several in a bin close to the culture hood to minimize arm and body motion that might waft unfiltered air into the hood. Always store pipettes in the same orientation to prevent accidentally opening them from the wrong end.
- *Sterile pipette tips.* Autoclave racks of pipette tips and keep at least one box of each size in the culture hood at all times. Do not remove from the hood after opening.
- *Sterile conical tubes (15 ml, 50 ml).* Purchase either in bulk or in disposable Styrofoam racks. Open the plastic sleeve only at one end and only in the hood. The plastic sleeve may be discarded if the rack is left permanently in the hood. If the rack needs to be removed from the hood to make room, roll the open end of the plastic sleeve closed and affix with tape before removing from the sterile environment.
- *Spray bottle with 70% ethanol.* Do not use pure ethanol (190–200 proof), as it evaporates quickly and is so not as effective at killing mold and bacteria as 70% ethanol.
- *Kimwipes.* Either large or small Kimwipes (Kimberly-Clark) or equivalent low lint wipe should be kept near but not within the cell culture hood. An acrylic Kimwipe box holder affixed to the culture hood above the sash is a convenient location.
- *Powder free gloves.* Powdered residue from the manufacturing process will contaminate culture media and cells. Keep powder-free, residue-free latex, vinyl, or nitrile gloves near the culture hood, but not within it.
- *1.5 ml microcentrifuge tubes with snap caps.* • *T25 tissue culture flasks, uncoated, with vented caps.* These 25 cm^2 surface area canted neck flasks are used for growing larvae in axenic growth media. The vented cap contains a 0.2 μm filter for sterile gas exchange. They are not required for embryonic or L1 stage cell culture.
- *Sodium hypochlorite (household bleach).* Only use bleach to sterilize glass or plastic. Halides such as bleach corrode metal. *Do not use* bleach to sterilize stainless steel or any other metal surfaces.

Appendix 1.4   Sterile Techniques for Cell Culture

Note: Open flames are no longer recommended for use inside of a class II laminar flow hood (Centers for Disease Control and Prevention, CDC). An open flame presents a fire hazard when used with 70% ethanol. Furthermore, heat disrupts the airflow pattern within the cabinet and can damage the HEPA filter.

1. Tie back long hair and remove any rings, watches, or bracelets. Wash both hands and wrists thoroughly with antibacterial soap.
2. Don a laboratory coat and powder free latex or vinyl gloves after washing and drying.
3. Spray gloves with 70% ethanol and dry with Kimwipes.
4. Change gloves after leaving or reentering the culture area.

Note: Do not touch your face, hair, pockets, clothes, or phone while working in the hood. Turn off your cell phone to avoid distractions. If you accidentally touch any potentially contaminated surface, decontaminate gloves with ethanol or change gloves depending on the extent of the potential contamination.

5. Before working in the culture hood, turn off the UV lamp, turn on the blower, and raise the sash to the working mark if the sash is adjustable.
6. Organize the work surface so that the area immediately in front is clear. Thoroughly spray the work surface inside the hood with 70% ethanol and wipe with Kimwipes.

Note: Disinfect often. When leaving the culture hood for more than 30 minutes or when changing operators, disinfect the work surface with 70% ethanol.

7. Disinfect items such as Pipet-Aids, bottles, and tubes with 70% ethanol and wipe with Kimwipes before placing them in the culture hood.
8. Move permanent residents of the hood such as sterile pipette boxes and racks for conical tubes to either side of the work surface when not in use.

Note: HEPA filters remove most particulate matter from air, but a small fraction (percent) of dust, bacteria, spores, etc., pass through. This percentage increases with filter age, so have the culture hood checked and certified yearly.

9. Organize the work surface of the culture hood. Move any permanent residents of the hood such as racks and pipette tip boxes to either side of the work surface.
10. Disinfect the culture hood work surface with 70% ethanol.
11. Disinfect the vacuum trap by aspirating a small amount of household bleach directly into the Tygon tubing. Follow with distilled water. Spray and wipe the tubing end with 70% ethanol. Discard liquid in the trap according to your institution's safety policies.
12. Lower the sash to its closed position (if adjustable), turn off the blower, and turn on the UV lamp.
13. Organize and disinfect any other open bench tops in the cell culture area with 70% ethanol.
14. If any at-hand stocks such as serological pipettes or gloves are low, refill the drawer or container. Properly dispose of sharps containers and trash when full.

Note: Be mindful of coworkers. Unlike your personal laboratory bench, cell culture areas are usually shared resources. Sloppiness can ruin your colleagues' experiments. When you are done, ensure that the cell culture area is tidy, organized, and clean. Remember that cleanup is an essential part of any experiment!

Appendix 1.5 Troubleshooting Immunofluorescence

Problem	Reason	Solution
Weak or no staining	Incorrect light source/filter	Check microscope
	Low exposure	Increase exposure time
	Fluorescent tag bleached	Avoid overexposure
		Store slide in dark
	Cells over-fixed	Reduce duration of fixation
		Perform antigen retrieval to unmask epitope
	Cells not permeabilized	If using formaldehyde, permeabilize cells with 0.2% Triton X-100.
	Tissue/cells dried out	Sample must be kept covered in liquid
	Not enough primary Ab	Use higher concentration of Ab
		Incubate longer
	Suitability of primary antibody	Confirm validation of antibody
		Western blot
	Protein tested not present	Run a +ve control
		Amplification step to maximize signal
High background	Autofluorescence	Check for autofluorescence
		Avoid glutaraldehyde fixative or wash with 0.1% sodium borohydride in PBS to remove free aldehyde groups
	Tissue too thick	Use thinner tissues
	Antibody concentration too high	Reduce concentration of primary and secondary antibody
	Nonspecific binding	Run a control with only secondary antibody, in case of staining change secondary
	Insufficient blocking	Increase incubation time
	Nonspecific staining	Multiple washing steps

Appendix 2   Laboratory Safety

Due to the wide variety of experiments listed in this text it would be cumbersome to roster each specific chemical danger here. Therefore, dangers inherent to each exercise are listed in the experiments in each chapter. The following safety precautions are a generalized list that are likely to be encountered in the exercises covered in the text. Individuals involved in the biochemical experimentation should familiarize themselves intimately with these precautions.

General Precautions

1. Follow the instructions and pay attention to all the steps from start to finish before beginning an experiment. Know the use of all the equipment in the lab before beginning the work.

2. The most important safety rule is to know the location of the safety equipment and how to use it. The equipment should be checked periodically to ensure that it is in working order. Remember the building evacuation protocol.

3. Wear safety goggles at all times in the laboratory. For biochemical experimentation regular eyeglasses do not provide sufficient protection from either chemical hazards or broken glassware. Recently, the American Chemical Society has approved the use of contact lenses but only when worn in combination with safety goggles. The contact/goggle combination is important because most modern eyewash stations are not able to remove chemicals trapped behind contacts.

4. Proper clothing should be worn in the laboratory at all times. Long sleeve shirts, long pants and full shoes are the best choice. Skin protection will be at a maximum if the aforementioned garments are covered with a full lab coat/apron.

5. Make use of the fume hoods for handling volatile and/or hazardous chemicals. When handling chemicals gloves should be worn to protect the hands.

6. Dispose of solid and liquid waste in containers, which are properly labeled. Notify the instructor if any of the waste containers are full or damaged. If you not sure where to dispose of the waste ask your instructor for help.

7. Get acquainted with the layout of the lab, paying special attention to the fire extinguishers, emergency eye wash stations, first aid kits and the nearest emergency phone. Knowledge of the location of this apparatus may help save your life and prevent injury to others.

8. Never eat or drink in the laboratory area. Contamination of food or drink can take place without your knowledge. Dropping a reagent bottle on the lab floor may cause a toxic substance to spray into your food or drink. Because the biochemistry lab usually involves long hours of analysis it is sometimes unavoidable for lab-time to overlap with meal-time. If you must eat or drink something during the laboratory period leave the food or drink outside the laboratory. A short break to eat or drink will not be detrimental to the outcome of your experiments.

9. Never sniff or taste chemicals in the lab as it could be very dangerous. The best way to know what is in the container is to label all containers before adding any chemicals.

10. Never experiment on yourself, you will never gain superpowers in doing so but only put yourself in danger.

11. Always be responsible in the lab. Never mix chemical randomly in order to avoid explosions, fire, or release of toxic gases.

12. The emergency contacts and phone numbers should be written and placed in proper locations in the lab.

13. If you are the last person to leave the lab, make sure to switch off all the lights, close all ignition sources and lock the doors.

General Laboratory Courtesy

Like most teaching laboratories, the biochemistry laboratory can be a confusing crowded place for the new student. A lack of experience with the chemicals involved in the biochemistry laboratory can cause time consuming mishaps. Therefore, all biochemistry laboratory students, experienced or inexperienced, should observe the following laboratory courtesies:

1. Prior to the laboratory period the student should read the experimental protocol thoroughly, noting any questions for the instructor. As confusing as a biochemistry laboratory is to the new student it becomes 10-fold more confusing when the student has no idea what to expect next.
2. When preparing reagents for your use from a common stock solution, be sure to return the stock solution to its proper storage place. Many chemicals used in biochemistry experiments degrade rapidly below 4°C. If you are preparing a mixture from a purchased chemical stock, check the label on the reagent bottle for the proper storage procedures.
3. After using common laboratory equipment, micropipetters, distilled water bottles, timers, etc., return them to their proper place immediately after cleaning. Many biochemistry laboratory courses do not have enough funding to provide equipment such as micropipetters to each student. Therefore, it is imperative that for events to flow smoothly during the experiments, common equipment be cleaned and returned as soon as possible.
4. Use only as much of the chemicals supplied to you as you need. In order to cut costs and produce less environmental waste many instructors prepare only enough of the common reagents for the experiment at hand. Use of excessive amounts of common reagents may cause a delay in the experiment for the others in the course while they wait for more reagents to be prepared by the instructor.
5. Never insert your pipet/micropipetter tip into a common reagent bottle. This practice can easily spread contamination throughout the laboratory, thus ruining many hours of work by yourself and other students.
6. After each lab period, clean your work area and any glassware that you used. After cleaning used glassware and rinsing with tap water rinse the glassware with distilled water and place in a strainer to dry overnight.

Appendix 3   Statistics

In the biochemistry laboratory, as in many other branches of chemistry, the statistical treatment of data is of the utmost importance for the accurate reporting of results. The unique nature of the biochemical sample places an even greater importance on said statistical processing. The biochemical sample is usually the result of many hours of chromatographic purification. The same sample usually degrades to an unusable status in a very short period of time and is more often than not at a very low concentration to begin. The biochemical sample characteristics listed above infer that characterization protocols must be performed quickly and repeated numerous times. Prior to the mention of the basic statistical analysis that will be used you will need to be familiar with the types of errors you will encounter in biochemical experimentation.

Statistical Terms and Definition

Accuracy: The closeness of an experimental measurement to the **true value**.

Precision: Is also sometimes called reproducibility, which is scattering of experimental value. The *precision* of a series of measurements refers to the closeness of the values obtained from the identical measurements of a quantity.

Errors in Biochemical Experimental Data

It would be impossible to explain the types of errors found in gathering biochemical data without asking the reader to keep in mind the definitions of *Precision* and *Accuracy*. With the above mentioned definitions at hand it is easier to delineate the following types of errors.

First, biochemical analysis can be affected by **random** (or **indeterminate**) **errors**. The effects of a random error can cause the results to be scattered around a mean value (the definition of mean will follow shortly). Ultimately, an indeterminate error is a reflection of the precision with which the data is measured. Most random errors arise in a system where the method of measurement is lengthened to its maximum sensitivity. The resulting random fluctuations in measurements are the effects of the random error contributions in total. In general, random errors of a measurement are the cumulative effects of many small random errors, which cannot be measured individually.

Second, **systematic** (or **determinate**) **errors** produce a mean value for a set of results that differs from an accepted value. Therefore, a determinate error causes the data from a series of measurements to vary either all high or low. Consequently, systematic errors are a reflection of the accuracy of the measurements. Systematic errors can be broken down into three categories: (a) *Instrumental errors* are the result of flaws in the instrumentation or in the system supplying power to the instrument. (b) *Method errors* are produced from abnormalities in chemical or physical behavior. (c) *Personal errors* are the product of carelessness on behalf of the experimenter. In general, systematic errors are the same for repeated measurements and are readily assigned a cause. The result of a systematic error is a *bias* in the biochemical data collected. More succinctly, all results are skewed in the same direction (higher/lower) and quantity.

Third, **gross errors** occur much less frequently than determinate or indeterminate errors. Gross errors are neither random nor systematic. The end result of a gross error is a data point with an extremely large degree of error (an *outlier*). The treatment of experimental data containing random, systematic and gross errors will be discussed in the following section.

Treatment of Biochemical Data Containing Error

Prior to the explanation of the statistical treatment of biochemical data it is important to understand the meaning of the term *Arithmetic* or *Sample Mean (x^{ave})*. In general, the x^{ave} is the mean of a small sample of the total population (n). The population being the total number of data points (usually N>20). Therefore, the x^{ave} is calculated as follows:

$$x^{ave} = (x_1 + x_2 + x_3 + \ldots x_n)/n \text{ or } = \Sigma x_i/n$$

At times in the reporting of your biochemical data you will be called upon to supply the instructor with the *percent error* in you calculation. Percent error is usually used in the teaching lab when it is necessary to make a comparison of students results to a known value. The percent error is calculated as follows:

$$\% \text{ error} = [|x^{ave} - x^{known}| \div x^{known}] \times 100$$

The type of error, which lends itself most readily to treatment by statistical methods is random or indeterminate error. If the reader will recall, from the previous section, random error is closely related to precision and accuracy. Therefore, most methods of statistical treatment for said error involves the proximity of the results to precision and accuracy. The statistical treatment most often used as a measure of the precision of biochemical data is *sample **standard deviation (SD)**. A related parameter, the **variance**, is defined as square of *standard deviation*.

$$SD = \left[\sum_{i=1}^{N} \left(x_1 - x^{ave} \right)^2 / (N-1) \right]^{\frac{1}{2}}$$

where,

x_i = the current value being manipulated

x^{ave} = the arithmetic or sample mean

N–1 = The number of degrees of freedom (the number of data points which are put into the calculation).

Note: If a population mean (μ, the mean value for the total population of data gathered) were used in the place of the sample mean, then N-1 is replaced by N, the total population of the data collected. N is usually used when the total number of data points is greater than 20. Therefore, the sample standard deviation (SD) would become the ***population standard deviation*** (σ); where:

$$\sigma = \left[\sum_{i=1}^{N} \left(x_i - \mu \right)^2 / N \right]^{\frac{1}{2}}$$

A related parameter, the *variance*, is defined as square of *standard deviation*.

$$V = \left[\sum_{i=1}^{N} \left(x_i - x^{ave} \right)^2 / (N-1) \right] \text{ and } SD = +\sqrt{V}$$

Systematic errors are, in general, more readily recognized and dealt with than their random error counterparts. When the student is trying to determine if an error in the biochemical data is a determinate or indeterminate error it is helpful to keep in mind that determinate errors may be either proportional or constant. Data containing a proportional error usually contain a sample with an interfering contaminate. That is the amount of error is directly proportional to the concentration of contaminate in the sample. Constant errors, on the other hand, can easily be detected if the error becomes larger as the concentration of analyte decreases.

One of the simplest ways to report error is standard error, which is the standard deviation of a group of averages. It is useful in estimating the precision of an average X, and helps decide how many significant figures to retain in an average value based on N data value.

$$S.E. (X) = S/\sqrt{N}$$

where X = average
S = standard deviation
N = set of values

In the biochemistry laboratory course, the types of systematic errors, which are the easiest for you, the student, to detect will be personal errors and instrumental errors. We have made it a priority to make you aware of any systematic method errors present in any of the experimental protocols, which you will perform. Any such errors that are present have not been removed for the sake of saving valuable laboratory time. When a method error is highlighted a correction for said error will follow. Generally, the circumvention of a method error is most easily performed by choosing a control sample, which contains a matrix identical to that of the analyte sample but without the analyte itself.

When confronting systematic personal errors it is best for the student to keep the following tips in mind. (1) *Detailed lab notes* can help you recognize mistakes. (2) *Planning your next move* in the lab will minimize the occurrence of mistakes; this means reading the total experimental protocol prior to the lab is a great idea. (3) *Ask your instructor for help* if you are not sure what is happening biochemically in the next step. Some students charge ahead without thinking each step through thoroughly. The result is a mistake, which will cost valuable lab time. The remaining systematic error, instrumental errors, can be easily avoided altogether. In order to avoid an instrumental error you must know something about the instrument you are using to perform the biochemical analysis. This is where asking your instructor detailed questions about the equipment you are using can save you time. Avoiding instrumental errors is as simple as performing a periodic calibration. The calibration process is needed due to the wear and tear placed on some fundamental pieces of laboratory equipment. The final segment, in the statistical treatment of biochemical data, involves the detection and treatment of data containing gross errors.

The detection of a particular type of error in biochemical data is a rather daunting task. Even biochemists with years of experience are generally unable to recognize most sources of error with just a glance of the data. The above statement holds true for all types of error except data containing gross error. If the biochemists' data contains an outlying value, a decision must be made. Should I retain or reject the outlying value? Unfortunately there is no ubiquitous rule that will allow for the rejection of data without the possibility of rejecting data that should be retained. The reverse of this statement also applies when treating outlying values. The most widely applied test in the rejection of suspected outlying values from small samples is the Q-test. With the Q-test as a tool a specific data point can be rejected with a confidence level of up to 99%. The Q-test formula is as follows:

$$Q_{exp} = |X_{suspected} - X_{nearest\ neighbor}|/Range$$

where
Q_{exp} is the result from the Q-test calculation for the outlier
$X_{suspected}$ is the suspected outlying value
$X_{nearest\ neighbor}$ is the sample value nearest to the $X_{suspected}$
Range is the absolute difference between the high and low sample values $|X_{high} - X_{low}|$

If the Q_{exp} value is greater than the $Q_{critical}$ value, then the outlying value may be rejected at the confidence level chosen for $Q_{critical}$, (see Table A3.1).

Table A3.1   Critical values for the rejection of Q_{exp}.

Q Table			
Number of Observations	**90% Confidence**	**95% Confidence**	**99% Confidence**
3	0.941	0.97	0.994
4	0.765	0.829	0.926
5	0.642	0.71	0.821
6	0.56	0.625	0.74
7	0.507	0.568	0.68
8	0.468	0.526	0.634
9	0.437	0.493	0.598
10	0.412	0.466	0.568

* Data is rejected if Qexp > Qcritical

For example, if the Q-test calculation yields a Q_{exp} value of 0.997, then you can be 99% confident that the result does not belong with the other data gathered in the sample.

A final test of your experimental data and the quality of your gathering technique will be the treatment of said data with the students T-test. The T-test is used to give a measure of precision for data that was gathered without the time or sample to determine the population standard deviation (σ). In its most general form the T-test provides for the comparison of an individual value to the population mean (μ) and the sample standard deviation (SD).

$$T = (x - \mu)/SD$$

Another form of the T-test equation allows for the comparison of a sample or arithmetic mean (x^{ave}) to the same population mean (μ), the sample standard deviation (SD), and the total population (N).

$$T = (x^{ave} - \mu)/(SD/N^{\frac{1}{2}})$$

The numerical results of the T-test are then compared to data collected for T at various levels of probability (Table A3.2). The various levels of probability are described in terms of **Confidence Intervals**. Confidence intervals are defined as the magnitude of the confidence limit interval around the arithmetic mean (x^{ave}) that probably contains the actual value of the population mean (μ).

Statistical hypotheses are stated in terms of two opposing statements, the null-hypothesis (Ho) and the alternative hypothesis (Ha). In general, the null-hypothesis states that there is significant difference between two quantities being compared. The alternative hypothesis may either be: directional (one-tailed), stating the way in which the two populations will differ, or nondirectional (two-tailed), not specifying the way in which two populations will differ. With the T-test we are comparing either a single sample or the arithmetic mean value to the population mean. The criteria for acceptance or rejection of the null-hypothesis are, as follows, in Table A3.3. From the table it follows that, if the probability that the x^{ave} differs from μ by chance alone is equal to 10% the result is insignificant, and the null-hypothesis is retained. If at any point in your comparison of data by the null-hypothesis the probability is observed to be between 5% and 1% or less than 1% the null-hypothesis is rejected and another hypothesis is adopted.

Table A3.2 T-values for various levels of probability.

Degree of Freedom (N–1)	Factors of Confidence Interval				
	80%	90%	95%	99%	99.90%
1	3.08	6.31	12.7	63.7	637
2	1.89	2.92	4.3	9.92	31.6
3	1.64	2.35	3.18	6.84	12.9
4	1.53	2.13	2.78	4.6	8.6
5	1.48	2.02	2.57	4.03	6.86
6	1.44	1.94	2.45	3.71	5.96
7	1.42	1.9	2.36	3.5	5.4
8	1.4	1.86	2.31	3.36	5.04
9	1.38	1.83	2.26	3.25	4.78
10	1.37	1.81	2.23	3.17	4.59
11	1.36	1.8	2.2	3.11	4.44
12	1.36	1.78	2.18	3.06	4.32
13	1.35	1.77	2.16	3.01	4.22
∞	1.19	1.64	1.96	2.58	3.29

Table A3.3 Standards for rejection/acceptance of the null-hypothesis.

Probability (P) (T-result x100)	Decision	Conclusion
$P \geq 10\%$	Insignificant result	Retain null-hypothesis
$10\% \geq P \geq 5\%$	Possibly significant result	No definite conclusion
$5\% \geq P \geq 1\%$	Significant result	Reject null-hypothesis
$P \leq 1\%$	Highly significant result	Definitely reject null-hypothesis

Probability and Significance

In a statistical world, the word significance has a specific and important definition. The difference between an observed and expected result is said to be statistically significant if, and only if:

1. Under the assumption that there is no true difference, the probability that the observed difference would be at least as large as that seen is less than or equal to 5% (0.05).
2. Conversely, under the assumption that there is no true difference, the probability that the observed difference would be smaller than that actually seen is greater than 95% (0.95).

Once the T-test is calculated, the investigator should be able to draw conclusion from it.

Log Scales

Data from studies, where relative or exponential changes are pervasive, also benefit from transformation to log scales. For example, transforming to a log scale is the standard way to obtain a straight line, from a slope that changes exponentially. This can make for a more straightforward presentation and can also simplify the statistical analysis. Thus, transforming 1, 10, 100, 1,000 into $\log_{10}$ gives us 0, 1, 2, 3. Which log base you choose does not particularly matter, although ten and two are quite intuitive, and therefore popular. The natural log (~2.718), however, has historical precedent within certain fields and may be considered standard. In some cases, back transformation (from log scale to linear) can be done after the statistical analysis to make the findings clearer to readers.

Correlation and Modeling

Modeling is an important form of analysis in genetics and molecular biology, while correlation is the co-variation of two variables. This method is mostly employed during cell sorting and the data is plotted using a scatterplot. The cells are fluorescently tagged and each cell is considered as one dot with associated fluorescence corresponding the x- and y-axis respectively. In the case of a positive correlation, the cloud of dots will trend up to the right. If there is a negative correlation, the dots will trend down to the right. If there is little or no correlation, the dots will generally show no obvious pattern. The closer the dots come to forming a unified tight line, the stronger is the correlation between the variables.

Useful Programs for Statistical Calculations

1. Microsoft Excel
2. Prism

Recommended Reading

- Motulsky, H. (2010). Intuitive Biostatistics: A Nonmathematical Guide to Statistical Thinking, Second Edition. New York: Oxford University Press.
- Triola M. F., and Triola M. M. (2006). Biostatistics for the Biological and Health Sciences. Boston: Pearson Addison-Wesley.
- Sokal R. R., and Rohlf, F. J. (2012). Biometry: The Principles and Practice of Statistics in Biological Research, Fourth Edition. New York: W. H. Freeman and Co.

Appendix 4 Significant Figures

In biochemistry, as in all other branches of chemistry, the reporting of data is, in many cases, as important as the experimentation, which took place to obtain the data. In our experience, in teaching the biochemistry laboratory course, we have found that many students feel that the strict adherence to reporting experimental data with the correct number of significant figures is a task only needed in the analytical chemistry laboratory. The lax attitude towards significant figures, scientific notation, accuracy and precision has caused much confusion for the students when reporting their experimental findings. Therefore, it is in the students' best interest to review the following rules regarding the basic principles for reporting experimental findings:

Number of Significant Figures

In general, the **number of significant figures** pertains to the number of digits recorded for the value of a calculated or a measured sum. Ultimately, the number of significant figures is an indication of the precision of the measurement or calculation (**precision** will be discussed in statistics section).

If, for example, a student weighs the mass of a biological sample to be 0.998, 0.997, and 0.999 g for 3 separate measurements, a total of 3 significant figures would result from each of the measurements (zeros here *are not* significant). The fluctuation in the third decimal place indicates that this number is an estimate and is an indication of the balance limit. If a less accurate balance were used the measurements may look something like 1.0, 1.0, and 1.0 g. The measurements on the crude balance would result in each of the measurements having 2 significant figures (zeros here *are* significant). The aforementioned example illustrates the problem for most students, "which zeros are significant and which are not." The rules for significant figures that follow should clarify any questions:

1. All digits are significant except zeros at the beginning of a number and possibly those at the end of a number (Rule 2 and 3 apply to terminal zeros).
2. All zeros, which terminate a number and are to the right of a decimal place are significant. For example, from our biological sample listed above, 1.0, 1.00, and 1.000 g. These examples contain 2, 3, and 4 significant figures respectfully.
3. Terminal zeros listed in a number without a decimal place may or may not be significant. For example, a biological sample mass of 10 g has 1 significant figure while a sample of 10. g has 2 significant figures.

When applying significant figure rules to calculations the following rules should be applied:

1. For *addition and subtraction*: the number of significant figures in the sum or difference should be equal to the number in the calculation with the smallest number of decimal places. For example, 10.6 + 0.421, the sum without significant figure consideration would be 11.021. Because 10.6 has only one digit after the decimal place the answer cannot have more than one. Therefore, the correct answer would be 11.0.
2. For *multiplication and division*: there can be no more significant figures in the product or quotient than there are in the number with the fewest number of significant digits. From the example above, without significant figure consideration the product of 10.0 x 0.421 would be 4.21. Since each of the numbers involved in the product contains 3 significant figures the answer of 4.21 with 3 significant figures is correct. If, on the other hand, the equation was 10 x 0.421, the correct answer would be 4. The single significant figure is correct because the first number in the equation contains only 1 significant figure.
3. Exact numbers have no effect on the number of significant figures in a calculation. Remember an **exact number** is one that involves no uncertainty. That is, an exact number arises when you count an item. For example, if you are calculating the average weight of an isolated protein in

5 fraction tubes and the total weight is 0.997 µg. The average protein per tube would be 0.997 µg/5 fractions = 0.199 µg/fraction and not 0.2 µg. This is because 5 is an exact number and has no bearing on the number of significant digits in the answer.

After the correct number of significant digits, have been determined the next step in reporting the correct answer to your biochemical experiment is rounding (off). The procedure of **rounding** encompasses the act of dropping any nonsignificant digits. The general rounding procedure is as follows:

1. If the digit directly to the right of the last significant digit is 5 or greater, round up the last digit to be retained by 1 and drop all the remaining digits to the right. Therefore, from the average protein content per fraction from above, if the raw answer were 0.1996 µg/fraction, then because the final digit is greater than 5 the last significant digit is rounded up by 1. The correct answer would then be 0.200 µg/fraction.
2. If the digit directly to the right of the last significant digit is 5 or less, simply drop all digits to the right of the last significant digit. From the same sample quoted above, if the raw answer were 0.1993 µg/fraction, then the final answer would be 0.199 µg/fraction. Because the digit to the right of the last significant digit is less than 5 it is simply dropped.

Scientific Notation

Many students in the biochemistry lab find it easier to remember which numbers are significant if they place their results in scientific notation format. Generally, scientific notation is placing a number in the form $Z. \times 10^n$. In this form Z. represents a single non-zero number followed by the decimal and n represents the integer number of places the decimal must be moved. If the decimal is moved 3 places to the right as in 0.00199 then n is negative and the correct scientific notation is 1.99×10^{-3}. Moving the decimal 3 places to the left as in 1990 would result in a positive n and a final answer of 1.99×10^3.

Appendix 5   Units in the Biochemistry Laboratory

In the biochemistry laboratory course there is a strong emphasis on the manner in which data is reported to the instructor. As you may remember from your freshman chemistry laboratory experience, keeping a close watch on the units of your results will help you when calculations must be performed via dimensional analysis. The system of units most readily recognized and used by biochemists the world over is the ***International System of Units* (SI)**. The SI system is rooted in 7 fundamental base units of measure (see Table A5.1). A description of the units, which are most regularly used in the biochemistry lab will follow. Biochemistry experiments and instrumentations mostly involve a range of different units. Students are required to know the multiple units and their prefix to report the quantities in conventional terms (Table A5.2).

Of the seven basic units listed in Table A5.1, the unit used most often in the biochemistry laboratory is the ***mole***. The mole and its multiple unit forms mmol, µmol and nmol are put to use in biochemistry whenever the amount of some chemical is to be determined/reported. Closely associated with the use of the mole quantity, is mass and its accompanying units. Prior to the description of mass and the most used multiple unit forms of mass it is important for the biochemistry student to be reminded of the difference between mass and weight. In general, the mass of an object is a uniform measure of the quantity (amount) of matter in an object. Weight, on the other hand, is the attraction affinity between an object and its environment (object's placement on earth). Recall that weight (W) can be expressed in the following formula:

$$W = mg$$

where,
m = the object mass
g = the force due to gravity

Table A5.1 SI system base units.

Physical Quantity	Unit Name	Abbreviation	Multiple Unit Form Most Used in the Biochemistry Lab
Mass	Kilogram	kg	g, mg, μg, ng
Length	Meter	m	mg, μg, nm
Time	Second	s	s, ms, μs, ns, ps
Temperature	Kelvin	K	°C
Amount	Mole	mol	mmol, μmol, nmol
Electric current	Ampere	A	
Radioactivity	Becquerel	Bq	

Table A5.2 SI system multiple unit form prefixes.

Quantity	Prefix	Symbol
10^{12}	tera	T
10^9	giga	G
10^6	mega	M
10^3	kilo	K
10^{-1}	deci	d
10^{-2}	centi	c
10^{-3}	milli	m
10^{-6}	micro	μ
10^{-9}	nano	n
10^{-12}	pico	p
10^{-15}	femto	f
10^{-18}	atto	a

Inclusion of the gravity term in the above equation indicates that objects at higher altitudes will weigh less than the same object at low altitudes, while the mass of the object remains the same. In the biochemistry lab, the mass multiple unit form that a student will most likely encounter will be increasingly small amounts from grams (g) to nanograms (ng). You will most often encounter g when weighing solids for making mixtures. The smaller quantities of mg, μg and ng will be encountered when the mass of an isolated product is tabulated.

The SI quantity for length is the meter. Units for length will most likely be used in this laboratory course when the determination of the migration distance on an electrophoretic gel is necessary. In the aforementioned distance determination the multiple unit form of the meter most used will be mm or cm. On other occasions the μm and nm will be the prominent unit of length. These extremely small units will most likely be the result of measurements on the molecular level, such as that found in fluorescence spectroscopy.

Time course measurements are a staple of biochemistry. Without the use of time the measurement of enzyme kinetic parameters and fluorescence lifetime would be impossible. In this course you will encounter time units in the minutes and seconds range when enzyme kinetic measurements are performed. In your biochemical experiences later in your careers you may be fortunate enough to perform fluorescence experiments where the object is the determination of the time the excited electron spends in the higher energy state. The time measurements in such experiments will be in the seconds range for phosphorescence and μs to ps range for fluorescence lifetimes.

Lastly, possibly the most important of the seven basic SI physical quantities, in terms of sample preparation and preservation, is temperature. The temperature unit most often used in the biochemistry laboratory is the degree centigrade (°C). Most proteins extracted for biochemical characterization are at extremely low concentrations. The actions of proteases and extremes in temperature can easily denature your isolated enzyme. It is of the utmost importance that a constant temperature (4°C) is established throughout the characterization procedures.

Appendix 6   Chapter Contributors

Chapter 1: Introduction ...   *Raj Kumar and Bal Ram Singh*
Chapter 2: Recombinant DNA and Protein Technology ...   *Raj Kumar and Bal Ram Singh*
Chapter 3: Enzyme Kinetics, Proteomics, and Mass Spectrometry ...   *Ghuncha Ambrin,*
                                                                              Raj Kumar and Bal Ram Singh
Chapter 4: Bioanalytical Techniques ...   *Raj Kumar and Bal Ram Singh*
Chapter 5: Molecular Biology ...   *Roshan Vijay Kukreja, Raj Kumar and Bal Ram Singh*
Chapter 6: Cell Culture ...   *Ghuncha Ambrin, Raj Kumar and Bal Ram Singh*
Chapter 7: Antibody Technology ...   *Ghuncha Ambrin, Raj Kumar and Bal Ram Singh*

Appendix 7   Online Resources

For the facilitation of students and readers relevant on-line resources have been listed below:

1. Protein structure prediction model including homology modeling, protein threading, and secondary structure prediction:
   http://www.scfbioiitd.res.in/bhageerath/bhageerath_h.jsp
   http://www.reading.ac.uk/bioinf/IntFOLD/

http://raptorx.uchicago.edu/
http://www.cbs.dtu.dk/services/CPHmodels/
https://arquivo.pt/wayback/20160514083149/http://toolkit.tuebingen.mpg.de/hhpred
https://toolkit.tuebingen.mpg.de/tools/hhpred
http://protein.ict.ac.cn/FALCON/
http://bioinf.cs.ucl.ac.uk/psipred/
https://www.predictprotein.org/

2. Protein yield and size:
   https://www.expasy.org/resources/search/keywords:gel%20electrophoresis

3. Western blot:
   https://www.licor.com/bio/image-studio-lite/

4. Antigen prediction tool:
   https://www.genscript.com/antigen-design.html
   http://tools.immuneepitope.org/bcell/
   https://www.expasy.org/resources/search/keywords:epitope

5. Epitope analysis and mapping tool:
   https://www.integralmolecular.com/epitope-mapping/?gclid=EAIaIQobChMIjcaZks-76wI
   VEovICh1NKwUHEAAYASAAEgIauvD_BwE
   http://tools.iedb.org/main/

6. ELISA software and data analysis:
   https://www.elisaanalysis.com/
   https://www.mybiosource.com/my_assay_data_analyzing_software

7. 3D view inside the cell:
   http://sciencenetlinks.com/tools/icell-app/
   https://edshelf.com/tool/3d-cell-simulation-and-stain-tool/

8. Construction of cell membrane:
   https://www.wisc-online.com/learn/natural-science/life-science/ap1101/construction-of-the-
   cell-membrane

9. Analysis of mitotic defects, segmentation, tracking, feature extraction:
   http://www.bioquant.uni-hd.de/bmcv/genomeresearch
   http://www.csie.ntu.edu.tw/~cjlin/libsvm
   https://github.com/bnoi/MAARS/tree/master/doc/demos

10. Confluency measurement and evaluation:
    https://opencirrus.org/
    http://www.samba.org/ftp/rsync/rsync.html
    https://doi.org/10.1371/journal.pone.0027672.g003
    https://doi.org/10.1371/journal.pone.0027672.g004
    https://doi.org/10.1371/journal.pone.0027672.t002

11. Enzyme kinetic analysis and rate analysis:
    https://icekat.herokuapp.com/icekat
    https://github.com/SmithLabMCW/icekat/blob/master/icekat/test.csv)

12. Designing enzymes:
    https://www.creative-biolabs.com/computer-aided-enzyme-design.html
    https://www.rosettacommons.org/software

13. Enzyme inhibition:
    https://www.microsoft.com/itit/p/easy-kinetics/9nx1f4q5fpg5?activetab=pivot:overviewtab
    https://github.com/ekin96/EasyKinetics

14. 2D gel electrophoresis:
    http://code.google.com/p/gel2de
    https://www.cleaverscientific.com/electrophoresis-products/samespots/

15. SDS-PAGE
    https://www.expasy.org/resources/search/keywords:gel%20electrophoresis
    http://www.gelanalyzer.com/?i=1

16. DNA/RNA modeling:
    http://www.vls3d.com/index.php/links/bioinformatics/3d-structure-prediction/protein-dna-rna-glycan-modeling
    http://haddock.chem.uu.nl/dna/dna.php
    http://www.rna123.com/
    http://en.wikipedia.org/wiki/List_of_RNA_structure_prediction_software
    http://openwetware.org/wiki/Wikiomics:RNA_secondary_structure_prediction

17. FTIR:
    https://www.protea.ltd.uk/freeftirsoftware#:~:text=Protea%20has%20developed%20the%20Protea,and%20manipulates%20mass%20spectra%20data.
    https://www.ssi.shimadzu.com/products/ftir-spectrophotometers/labsolutions-ir-software-options.html
    https://www.essentialftir.com/

18. Vector design:
    https://www.snapgene.com/snapgene-viewer/
    http://serialbasics.free.fr/Serial_Cloner.html
    http://www.addgene.org/analyze-sequence
    http://www.acaclone.com

19. Circular dichroism (CD) tools:
    http://www.cdtools.cryst.bbk.ac.uk.
    https://dev.mysql.com/downloads/windows/installer/5.7.html.

Index

Color Plates

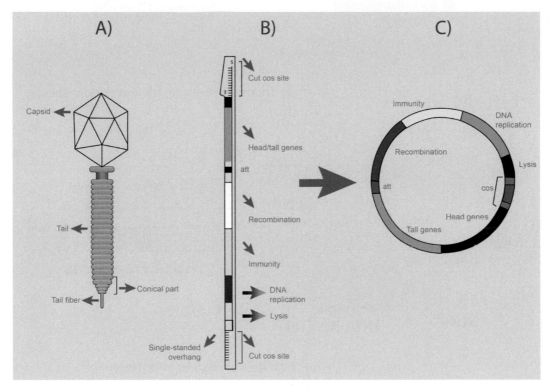

Fig. 2.3 (A) Structure of Lambda bacteriophage. They have an isomeric head (Capsid: ~ 55 nm), tail tube (~ 135 nm), conical region (~ 15 nm) and tail fiber (~ 23 nm). (B) DNA organization in bacteriophage head. (C) At the cos site, at both ends, DNA is circularized and the phase starts replicating. [Page 23]

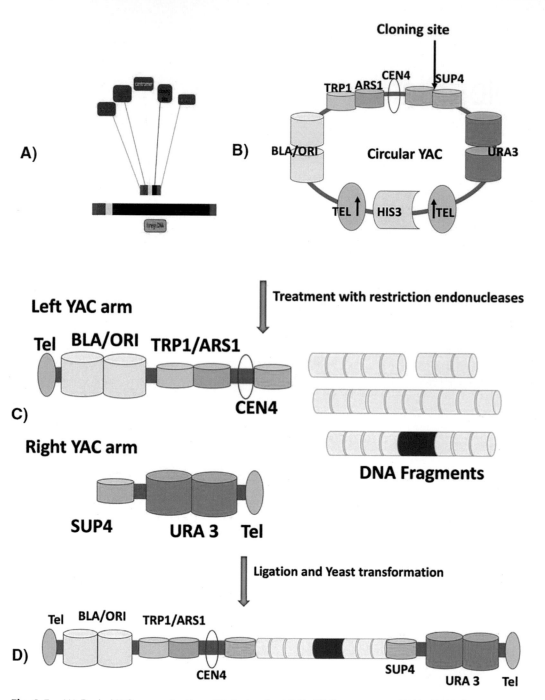

Fig. 2.5 (A) Basic YACs organization. (B) A circular YAC. (C) From source DNA, DNA fragments with compatible ends are designed and prepared. Using restriction endonucleases, YAC vector is digested. The digested vectors are separated into two chromosomal arms: TRP1 on the left and URA3 on the right arm. (D) Ligation of the separated chromosomal arms is done with DNA and transformed into an appropriate yeast strain. [Page 26]

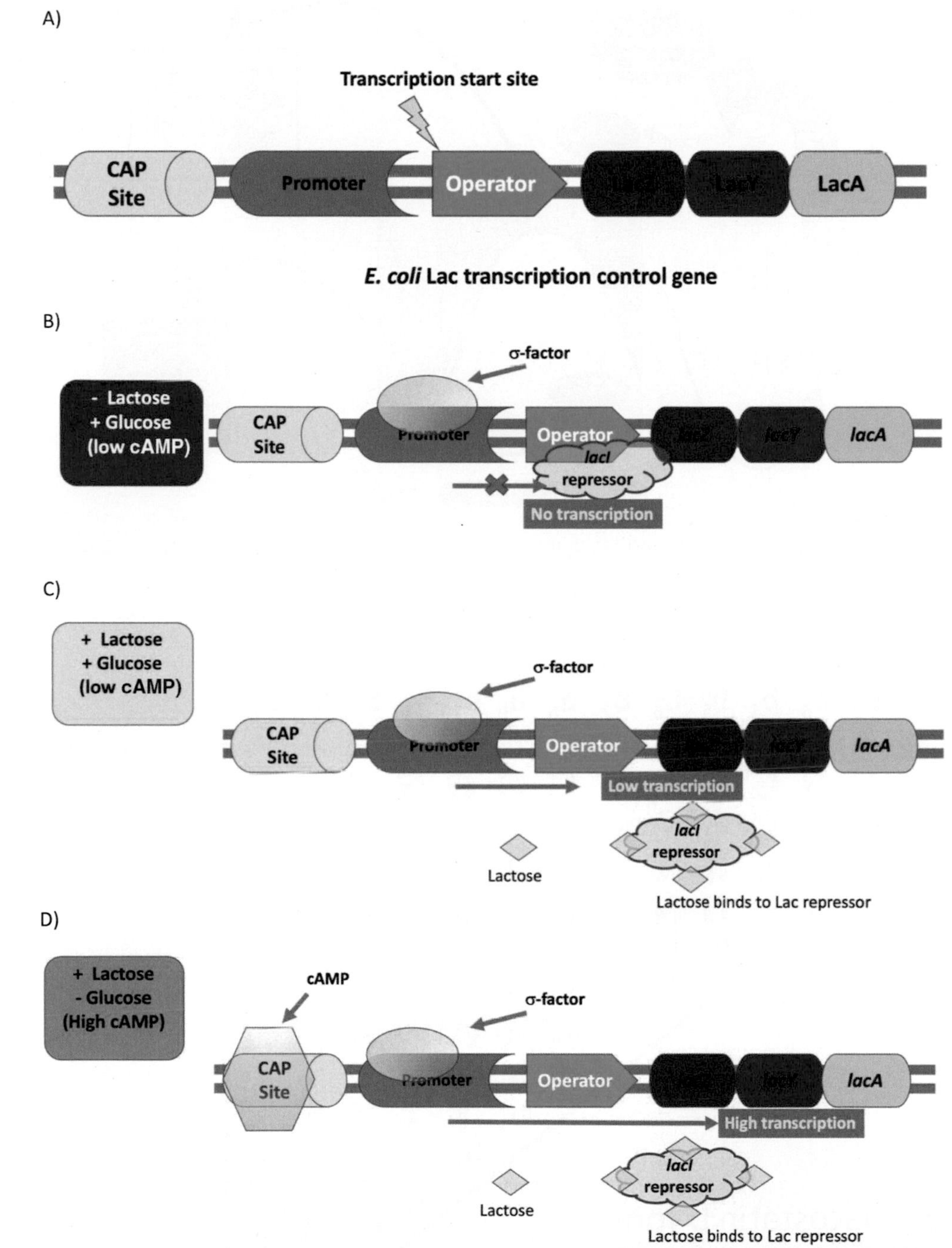

Fig. 2.10 (A) Lac promoter system. (B) When there is no lactose, the lac repressor binds to the operator, so no mRNA transcription. (C) With both glucose and lactose present, σ-factor binds to the promoter region resulting in low mRNA transcription. (D) In presence of lactose (no glucose) both catabolite gene activator protein and σ-factor bind to the promoter and CAP binding site resulting in high mRNA transcription. σ-factor is a transcription initiation factor. [Page 33]

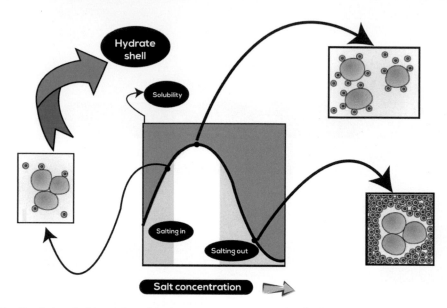

Fig. 2.15   Depicting "salting in" and "salting out" processes. Blue balls represent solvated ions of salt. [Page 43]

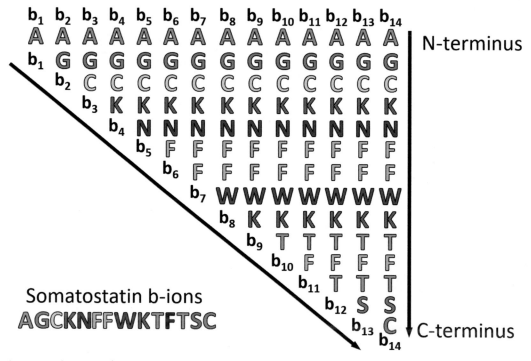

Fig. 3.26   *b – ions* of somatostatin. [Page 96]

Somatostatin b-ions

AGCKN FFWKTFTSC

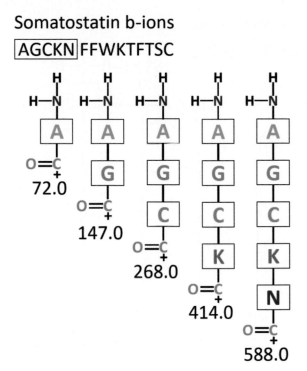

Fig. 3.27 Formation of *b – ions*. [Page 97]

Somatostatin y-ions

AGCKNFFWKTFTSC

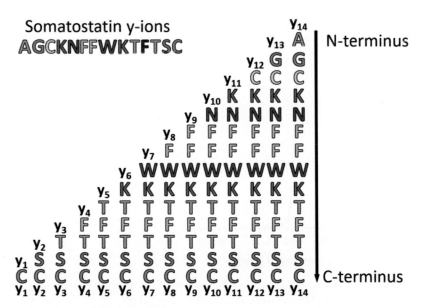

Fig. 3.28 *y – ions* of somatostatin. [Page 97}

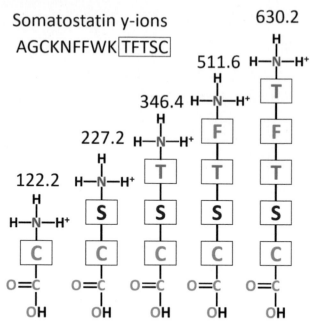

Fig. 3.29 Formation of *y – ions* of somatostatin. [Page 98]

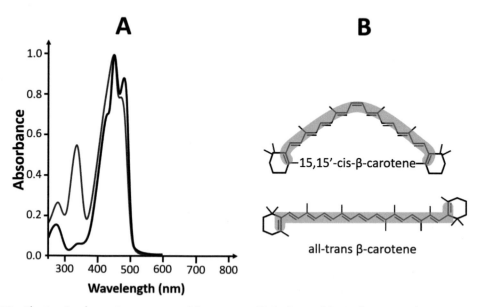

Fig. 4.16 Electronic absorption spectra of β-carotene (A) in linear (blue) all trans and 15,15-cis (red) structure forms (B) (Adopted from Fiedor et al., 2016). [Page 118]

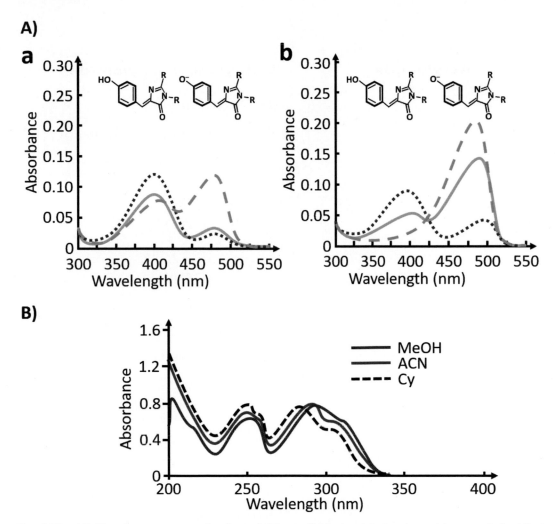

Fig. 4.30 (A) Absorbance spectra of unbound (*blue, solid line*), minimizer-bound (*green, dashed line*) or enhancer-bound (*red, dotted line*) wt GFP (a) or eGFP (b). The absorption at 395 nm corresponds to the protonated chromophore and absorption at 475 nm to the anionic chromophore. Both enhancer and minimizer affected the absorption of deprotonated form (Kirchoffer et al., 2010, Nature Structural and Molecular Biology, 17, 133–138). (B) Absorbance spectra of Flavones in methanol (red), acetonitrile (ACN, blue), and cyclohexane (Cy, black). Both hydrogen bond donating ability and non-specific dipolar interaction can affect absorption spectra (Sancho et al., 2011). [Page 126]

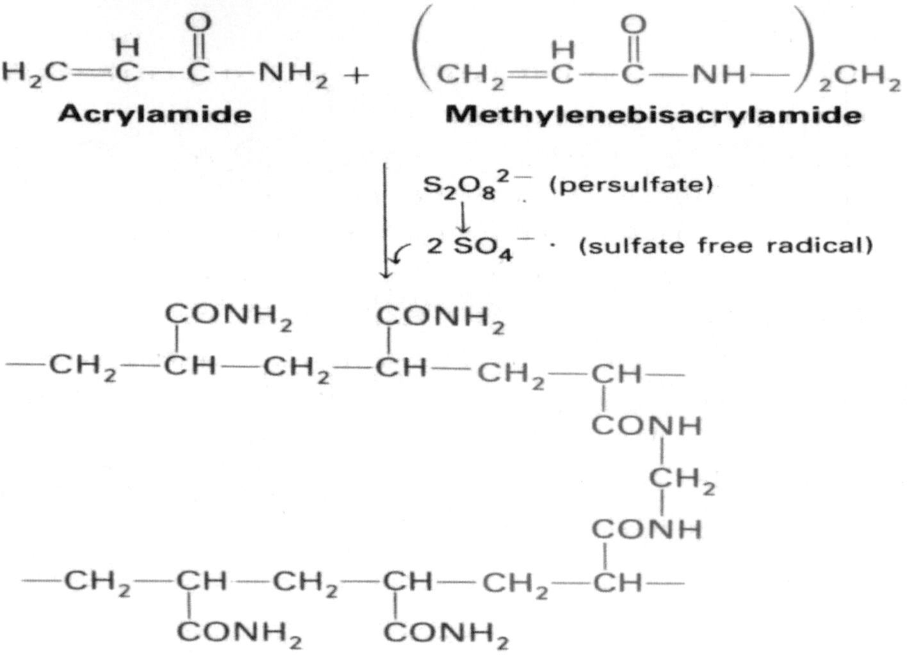

$$H_2C{=}C{-}C{-}NH_2 \ + \ \left(CH_2{=}C{-}C{-}NH{-} \right)_2 CH_2$$

Acrylamide   **Methylenebisacrylamide**

$S_2O_8{}^{2-}$ (persulfate)

$2\ SO_4{}^- \cdot$ (sulfate free radical)

$$
\begin{array}{c}
CONH_2 \qquad\quad CONH_2 \\
-CH_2{-}CH{-}CH_2{-}CH{-}CH_2{-}CH{-} \\
\qquad\qquad\qquad\qquad\qquad\quad CONH \\
\qquad\qquad\qquad\qquad\qquad\quad CH_2 \\
\qquad\qquad\qquad\qquad\qquad\quad CONH \\
-CH_2{-}CH{-}CH_2{-}CH{-}CH_2{-}CH{-} \\
\qquad CONH_2 \qquad\quad CONH_2
\end{array}
$$

Fig. 4.49 Formation of polyacrylamide gel. The pore size can be controlled by adjusting the concentration of activated monomer (red) and cross-linker (green). [Page 157]

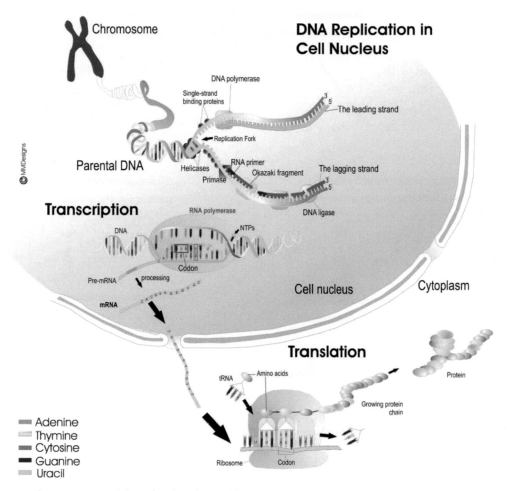

Fig. 5.13 Schematic view of the role of nucleic acids in transmission of genetic information. [Page 185]

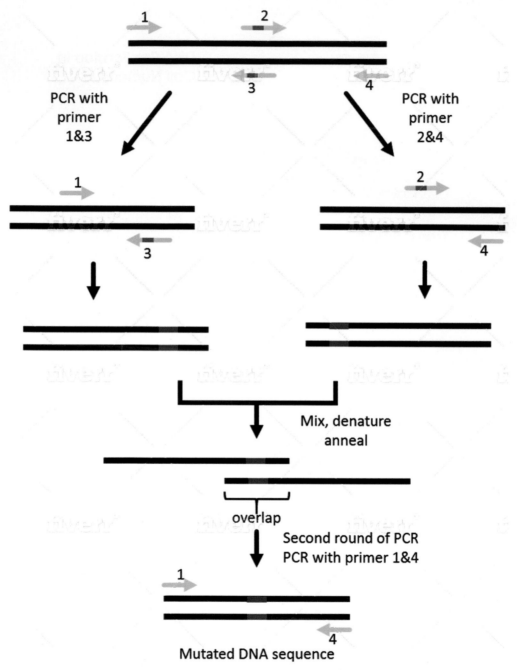

Fig. 5.17 PCR-based mutagenesis. Two external primers (1 and 4) that are complementary to the forward and reverse DNA strands, respectively, and two internal primers (2 and 3) that contain the desired mutations are used in the two PCR reactions that are carried out in separate tubes under the same reaction conditions. The products of the two reactions are allowed to mix, denature, and reanneal where some strands from the first PCR product anneal with those obtained from the second PCR reaction leading to regions of overlap corresponding to the sequences of primers 2 and 3. Subsequent PCR reactions lead to amplification of the full length fragment of the mutated DNA. [Page 200]

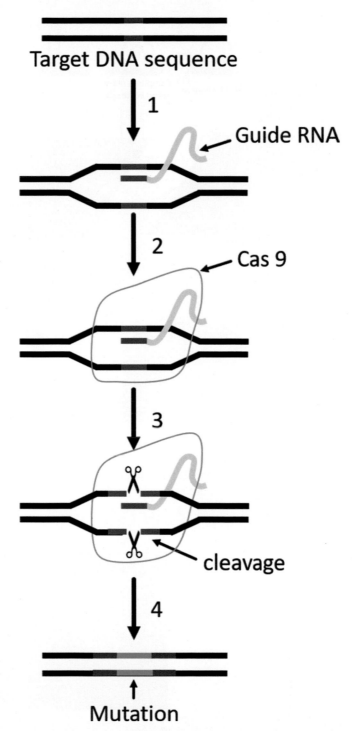

Fig. 5.18 Mechanism of CRISPR/Cas9 genome editing. This technology uses a short guide RNA molecule that directs the Cas-9 enzyme to a specific region of the genomic DNA resulting in a double-strand cut/break. The double-strand break is then repaired by the host cell leading to introduction of desired changes to the fragment of interest. [Page 202]

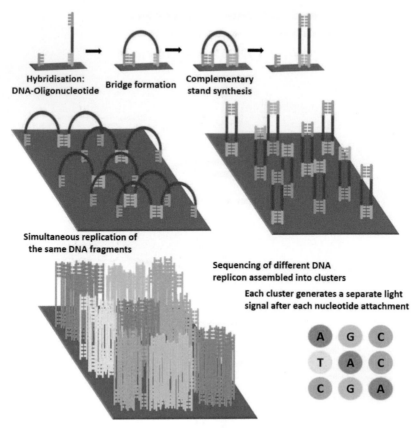

Fig. 5.32 Next generation sequencing on an Illumina platform. DNA fragments to be sequenced are amplified and bound to a flow cell generating clusters with about 1000 copies of each fragment. Upon nucleotide incorporation, the fluorescence signal corresponding to each base is measured and the imaging of tens of millions of clusters is carried out in parallel resulting in a rapid and cost-effective sequencing of the entire genome. [Page 221]

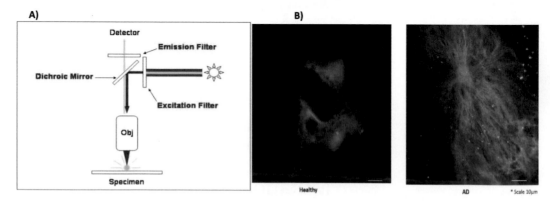

Fig. 6.13 (A) Schematic diagram of a fluorescence microscope. (B) Fluorescent image of nonactivated and activated astrocyte in healthy and AD (Alzheimer disease) model. Protein was tagged with Alexa fluor 488 dye (green) and nucleus was tagged with DAPI (4′,6-diamidino-2-phenylindole; blue). [Page 271]

A)

B)

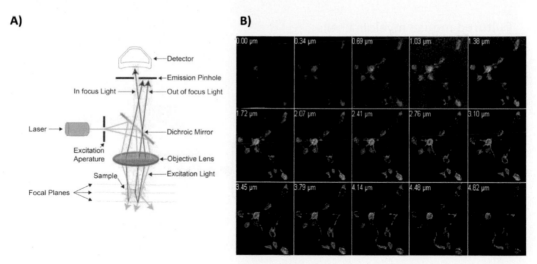

Fig. 6.14 (A) Diagram of a confocal microscope. (B) Z-stack image of SHSY-5Y cell demonstrating internalization of a protein (green). Z-stack feature of confocal microscopy provides images of a cell at different depths (one end to the other). (Adopted from Kumar et al., 2012). [Page 271]

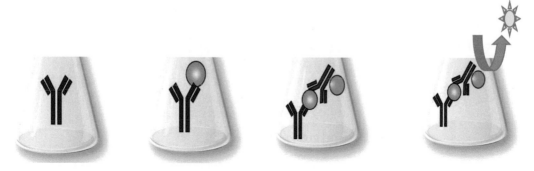

Fig. 7.6 Overview of direct sandwich ELISA. Capture antibody is in red while detection antibody is in blue, with antigen in the middle (sandwiched between the two antibodies). [Page 291]

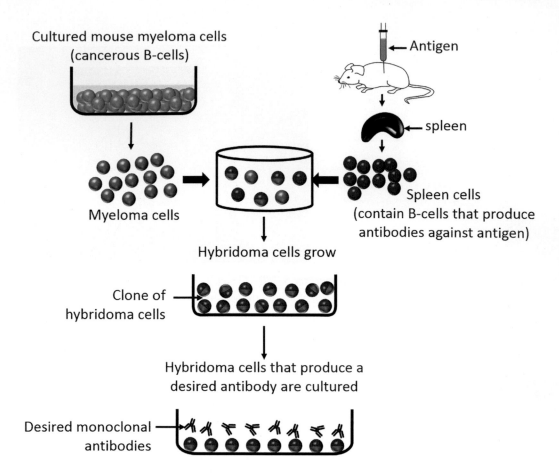

Production of monoclonal antibodies.

Fig. 7.20   Steps to produce monoclonal antibodies. [Page 312]

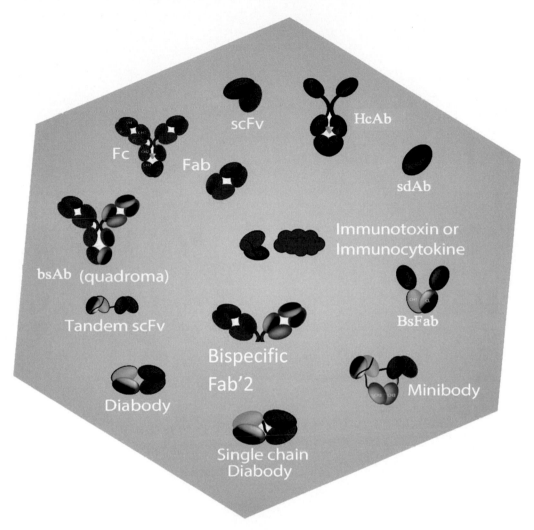

Fig. 7.22 Antibody fragments with therapeutic potential. [Page 315]